2011
YEAR BOOK OF
ORTHOPEDICS®

The 2011 Year Book Series

Year Book of Anesthesiology and Pain Management™: Drs Chestnut, Abram, Black, Gravlee, Lien, Mathru, and Roizen

Year Book of Cardiology®: Drs Gersh, Cheitlin, Elliott, Gold, Graham, and Thourani

Year Book of Critical Care Medicine®: Drs Dellinger, Parrillo, Balk, Dorman, Dries, and Zanotti-Cavazzoni

Year Book of Dermatology and Dermatologic Surgery™: Dr Del Rosso

Year Book of Diagnostic Radiology®: Drs Osborn, Abbara, Elster, Manaster, Oestreich, Offiah, Rosado de Christenson, Stephens, and Walker

Year Book of Emergency Medicine®: Drs Hamilton, Bruno, Handly, Mullin, Quintana, and Ramoska

Year Book of Endocrinology®: Drs Schott, Apovian, Clarke, Eugster, Ludlam, Meikle, Schinner, Schteingart, and Toth

Year Book of Gastroenterology™: Drs Talley, DeVault, Harnois, Murray, Pearson, Philcox, Picco, and Smith

Year Book of Hand and Upper Limb Surgery®: Drs Yao and Steinmann

Year Book of Medicine®: Drs Barker, Garrick, Gersh, Khardori, LeRoith, Seo, Talley, and Thigpen

Year Book of Neonatal and Perinatal Medicine®: Drs Fanaroff, Benitz, Donn, Neu, Papile, Polin, and van Marter

Year Book of Neurology and Neurosurgery®: Drs Klimo and Rabinstein

Year Book of Obstetrics, Gynecology, and Women's Health®: Drs Dungan and Shulman

Year Book of Oncology®: Drs Arceci, Bauer, Chiorean, Gordon, Lawton, Murphy, Thigpen, and Tsao

Year Book of Ophthalmology®: Drs Rapuano, Cohen, Flanders, Hammersmith, Milman, Myers, Nelson, Penne, Pyfer, Sergott, Shields, and Vander

Year Book of Orthopedics®: Drs Morrey, Beauchamp, Huddleston, Swiontkowski, and Trigg

Year Book of Otolaryngology-Head and Neck Surgery®: Drs Sindwani, Balough, Franco, Gapany, and Mitchell

Year Book of Pathology and Laboratory Medicine®: Drs Raab, Parwani, Bejarano, and Bissell

Year Book of Pediatrics®: Dr Stockman

Year Book of Plastic and Aesthetic Surgery™: Drs Miller, Gosain, Gurtner, Gutowski, Ruberg, Salisbury, and Smith

Year Book of Psychiatry and Applied Mental Health®: Drs Talbott, Ballenger, Buckley, Frances, Krupnick, and Mack

Year Book of Pulmonary Disease®: Drs Barker, Jones, Maurer, Raza, Tanoue, and Willsie

Year Book of Sports Medicine®: Drs Shephard, Cantu, Feldman, Jankowski, Khan, Lebrun, Nieman, Pierrynowski, and Rowland

Year Book of Surgery®: Drs Copeland, Behrns, Daly, Eberlein, Fahey, Huber, Klodell, Mozingo, and Pruett

Year Book of Urology®: Drs Andriole and Coplen

Year Book of Vascular Surgery®: Drs Moneta, Gillespie, Starnes, and Watkins

2011

The Year Book of ORTHOPEDICS®

Editor-in-Chief
Bernard F. Morrey, MD
Professor of Orthopedics, Mayo Graduate School of Medicine; Professor of Orthopedics, University of Texas, Health Science Center, San Antonio, Texas

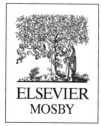

ELSEVIER
MOSBY

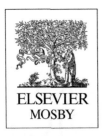

ELSEVIER
MOSBY

Vice President, Continuity: Kimberly Murphy
Developmental Editor: Teia Stone
Production Supervisor, Electronic Year Books: Donna M. Skelton
Electronic Article Manager: Mike Sheets
Illustrations and Permissions Coordinator: Dawn Vohsen

Composition by TNQ Books and Journals Pvt Ltd, India

Editorial Office:
Elsevier, Inc.
Suite 1800
1600 John F. Kennedy Blvd
Philadelphia, PA 19103-2899

International Standard Serial Number: 0276-1092
International Standard Book Number: 978-0-323-08422-2

Printed and bound by CPI Group (UK) Ltd, Croydon, CR0 4YY

Transferred to Digital Print 2011

Editorial Board

Table of Contents

EDITORIAL BOARD vii

JOURNALS REPRESENTED xi

INTRODUCTION xiii

1. General Orthopedics 1

    Introduction 1

2. Basic Science 29

    Introduction 29

3. Trauma and Amputation 41

    Introduction 41

    General Topics 41

    Femur Fractures 57

    Early Fracture Fixation 70

    Femur 73

    Pelvic and Acetabular Fractures 78

    Hip Fracture 81

    Foot and Ankle Fractures 88

    Tibia Fractures 96

    Upper Extremity 97

    Impact on Outcome 122

    Amputation Surgery: Outcome 123

4. Total Hip Arthroplasty 127

    Introduction 127

5. Total Knee Arthroplasty 155

    Introduction 155

6. Shoulder 173

    Introduction 173

7. Elbow 187

    Introduction 187

8. Sports Medicine 197

    Introduction 197

9. Foot and Ankle.................................... 225

    Introduction..................................... 225

10. Forearm, Wrist, and Hand 241

    Introduction..................................... 241

    Evaluation and Diagnosis.......................... 241

    Forearm and Wrist............................... 249

    Hand 260

    Nerve.. 266

11. Orthopedic Oncology............................. 271

    Introduction..................................... 271

    Biopsy 271

    Radiation....................................... 274

    Radiology....................................... 275

    Reconstruction Techniques......................... 277

    Tumor General.................................. 284

    Tumor Reconstruction 288

    Tumor Treatment................................ 296

12. Spine... 313

    Introduction..................................... 313

    ARTICLE INDEX.................................... 349

    AUTHOR INDEX.................................... 361

Journals Represented

Journals represented in this YEAR BOOK are listed below.

Acta Orthopaedica
American Journal of Clinical Pathology
American Journal of Infection Control
American Journal of Sports Medicine
American Journal of Surgery
Anesthesiology
Annals of the Rheumatic Diseases
Annals of Vascular Surgery
Arthroscopy
British Journal of Sports Medicine
Clinical Nuclear Medicine
Clinical Orthopaedics and Related Research
Clinical Radiology
European Journal of Cancer
European Journal of Radiology
Foot & Ankle International
Journal of Applied Physiology
Journal of Bone and Joint Surgery (American Volume)
Journal of Bone and Joint Surgery (British Volume)
Journal of Clinical Endocrinology & Metabolism
Journal of Emergency Medicine
Journal of Hand Surgery
Journal of Orthopaedic Research
Journal of Orthopaedic Trauma
Journal of Pain
Journal of Pediatric Orthopaedics
Journal of Rheumatology
Journal of Surgical Research
Journal of the American Medical Association
Journal of Trauma
Injury
International Journal of Obesity
International Journal of Radiation Oncology Biology Physics
International Journal of Sports Medicine
Journal of Hand Surgery
Journal of Trauma
Laryngoscope
Mayo Clinic Proceedings
New England Journal of Medicine
Orthopedics
Plastic and Reconstructive Surgery
Public Library of Science One
Radiology
Scandinavian Journal of Rheumatology

Spine
Spine Journal
Sports Medicine
Transplantation

STANDARD ABBREVIATIONS

The following terms are abbreviated in this edition: acquired immunodeficiency syndrome (AIDS), anterior cruciate ligament (ACL), anteroposterior (AP), avascular necrosis (AVN), cardiopulmonary resuscitation (CPR), central nervous system (CNS), cerebrospinal fluid (CSF), computed tomography (CT), deoxyribonucleic acid (DNA), electrocardiography (ECG), health maintenance organization (HMO), human immunodeficiency virus (HIV), intensive care unit (ICU), intramuscular (IM), intravenous (IV), magnetic resonance (MR) imaging (MRI), range of motion (ROM), ribonucleic acid (RNA), total hip arthroplasty (THA), total knee arthroplasty (TKA), ultrasound (US), and ultraviolet (UV).

NOTE

The YEAR BOOK OF ORTHOPEDICS® is a literature survey service providing abstracts of articles published in the professional literature. Every effort is made to assure the accuracy of the information presented in these pages. Neither the editors nor the publisher of the YEAR BOOK OF ORTHOPEDICS® can be responsible for errors in the original materials. The editors' comments are their own opinions. Mention of specific products within this publication does not constitute endorsement.

To facilitate the use of the YEAR BOOK OF ORTHOPEDICS® as a reference tool, all illustrations and tables included in this publication are now identified as they appear in the original article. This change is meant to help the reader recognize that any illustration or table appearing in the YEAR BOOK OF ORTHOPEDICS® may be only one of many in the original article. For this reason, figure and table numbers will often appear to be out of sequence within the YEAR BOOK OF ORTHOPEDICS®.

Introduction

This year's volume of the YEAR BOOK represents the ongoing transition from the hardbound written text to the electronic environment. Although there are substantive challenges in transitioning to the real-time electronic environment, the advantages will be increasingly realized with subsequent editions of the YEAR BOOK. We are in the process of reassessing the most efficient manner in which the material may be organized, particularly from a real-time continuous-flow perspective. Next year's volume, therefore, should be even better than this one; yet we are quite pleased with the selections and content of this year's edition. As with prior volumes, the editors have spent a good deal of time reviewing the spectrum of orthopedic literature to select the most relevant and timely contributions. With the evolving processes, this has meant we review about 25% more titles than in the past. As in the past, my personal perspective—as well as my colleagues—is a focus principally on a general orthopedic–type practice. I believe the ongoing value of the YEAR BOOK, therefore, is characterized by individuals carefully reviewing and selecting those topics that are felt to be the most relevant. Also, we are hopefully providing additional value with comments that are designed to place the work in the context of previous literature and our current practice. I have personally benefited from reviewing the spectrum of orthopedic literature in an effort to sort out the most relevant and timely contributions. It is hoped that as our manner of learning and the utility of the YEAR BOOK continues to evolve, this year's contribution will be recognized as valuable to the reader. We are particularly looking forward to the challenges of improvement and innovation in the years to come.

Bernard F. Morrey, MD

1 General Orthopedics

Introduction

General orthopedics is a difficult category today since so much, if not all of our specialty, can be stratified according to subspecialization. Nonetheless, there are several interesting articles covering a wide array of topics that have been included in the general section. Some of these, of necessity, do relate to joint replacement arthroplasty, such as the impact on outcome of surgeon familiarity, case volume, etc. In addition, as always, issues with regard to thrombophlebitis are generally studied in joint replacement patients, but these are also of interest from a general orthopedic practice perspective. The emerging concepts of hip arthritis termed *femoral acetabular impingement* (FAI) have been included in the general section this year. Such reports provide the surgeon with an awareness of these emerging and increasingly accepted views as to etiology of many of those with osteoarthritis of the hip occurring at a relatively young age. General topics regarding the knee are focused on patellofemoral joint; although this might be considered a sports topic, it is one that plagues the general orthopedic surgeon and therefore is included in this section. Overall, I enjoy reviewing the general section and have included articles that represent a cross-section of our specialty that are clinically relevant today.

Bernard F. Morrey, MD

Meta-Analysis Comparing Arthroplasty with Internal Fixation for Displaced Femoral Neck Fracture in the Elderly

Dai Z, Li Y, Jiang D (Chongqing Med Univ, China)
J Surg Res 165:68-74, 2011

Background.—The treatment of displaced femoral neck fracture includes internal fixation and arthroplasty. However, which is the best surgical treatment for the elderly patient with displaced femoral neck fractures has been controversial. Our objective was to compare the clinical effects of internal fixation with that of arthroplasty for displaced femoral neck fracture in the elderly (≥60 y of age).

Materials and Methods.—We searched for all randomized controlled trials of hip arthroplasty *versus* internal fixation for displaced femoral neck fractures in the elderly by electronically searching PUBMED (1966 to December, 2008), MEDILINE (1966 to December, 2008) and manually searching grey literatures. The quality of the trials was assessed and meta-analyses were conducted using the Cochrane Collaboration's RevMan 4.2 software.

Results.—Nineteen published randomized controlled trials involving a total of 3505 patients were suitable for inclusion in the review. The combined results of meta-analyses showed no significant difference in mortality at 1 y postoperatively between the two methods. However, compared with internal fixation, arthroplasty could reduce the rate of reoperations and the major method-related complications.

Conclusions.—Compared with internal fixation, arthroplasty can not only reduce the surgical revision, but also decrease the incidence of complications, and does not increase mortality. The present meta-analysis shows that there is an evidence base to support arthroplasty as a primary treatment for displaced femoral neck fractures in the elderly.

▶ As I have indicated before, I am drawn to meta-analyses that address a particularly important and controversial topic. Management of the femoral neck fracture certainly qualifies. Of note is that this article originated from China. Interesting. In the United States, we have already accepted the recommendation to treat with arthroplasty. The reader should note that the study ignores the major question we ask: hemi or total replacement? In this study, both were included without distinction. The major remaining question is the cost-effectiveness of the treatment. Arthroplasty will be shown to be cost-effective, but the hemi replacement, especially the bipolar device, may emerge as the treatment of choice.

B. F. Morrey, MD

Cost-effectiveness analyses of elective orthopaedic surgical procedures in patients with inflammatory arthropathies
Osnes-Ringen H, Kvamme MK, Kristiansen IS, et al (Diakonhjemmet Hosp, Oslo, Norway; Univ of Oslo, Norway; et al)
Scand J Rheumatol 40:108-115, 2011

Objective.—To examine the costs per quality-adjusted life year (QALY) gained for surgical interventions in patients with inflammatory arthropathies, and to compare the costs per QALY gained for replacement versus non-replacement surgical interventions.

Methods.—In total, 248 patients [mean age 57 (SD 13) years, 77% female] with inflammatory arthropathies underwent orthopaedic surgical treatment and responded to mail surveys at baseline and during follow-up (3, 6, 9, and 12 months). Questionnaires included the quality-of-life EuroQol-5D (EQ-5D) and Short Form-6D (SF-6D) utility scores. The health benefit from surgery was subsequently translated into QALYs. The

TABLE 1.—Location of Surgical Procedures Performed in 248 Patients with Inflammatory Arthropathies

Joint	Replacement Surgery n = 61 (24%)	Non-Replacement Surgery n = 187 (76%)
Shoulder	6	18
Elbow	9	5
Hand/fingers	0	70
Hip	19	0
Knee	14	9
Ankle/foot	13	85

direct treatment costs in the first year were, for each patient, derived from the hospital's cost per patient accounting system (KOSPA). The costs per QALY were estimated and future costs and benefits were discounted at 4%.

Results.—Improvement in utility at 1-year follow-up was 0.10 with EQ-5D and 0.03 with SF-6D (p < 0.05). The estimated 10-year cost per QALY gained was EUR 5000 for hip replacement surgery (EUR18 600 using SF-6D) and EUR 10 500 (EUR 48 500 using SF-6D) for all replacement procedures. The 5-year cost per QALY was EUR 17 800 for non-replacement surgical procedures measured by EQ-5D (SF-6D: EUR 67 500).

Conclusions.—Elective orthopaedic surgery in patients with inflammatory arthropathies was cost-effective when measured with EQ-5D, and some procedures were also cost-effective when SF-6D was used in the economic evaluations. Hip replacement surgery was most cost-effective, irrespective of the method of analysis (Table 1).

▶ This is a rather sophisticated analysis of not just the cost-effectiveness of joint replacement, but the cost-effectiveness of orthopedic intervention, in general, for those with inflammatory arthritis (Table 1). The findings are important, as they confirm other studies from other countries. Hence, whenever this question has been asked, over time and place, the answer is always the same. Orthopedic procedures are cost effective, and, as confirmed here, total hip replacement is the most cost effective of all.

B. F. Morrey, MD

Do "Premium" Joint Implants Add Value?: Analysis of High Cost Joint Implants in a Community Registry
Gioe TJ, Sharma A, Tatman P, et al (Univ of Minnesota Med School, Minneapolis; HealthEast Hosps, St Paul, MN)
Clin Orthop Relat Res 469:48-54, 2011

Background.—Numerous joint implant options of varying cost are available to the surgeon, but it is unclear whether more costly implants add value in terms of function or longevity.

Questions/Purposes.—We evaluated registry survival of higher-cost "premium" knee and hip components compared to lower-priced standard components.

Methods.—Premium TKA components were defined as mobile-bearing designs, high-flexion designs, oxidized-zirconium designs, those including moderately crosslinked polyethylene inserts, or some combination. Premium THAs included ceramic-on-ceramic, metal-on-metal, and ceramic-on-highly crosslinked polyethylene designs. We compared 3462 standard TKAs to 2806 premium TKAs and 868 standard THAs to 1311 premium THAs using standard statistical methods.

Results.—The cost of the premium implants was on average approximately $1000 higher than the standard implants. There was no difference in the cumulative revision rate at 7—8 years between premium and standard TKAs or THAs.

Conclusions.—In this time frame, premium implants did not demonstrate better survival than standard implants. Revision indications for TKA did not differ, and infection and instability remained contributors. Longer followup is necessary to demonstrate whether premium implants add value in younger patient groups.

Level of Evidence.—Level III, therapeutic study. See Guidelines for Authors for a complete description of levels of evidence.

▶ As is obvious, I gravitate to these kinds of studies. I strongly feel that the orthopedic community must become aware of the cost-effectiveness, or ineffectiveness, of our choices. This nice study, once again, fails to document improved outcomes with more expensive high-tech designs. This is true for both total knee (Fig 1 in the original article) and total hip implant designs (Fig 2 in the original article). So why do we persist in choosing such devices? First, we think that they are better; second, we are not too concerned about price; and finally, we may not believe the data. Regardless, unless we pay more attention to this issue, someone or something will be making the implant choices for us in the future.

B. F. Morrey, MD

IOC consensus paper on the use of platelet-rich plasma in sports medicine
Engebretsen L, Steffen K, Alsousou J, et al (IOC Med Commission, Lausanne, Switzerland; Univ of Oxford, UK; et al)
Br J Sports Med 44:1072-1081, 2010

Background.—Platelet-rich plasma (PRP) is widely used to treat musculoskeletal injuries in sports even in the absence of robust clinical studies supporting that use. The International Olympic Committee (IOC) assembled an expert group in May 2010 to review the present state of PRP use for athletes; to provide recommendations for clinicians, athletes, and sports governing bodies; to review the evidence for the clinical effectiveness of

PRP, its ergogenic potential, and its safety; and to try to reconcile disparities between its use and current evidence.

Basic Science.—PRP is a volume of the plasma fraction of autologous blood that has an increased concentration of platelets, thereby serving as a source for autologous platelets. Platelets contain many growth factors involved in healing injured tissues. PRP is used to facilitate the application of autologous plasma and platelet-derived proteins and develop a fibrin scaffold at the desired location that can be used as a matrix for cell growth and differentiation, necessary for the repair process. Research on how PRP influences the inflammation and repair of connective tissue and skeletal muscle remains limited. Several techniques can be used to prepare PRP, and there is currently no standardization of preparation or use. The different preparation methods yield different platelet concentrations and may produce products with varying biology, amount and type of growth factors, and potential uses. A classification system for the different PRPs should be developed for use in research and treatment scenarios.

Clinical Use.—PRP is used especially for elite athletes who are highly motivated to return quickly to competition. For sports injuries it is usually injected in a fluid form under ultrasound guidance. Platelets begin actively secreting proteins within 10 minutes of clotting, with over 95% of the pre-synthesized growth factors secreted within 1 hour. The platelets then synthesize and secrete more growth factors for the next several days. PRP is used to promote tissue healing and implant integration, control blood loss, and exert an antibacterial effect. The tissue-specific effects of PRP depend on the underlying cellular and molecular processes for that tissue's healing, which can differ widely. PRP can be injected inactivated and then activated by providing calcium chloride and autologous prepared thrombin or soluble type 1 collagen. Alternatively, the local environment may provide the activation impetus. PRP may enhance mesenchymal stem cell proliferation and migration but may also limit cell differentiation into the appropriate lineage. Although it is widely used for these applications, little evidence supports the use of PRP for muscle injuries, tendon injuries, or cartilage injuries or in regenerative roles. The World Anti-Doping Agency permits the use of PRP via all routes of administration.

Conclusions.—The evidence on PRP has been drawn from studies whose methodologies make them difficult to interpret and extrapolate to firm guidelines for use in human athletes. Current evidence supports PRP use as safe, but suggests a cautious approach for athletic injury applications. It may have a future use in the prophylaxis of infection and as an adjuvant to normal treatment regimens. Further work in basic science combined with well-designed randomized clinical trials is needed to document PRP's efficacy or lack thereof.

▶ Is there anything hotter in orthopedics than platelet-rich plasma (PRP)? This review, a consensus article, boasts 22 authors and over 90 references, so it is worth reading in its entirety. The authors also do a nice job discussing the drivers: theory predicated on enhanced growth factor activation, patient perception, and safety. However, the complexity surrounds a different potential response as a function of tissue type, that is, bone, tendon muscle, etc. The preparation of the PRP also is complex and introduces numerous additional variables. Finally, the paucity of good, prospective, randomized studies all justify the caution these authors recommend when offering this treatment to our patients.

B. F. Morrey, MD

Improving Injection Accuracy of the Elbow, Knee, and Shoulder: Does Injection Site and Imaging Make a Difference? A Systematic Review
Daley EL, Bajaj S, Bisson LJ, et al (Rush Univ Med Ctr, Chicago, IL; Univ of Buffalo, NY)
Am J Sports Med 39:656-662, 2011

Background.—Joint injections and aspirations are used to reduce joint pain and decrease inflammation. The efficacy of these injections is diminished when they are placed inadvertently in the wrong location or compartment. The purpose of this study was to determine whether the use of varying sites or imaging techniques affects the rate of accurate needle placement in aspiration and injection in the shoulder, elbow, and knee.

Hypotheses.—(1) Accuracy rates of different joint injection sites will demonstrate variability. (2) Injection accuracy rates will be improved when performed with concomitant imaging.

Study Design.—Systematic review of the literature.

Methods.—Studies reporting injection accuracy based on image verification were identified through a systematic search of the English literature. Accuracy rates were compared for currently accepted injection sites in the shoulder, elbow, and knee. In addition, accuracy rates with and without imaging of these joints were compared.

Results.—In the glenohumeral joint, there is a statistically higher accuracy rate with the posterior approach when compared with the anterior approach (85% vs 45%). Injection site selection did not affect accuracy for the subacromial space, acromioclavicular joint, elbow, or knee. The use of imaging improved injection accuracy in the glenohumeral joint (95% vs 79%), subacromial space (100% vs 63%), acromioclavicular joint (100% vs 45%), and knee (99% vs 79%).

Conclusion.—Injection accuracy rates are significantly higher for the posterior approach compared with the anterior approach for the glenohumeral joint. Similarly, the accuracy rates are also higher when imaging is used in conjunction with injection of the glenohumeral joint, subacromial space, acromioclavicular joint, and knee.

▶ This is an attractive article, as it uses a methodology that I find intriguing (Fig 1 in the original article). In addition, it addresses a question frequently asked, or at least considered. Finally, it is especially relevant from a cost-effective perspective. The surprising finding is the increased accuracy of image-guided knee injections. For me, this is of concern because of the increased cost. I can accept this for the shoulder. And, of course, in those with effusion, an experienced surgeon should be able to accurately inject or aspirate the knee 100% of the time. I also would agree with the literature indicating that the elbow does not typically benefit from imaging for injection/aspiration.

B. F. Morrey, MD

A Proximal Strengthening Program Improves Pain, Function, and Biomechanics in Women With Patellofemoral Pain Syndrome

Earl JE, Hoch AZ (Univ of Wisconsin—Milwaukee and the Med College of Wisconsin)
Am J Sports Med 39:154-163, 2011

Background.—It is hypothesized that patients with patellofemoral pain syndrome (PFPS) have hip and core muscle weakness leading to dynamic malalignment of the lower extremity. Thus, hip strengthening is a common PFPS treatment approach.

Purpose.—To determine changes in hip strength, core endurance, lower extremity biomechanics, and patient outcomes after proximally focused rehabilitation for PFPS patients.

Study Design.—Case series; Level of evidence, 4.

Methods.—Nineteen women (age, 22.68 ± 7.19 years; height, 1.64 ± 0.07 m; mass, 60.2 ± 7.35 kg) with PFPS participated in an 8-week program to strengthen the hip and core muscles and improve dynamic malalignment. Paired t tests were used to compare the dependent variables between prerehabilitation and postrehabilitation. The dependent variables were pain; functional ability; isometric hip abduction and external rotation strength; anterior, lateral, and posterior core endurance; joint range of motion (ROM; rearfoot eversion, knee abduction and internal rotation, and hip adduction and internal rotation); and peak internal joint moments (rearfoot inversion, knee abduction, and hip abduction and external rotation) during the stance phase of running.

Results.—Significant improvements in pain, functional ability, lateral core endurance, hip abduction, and hip external rotation strength were observed. There was also a significant reduction in the knee abduction moment during running, although there were no significant changes in joint ROM.

Conclusion.—An 8-week rehabilitation program focusing on strengthening and improving neuromuscular control of the hip and core musculature produces positive patient outcomes, improves hip and core muscle strength, and reduces the knee abduction moment, which is associated with developing PFPS.

▶ In spite of the fact that the orthopedic surgeon is dependent on physical therapy for the management of many conditions, there are relatively few studies that document its effectiveness. This contribution is of value, as it addresses a very common problem—knee pain. The study is well conceived and executed. It is encouraging to find that the strength program described herein does in fact improve knee symptoms. Of note is the inclusion of core body-strengthening exercises. This program should be seriously considered for those with patello-femoral knee pain.

B. F. Morrey, MD

Co-existent medial collateral ligament injury seen following transient patellar dislocation: observations at magnetic resonance imaging
Quinlan JF, Farrelly C, Kelly G, et al (Cappagh Natl Orthopaedic Hosp, Finglas, Dublin, Republic of Ireland; Univ College Dublin, Belfield, Republic of Ireland)
Br J Sports Med 44:411-414, 2010

This study reports on a series of patients who were diagnosed as having had a transient lateral patellar dislocation by magnetic resonance imaging (MRI). The images were reviewed with specific reference to the medial collateral ligament (MCL), a heretofore undescribed concomitant injury. Eighty patients were diagnosed on MRI as having had transient lateral patellar dislocation. Their mean age was 23.9 years (SD 7.5). Forty patients (50.0%) had co-existent MCL injuries. These injuries were classified as grade 1 (n = 20), grade 2 (n = 17) and grade 3 (n = 3). These results suggest that MCL injury commonly accompanies transient lateral patella dislocation, most likely due to a shared valgus injury. It appears to occur more commonly in male patients and if unidentified may explain both delayed recovery and persistent morbidity in more severe cases. In this setting, without specifically excluding co-existent MCL injury, the current vogue for early rehabilitation should be adopted with caution.

▶ This would appear to be another of a series of publications in which sophisticated imaging offers a broader definition of pathology than is clinically suspected. Who would ever guess that lateral patellar instability is associated with injury to the medial collateral ligament (MCL) in 50% of patients? This is particularly true because the MRI diagnosis allows for subclinical subluxation to be included in the cohort. The suggestion to go carefully with rehabilitation would seem to be warranted if a clinical examination, not performed by radiologists, reveals MCL pain. Lacking this finding, the imaging diagnosis would seem to have little clinical utility.

B. F. Morrey, MD

A clinical prediction rule for identifying patients with patellofemoral pain who are likely to benefit from foot orthoses: a preliminary determination
Vicenzino B, Collins N, Cleland J, et al (The Univ of Queensland, Brisbane, Australia; Franklin Pierce Univ, Concord, NH)
Br J Sports Med 44:862-866, 2010

Objective.—To develop a clinical prediction rule to identify patients with patellofemoral pain (PFP) who are more likely to benefit from foot orthoses.

Design.—Posthoc analysis of one treatment arm of a randomised clinical trial.

Setting.—Single-centre trial in a community setting in Brisbane, Australia.

Participants.—42 participants (mean age 27.9 years) with a clinical diagnosis of PFP (median duration 36 months).

Interventions.—Foot orthoses fitted by a physiotherapist.

Main Outcome Measures.—Five-point global improvement scale at 12-week follow-up, dichotomised with marked improvement equalling success.

Results.—Potential predictor variables identified by univariate analyses were age, height, pain severity, anterior knee pain scale score, functional index questionnaire score, foot morphometry (arch height ratio, midfoot width difference from non-weight bearing to weight bearing) and overall orthoses comfort. Parsimonious fitting of these variables to a model that explained success with orthoses identified the following: age (>25 years), height (<165 cm), worst pain visual analogue scale (<53.25 mm) and a difference in mid-foot width from non-weight bearing to weight bearing (>10.96 mm). The pretest success rate of 40% increased to 86% if the patient exhibited three of these variables (positive likelihood ratio 8.8; 95% CI 1.2 to 66.9).

Conclusion.—Post-hoc analysis identified age, height, pain severity and mid-foot morphometry as possible predictors of successful treatment of PFP with foot orthoses, thereby providing practitioners with information for prescribing foot orthoses in PFP and stimulating further research.

▶ Because patellofemoral pain is such a ubiquitous problem, insight into effective, evidence-based, nonoperative treatment is of tremendous value. This interesting study offers a relatively inexpensive solution to the problem but then offers the specific added value of defining those patient characteristics that will identify those with the greatest likelihood of benefiting from this treatment. It is uncommon that we could indicate a patient greater than 25 years, taller than 5 feet 6 inches, moderate pain, and limited splaying of the midfoot with weight bearing has an 85% chance of a favorable result with the foot arthrosis. The key is to apply this knowledge, but to these authors I say—bravo.

B. F. Morrey, MD

Anatomy of Lateral Patellar Instability: Trochlear Dysplasia and Tibial Tubercle–Trochlear Groove Distance Is More Pronounced in Women Who Dislocate the Patella

Balcarek P, Jung K, Ammon J, et al (Univ Medicine, Göttingen, Germany)
Am J Sports Med 38:2320-2327, 2010

Background.—A trend toward young women being at greatest risk for primary and recurrent dislocation of the patella is evident in the current literature. However, a causative factor is missing, and differences in the anatomical risk factors between men and women are less defined.

Purpose.—To identify differences between the sexes in the anatomy of lateral patellar instability.

Study Design.—Case control study; Level of evidence, 3.

Methods.—Knee magnetic resonance images were collected from 100 patients treated for lateral patellar instability. Images were obtained from 157 patients without patellar instability who served as controls. Using 2-way analyses of variance, the influence of patellar dislocation, gender, and their interaction were analyzed with regard to sulcus angle, trochlear depth, trochlear asymmetry, patellar height, and the tibial tubercle–trochlear groove (TT-TG) distance. Mechanisms of injury of first-time dislocations were divided into high-risk, low-risk, and no-risk pivoting activities and direct hits.

Results.—For all response variables, a significant effect was observed for the incidence of patellar dislocation (all $P < .01$). In addition, sulcus angle, trochlear asymmetry, and trochlear depth depended significantly on gender (all $P < .01$) but patellar height did not ($P = .13$). A significant interaction between patellar dislocation and gender was observed for the TT-TG distance ($P = .02$). The mean difference in TT-TG distance between study and control groups was 4.1 mm for women ($P < .01$) and 1.6 mm for men ($P = .05$). Low-risk and no-risk pivoting injuries were most common in women, whereas first-time dislocations in men occurred mostly during high-risk pivoting activities ($P < .01$).

Conclusion.—The data from this study indicate that trochlear dysplasia and the TT-TG distance is more prominent in women who dislocate the patella. Both factors might contribute to an increased risk of lateral patellar instability in the female patient as illustrated by the fact that dislocations occurred most often during low-risk or no-risk pivoting activities in women.

▶ I seem to be drawn at the present time to those studies that involve the patellofemoral joint. I don't know why, other than it is a common yet poorly understood and treated entity. That the occurrence is associated with a type of trochlear dysplasia is noteworthy, as is the tubercle/grove dimension. The latter would seem to be a variant or at least related to patella alta. Regardless, the findings are clear. Trochlear dysplasia plays a major role in the entity, and this occurs more common in females. What is the value to the clinician? If this is recognized, then surgical intervention would seem to be indicated sooner, rather than later.

B. F. Morrey, MD

A Prospective Study of 80,000 Total Joint and 5000 Anterior Cruciate Ligament Reconstruction Procedures in a Community-Based Registry in the United States
Paxton EW, Namba RS, Maletis GB, et al (Southern California Permanente Med Group, San Diego, CA; Southern California Permanente Med Group, Irvine, CA; Southern California Permanente Med Group, Baldwin Park, CA; et al)
J Bone Joint Surg Am 92:117-132, 2010

Background.—Total joint replacement is among the most costly health procedures, yet the demand is expected to increase because of advances in medical technology and a population that is more obese and older. The ability to monitor total joint outcomes nationwide could identify procedures and implants with higher revision rates. This in turn could prompt improved methods or products and lead to better patient care. The Swedish Hip Register has led to changes in clinical practice based on its storehouse of data. Currently the United States has no mechanism to collect data on implanted orthopedic devices. A community total joint replacement registry was set up in 2001 and now has been implemented in 50 hospitals in six geographic regions. Its goals are to monitor revisions, reoperations, and complications; immediately identify and notify patients and surgeons about implant recalls or advisories; identify patients at risk for revisions and complications; assess the clinical effectiveness of implants and techniques; and provide a framework for more comprehensive clinical research studies. The data obtained were analyzed, the impact of the registry was assessed, and information relative to anterior cruciate ligament reconstruction was presented.

Methods.—The total joint replacement data analyzed dated from April 2001 to March 2008. The information on anterior cruciate ligament reconstruction was gathered between February 2005 and June 2008. Data included patient characteristics and outcomes, hospital- and surgeon-related variables, and implant characteristics.

Results.—The total joint registry documented cumulative total joint survival rates of 97.1% for knee arthroplasty and 97.3% for hip arthroplasty at 5.5 years. These rates are similar to those of other national registries. Important independent risk factors for aseptic revision after total hip arthoplasty were geographical region, female gender, lower annual surgeon case volume, use of a conventional insert, and a femoral head of 28 mm or less. Use of the uncemented technique had a higher relative risk of revision than use of hybrid fixation. Larger femoral head size carried a lower risk for revision surgery. Important independent risk factors for aseptic revision after total knee arthroplasty were geographic region, younger patient age, higher ASA score, diabetes, uncemented fixation, and a mobile-bearing design.

Feedback to surgeons positively influenced clinical practice. Fewer procedures are done with unicompartmental knee arthroplasty or uncemented techniques and fewer small femoral head sizes are being used. Specific surgeon profiles are also provided confidentially to participating surgeons for use in practice assessment and to compare their revision and complication rates with those found regionally. Eight recalls and advisories were tracked and monitored during the study. The identification of defective devices was facilitated. A comparative effectiveness of implants allowed the best ones to be selected in value-based contracting. Lists of patients due for follow-up were generated and e-mailed to providers for telephone or e-mail contact, avoiding clinic visits.

The anterior cruciate ligament reconstruction registry reported a revision rate of 0.6% and a reoperation rate of 4.4% over the 4-year period. Different survival rates were associated with the three graft types. The reasons for reoperation on the index knee were found to be meniscal injury, stiffness, and infections. Such reoperations were three times more likely than reoperation on the contralateral knee, which most commonly underwent ligament reconstruction and meniscal surgery. Among female patients, contralateral reoperations were more likely to be for ligament injuries, but for male patients they were more likely to be for meniscal injuries. The effect of differences in postoperative rehabilitation protocols and other factors at various centers was identified as a target for study. Removal of fixation hardware is an additional cause of reoperation, and specific implant designs or materials are being studied to determine if some have a lower reoperation rate. Anterior cruciate ligament reconstruction is most common among young women age 14 to 17 years, so this group should be targeted for injury prevention interventions. Longer time from injury to surgery carries an increased rate of medial meniscal injury, which bears study. Overall the rates of deep vein thrombosis and pulmonary embolism associated with anterior cruciate ligament reconstruction are low.

Conclusions.—Registries offer an alternative to comparative research when it is impractical or unethical and when it would require long-term follow-up with large samples to reveal rare complications. Generalities can be developed from registries' real-world results more readily than from the results of randomized controlled trials. Registries can change clinical practices, augment safety, provide cost-effective results, and identify research topics and approaches. A national US registry to monitor device performance would be useful. Establishing a network of institutional and regional registries may permit the development of a US national registry (Fig 1).

▶ Most surgeons in this country are well familiar with the existence of joint replacement registries that have been established around the world, being popularized from the work of investigators in Scandinavia. We commend the

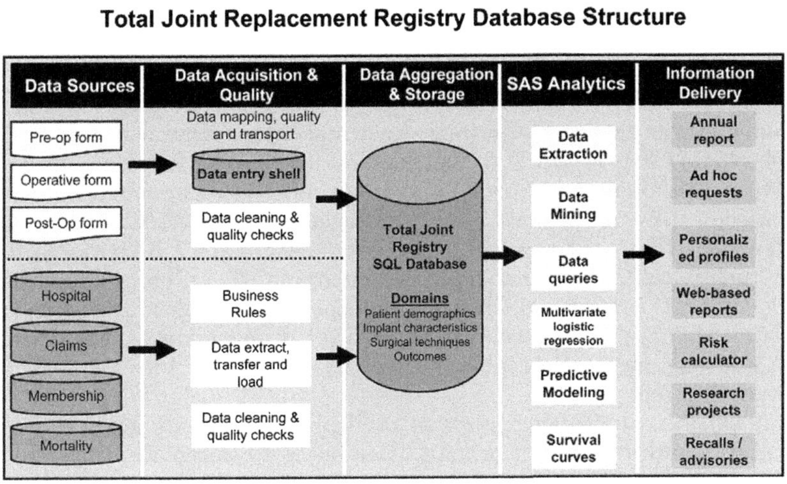

Total Joint Replacement Registry Database Structure

FIGURE 1.—Total joint replacement registry database structure. SAS = SAS software (version 9.1.3; SAS Institute, Cary, North Carolina). (Reprinted from Paxton EW, Namba RS, Maletis GB, et al. A prospective study of 80,000 total joint and 5000 anterior cruciate ligament reconstruction procedures in a community-based registry in the United States. *J Bone Joint Surg Am.* 2010;92:117-132. Reprinted with permission from the Journal of Bone and Joint Surgery, Inc.)

Permanente group for initiating and funding the registry/database approach to better understand their practice. This report offers insight into the clinical detail the group has defined as necessary to take full advantage of data-gathering efforts. The reader should know that the American Academy of Orthopaedic Surgeons is actively pursuing steps to allow the entire country to participate in a similar data-gathering effort. Depending on the detail of the data (Fig 1), the value to the clinician regarding decision making can be enormous. The reader is encouraged to read this full article.

B. F. Morrey, MD

Is Physical Activity a Risk Factor for Primary Knee or Hip Replacement Due to Osteoarthritis? A Prospective Cohort Study
Wang Y, Simpson JA, Wluka AE, et al (Monash Univ, Melbourne, Australia; Univ of Melbourne, Carlton, Australia; The Cancer Council Victoria, Carlton, Australia; et al)
J Rheumatol 38:350-357, 2011

Objective.—To estimate prospectively any association between measures of physical activity and the risk of either primary knee or hip replacement due to osteoarthritis (OA).

Methods.—Eligible subjects (n = 39,023) were selected from participants in a prospective cohort study recruited 1990-1994. Primary knee and hip replacement for OA during 2001-2005 was determined by linking the cohort records to the National Joint Replacement Registry. A total physical activity level was computed, incorporating both intensity and frequency for different forms of physical activity obtained by questionnaire at baseline attendance.

Results.—There was a dose-response relationship between total physical activity level and the risk of primary knee replacement [hazards ratio (HR) 1.04, 95% CI 1.01−1.07 for an increase of 1 level in total physical activity]. Although vigorous activity frequency was associated with an increased risk of primary knee replacement (HR 1.42, 95% CI 1.08−1.86) for 1−2 times/week and HR 1.24 (95% CI 0.90−1.71) for ≥ 3 times/week), the p for trend was marginal (continuous HR 1.08, 95% CI 1.00−1.16, p = 0.05). The frequency of less vigorous activity or walking was not associated with the risk of primary knee replacement, nor was any measure of physical activity associated with the risk of primary hip replacement.

Conclusion.—Increasing levels of total physical activity are positively associated with the risk of primary knee but not hip replacement due to OA. Physical activity might affect the knee and hip joints differently depending on the preexisting health status and anatomy of the joint, as well as the sort of physical activity performed (Tables 3 and 4).

▶ This is an excellent example of health science research. It does answer one question, but not another: Is physical activity a causative factor, or at least

TABLE 3.—Association Between Physical Activity and Risk of Primary Knee Replacement

	Total Population, n = 39,023 Hazard Ratio (95% CI)[†]	p[†]	Sensitivity Analysis on Participants with Complete 2nd Followup Data, n = 27,323 Hazard Ratio (95% CI)[†]	p[†]
Total physical activity level				
None (0)	1.00		1.00	
Low (> 0−3)	1.16 (0.88, 1.52)	0.28	1.17 (0.85, 1.62)	0.33
Moderate (> 3−4)	1.13 (0.87, 1.46)	0.35	1.08 (0.79, 1.47)	0.64
High (> 4)	1.46 (1.13, 1.87)	0.003	1.47 (1.09, 1.96)	0.01
Trend test	1.04 (1.01, 1.07)	0.003	1.04 (1.01, 1.08)	0.01
Vigorous activity*				
None at all	1.00		1.00	
1−2 times/week	1.42 (1.08, 1.86)	0.01	1.43 (1.06, 1.94)	0.02
≥ 3 times/week	1.24 (0.90, 1.71)	0.19	1.44 (1.02, 2.04)	0.04
Trend test	1.08 (1.00, 1.16)	0.05	1.11 (1.02, 1.21)	0.01
Less vigorous activity*,††				
None at all	1.00		1.00	
1−2 times/week	1.09 (0.85, 1.40)	0.49	1.17 (0.88, 1.56)	0.28
≥ 3 times/week	1.19 (0.94, 1.52)	0.16	1.11 (0.83, 1.49)	0.49
Trend test	1.05 (0.98, 1.11)	0.15	1.03 (0.96, 1.11)	0.43
Walking*,††				
None at all	1.00		1.00	
1−2 times/week	1.01 (0.77, 1.32)	0.95	0.95 (0.69, 1.31)	0.75
≥ 3 times/week	1.09 (0.89, 1.35)	0.41	1.04 (0.81, 1.33)	0.79
Trend test	1.02 (0.97, 1.08)	0.40	1.01 (0.95, 1.08)	0.75

†Adjusted for age, gender, body mass index, country of birth, occupational physical activity, and education level.
*Weekly frequency of physical activity undertaken for at least 20 minutes.
††Analysis excluding those reporting vigorous activity.

TABLE 4.—Association Between Physical Activity and Risk of Primary Hip Replacement

	Total Population, n = 39,023 Hazard Ratio (95% CI)[†]	p[†]	Sensitivity Analysis on Participants with Complete 2nd Followup Data, n = 27,323 Hazard Ratio (95% CI)[†]	p[†]
Total physical activity level				
None (0)	1.00		1.00	
Low (> 0–3)	0.76 (0.56, 1.03)	0.07	0.71 (0.50, 1.02)	0.07
Moderate (> 3–4)	0.89 (0.67, 1.16)	0.38	0.84 (0.61, 1.17)	0.30
High (> 4)	1.09 (0.84, 1.41)	0.52	1.13 (0.84, 1.52)	0.42
Trend test*	1.03 (1.00, 1.06)	0.09	NA	NA
Vigorous activity**				
None at all	1.00		1.00	
1–2 times/week	1.11 (0.83, 1.48)	0.49	1.19 (0.87, 1.63)	0.27
≥ 3 times/week	1.27 (0.94, 1.73)	0.12	1.32 (0.95, 1.86)	0.10
Trend test	1.06 (0.99, 1.14)	0.11	1.08 (0.99, 1.17)	0.07
Less vigorous activity**,††				
None at all	1.00		1.00	
1–2 times/week	1.04 (0.80, 1.36)	0.76	1.04 (0.76, 1.42)	0.82
≥ 3 times/week	1.09 (0.83, 1.41)	0.55	1.10 (0.81, 1.50)	0.54
Trend test	1.02 (0.96, 1.09)	0.54	1.02 (0.95, 1.11)	0.54
Walking**,††				
None at all	1.00		1.00	
1–2 times/week	0.75 (0.55, 1.03)	0.07	0.71 (0.49, 1.03)	0.07
≥ 3 times/week	0.97 (0.77, 1.21)	0.78	0.96 (0.74, 1.25)	0.77
Trend test*	1.00 (0.94, 1.06)	0.93	NA	NA

*No evidence of linear association found between total physical activity level or walking and the risk of hip replacement (likelihood ratio test, p = 0.05), thus no trend test results presented.
†Adjusted for age, gender, body mass index, country of birth, occupational physical activity, and education level.
**Weekly frequency of physical activity undertaken for at least 20 minutes.
††Analysis excluding those reporting vigorous activity. NA: not applicable.

associated with increased arthritis? Yes for the knee, and no for the hip (Tables 3 and 4). But this large database does not allow insight as to the most likely causative difference, which is injury. So it is easy to hypothesize that the reason the knee is correlated to arthritis leading to joint replacement is because of injury that occurs with activity. Regardless of the explanation, the association seems clearly defined.

B. F. Morrey, MD

Arthroscopic femoral osteochondroplasty for cam lesions with isolated acetabular chondral damage
Haviv B, Singh PJ, Takla A, et al (St Vincents and Mercy Private Hosp, Melbourne, Victoria, Australia)
J Bone Joint Surg [Br] 92-B:629-633, 2010

This study evaluates the outcome of arthroscopic femoral osteochon-droplasty for cam lesions of the hip in the absence of additional pathology other than acetabular chondral lesions. We retrospectively reviewed 166 patients (170 hips) who were categorised according to three different grades of chondral damage. The outcome was assessed in each grade using the modified Harris Hip Score (MHHS) and the Non-Arthritic Hip Score (NAHS).

Overall, at the last follow-up (mean 22 months, 12 to 72), the mean MHHS had improved by 15.3 points (95% confidence interval (CI), 8.9 to 21.7) and the mean NAHS by 15 points (95% CI, 9.4 to 20.5). Significantly better results were observed in hips with less severe chondral damage. Microfracture in limited chondral lesions showed superior results.

Arthroscopic femoral osteochondroplasty for cam impingement with microfracture in selected cases is beneficial. The outcome correlates with the severity of acetabular chondral damage (Figs 1b and 2a).

▶ The value of and reason for including this experience is that it serves to further introduce the concept of impingement as a precursor of hip arthritis (Fig 1b) and offers a relatively large experience with one of the emerging or at least investigated treatment options, arthroscopic hip debridement (Fig 2a). In spite of the obvious weaknesses of no control group and very short-term follow-up, it is important to recognize the relatively favorable early outcomes because the alternative is to sit back and wait for the natural progression of untreated disease. It is not surprising to learn that less severe lesions did better than more severe ones. As an aside, I find it particularly interesting to observe

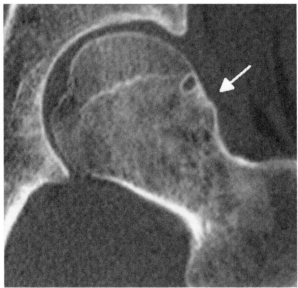

Fig. 1b

FIGURE 1.—CT scans of the anterolateral cam femoroacetabular impingement of the left hip showing. b) a coronal CT scan reconstruction (arrow). (Reprinted from Haviv B, Singh PJ, Takla A, et al. Arthroscopic femoral osteochondroplasty for cam lesions with isolated acetabular chondral damage. *J Bone Joint Surg [Br]*. 2010;92-B:629-633. Reproduced with permission and copyright © of the British Editorial Society of Bone and Joint Surgery.)

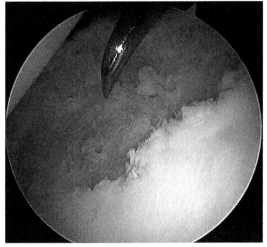

Fig. 2a

FIGURE 2.—Intra-operative photographs of microfracture of a chondral defect showing. a) a micro-fracture awl used to make multiple holes perpendicular to the subchondral bone. (Reprinted from Haviv B, Singh PJ, Takla A, et al. Arthroscopic femoral osteochondroplasty for cam lesions with isolated acetabular chondral damage. *J Bone Joint Surg [Br]*. 2010;92-B:629-633. Reproduced with permission and copyright © of the British Editorial Society of Bone and Joint Surgery.)

the significant strides that have been made with hip arthroscopy, as a treatment modality, since the advent of the recognition of this disease state.

B. F. Morrey, MD

Open Surgical Dislocation Versus Arthroscopy for Femoroacetabular Impingement: A Comparison of Clinical Outcomes
Botser IB, Smith TW Jr, Nasser R, et al (Hinsdale Orthopaedics Associates, IL)
Arthroscopy 27:270-278, 2011

Purpose.—Over the last decade, the surgical treatment of femoroacetabular impingement (FAI) has evolved as surgical techniques through arthroscopy, open surgical dislocation, and combined approaches have been developed. The purpose of this systematic review was to evaluate and compare the clinical results of available surgical approaches for FAI.

Methods.—A review of the literature was performed through the PubMed database and related articles' reference lists. Inclusion criteria were (1) all patients treated for FAI, (2) Level I, II, III, or IV study design, and (3) written in the English language. Case reports and studies involving patients with acetabular dysplasia were excluded.

Results.—Overall, 1,299 articles fit our keyword search criteria. Of these, 26 articles reported clinical outcomes, using 3 surgical modalities: open surgical dislocation, arthroscopic, and combined approaches. In

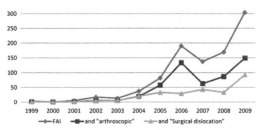

FIGURE 1.—Search results in Google Scholar for number of articles containing the term "femoroace-tabular impingement" by year. Separate numbers for search terms "femoroacetabular impingement and arthroscopic" and "femoroacetabular impingement and surgical dislocation" are shown in red and green, respectively. (Reprinted from Botser IB, Smith TW Jr, Nasser R, et al. Open surgical dislocation versus arthroscopy for femoroacetabular impingement: a comparison of clinical outcomes. *Arthroscopy.* 2011;27:270-278, Copyright 2011, with permission from the Arthroscopy Association of North America.)

compiling the data in these articles, we analyzed the outcomes of a total 1,462 hips in 1,409 patients. The most published surgical method was arthroscopy, which included 62% of the patients. Labral repair was performed more frequently in open surgical dislocation (45%) and combined approach (41%) procedures than in arthroscopies (23%). Mean improvement in the modified Harris hip score after surgery was 26.4 for arthroscopy, 20.5 for open surgical dislocation, and 12.3 for the combined approach. A higher rate of return to sport was reported for arthroscopy in professional athletes than for open surgical dislocation. Overall complication rates were 1.7% for the arthroscopic group, 9.2% for the open surgical dislocation group, and 16% in the combined approach group.

Conclusions.—All 3 surgical approaches led to consistent improvements in patient outcomes. Because a wide variety of subjective hip questionnaires were used, direct comparisons could not be made in many cases, and none of the approaches could be clearly shown to be superior to the others. However, it seems that, overall, the arthroscopic method had the lowest complication and fastest rehabilitation rate (Fig 1).

▶ The authors are addressing a very hot topic in orthopedics. The very existence of impingement as a cause of early hip arthritis is of recent origin. That there are 1300 articles on this subject according to the authors' review is truly amazing. The exponential increase in recognition is paralleled by the increase in articles dealing with treatment (Fig 1). This and other recent reviews are arriving at the same conclusion, marginally better outcomes with arthroscopic intervention. One major reason is a markedly lower complication rate. The only requirement is expertise with the arthroscopic procedure, which is not a simple task. We will see a growth in this competency in the future driven by this pathology and the awareness that arthroscopy is the optimal management procedure.

B. F. Morrey, MD

Comparative Systematic Review of the Open Dislocation, Mini-Open, and Arthroscopic Surgeries for Femoroacetabular Impingement

Matsuda DK, Carlisle JC, Arthurs SC, et al (Kaiser Permanente West Los Angeles Med Ctr, CA; Steadman Philippon Res Inst Vail, CO; Permanente Federation, Oakland, CA)

Arthroscopy 27:252-269, 2011

Purpose.—To analyze the current approaches to the surgical management of symptomatic femoroacetabular impingement (FAI).

Methods.—Thirteen relevant queries were used in four search engines (PubMed, EMBASE, Ovid, and the Cochrane Review) with a resultant 5,856 articles. Eighteen peer-reviewed treatment outcome studies met the inclusion criteria with minimum 1-year follow-up of the surgical

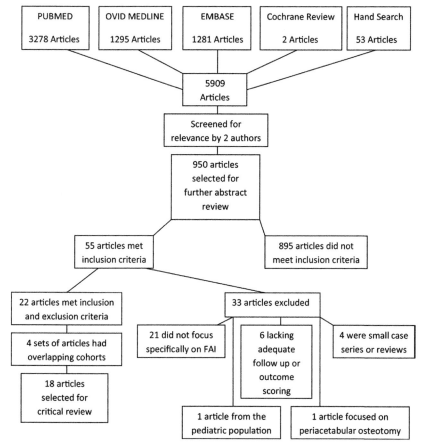

FIGURE 1.—Flowchart of methodology. (Reprinted from Matsuda DK, Carlisle JC, Arthurs SC, et al. Comparative systematic review of the open dislocation, mini-open, and arthroscopic surgeries for femoroacetabular impingement. *Arthroscopy.* 2011;27:252-269, Copyright 2011, with permission from the Arthroscopy Association of North America.)

treatment of skeletal pathoanatomy and associated chondrolabral pathology in skeletally mature patients with FAI.

Results.—There were 6 open surgical dislocation, 4 mini-open, and 8 arthroscopic studies, all with Levels of Evidence III or IV. The only prospective studies were in the arthroscopic category. Outcome data were extracted and analyzed with respect to surgical efficacy, failure rates, and complications.

Conclusions.—The open dislocation, mini-open, and arthroscopic methods for treating symptomatic FAI are effective in improving pain and function in short-term to midterm studies and are relatively safe procedures. The historical gold standard of open dislocation surgery had a comparatively high major complication rate primarily because of trochanteric osteotomy—related issues. The mini-open method showed comparable efficacy but a significant incidence of iatrogenic injury to the lateral femoral cutaneous nerve in some studies. The arthroscopic method had surgical outcomes equal to or better than the other methods with a lower rate of major complications when performed by experienced surgeons (Fig 1).

▶ As may be obvious, I do gravitate to the evidence-based literature reviews (Fig 1). This one was selected because it is an early review of a currently evolving aspect of our profession. Subtle dysplasia, manifesting as impingement, is evolving as a major diagnostic and therapeutic challenge for the orthopedic surgeon. The reason it is so critical is that early diagnosis, and effective intervention, may alter the natural history in the young patient, that is, total hip replacement. All 3 modalities, open dislocation and debridement, mini-open, and arthroscopic techniques are currently considered acceptable. Yet the conclusions of this review are clear. Arthroscopic intervention is as effective, if not more so than the others, and has the lowest complication rate. But this is true only with those experienced in hip arthroscopy.

B. F. Morrey, MD

Assessment of peritrochanteric high T2 signal depending on the age and gender of the patients
Haliloglu N, Inceoglu D, Sahin G (Ankara Univ School of Medicine, Turkey)
Eur J Radiol 75:64-66, 2010

Introduction.—The aim of this study is to evaluate the incidence of peritrochanteric high T2 signal (peritrochanteric edema, peritendinitis) on routine MR imaging studies and to determine whether reporting peritrochanteric edema is always clinically relevant depending on the age and gender of the patients.

Materials and Methods.—We evaluated 79 consecutive bilateral hip MR images performed in our department between January 2006 and December 2006 (57 female, 22 male patients, mean age 49 years). Each study was evaluated for areas of T2 hyperintensity representing edema around the greater trochanter. Patients with a known fracture, tumor, history of radiation therapy, history of hip surgery and prothesis were excluded from the study. Patients with signal intensity alterations within the thickened gluteus medius/minimus tendons (tendinitis) or peritrochanteric bursal fluid accumulation (bursitis) were also excluded. All patients were scanned with our routine MR imaging protocol for hip imaging.

Results.—In 55 of the 79 patients (70%) peritrochanteric edema was detected on MR images and 52 of these 55 patients (95%) had these changes on both hips. The median age was 56 years for the patients with peritrochanteric edema and 35.5 years for the patients without peritrochanteric edema. There was statistical significance between the median ages of the patients and a significant increased risk of peritrochanteric edema was found over 40 years of age. There was no significant difference between male and female patients.

Conclusion.—Bilateral peritrochanteric high T2 signal may be a part of the degeneration process and we suggest that it may not be necessarily reported if the clinical findings do not support greater trochanteric pain syndrome (Fig 2c).

▶ Degeneration of the attachment of the gluteus medius and minimus is a serious problem that can adversely affect an otherwise successful hip replacement. This is clearly an example of a lesion that has seen us more often than we have seen it. Because the diagnosis is by clinical assessment and MRI, this is an interesting study that reveals some physiologic changes at the greater trochanter far in excess of what is recognized clinically. There may be truth but certainly no data to support the observation that this finding, Fig 2c, is

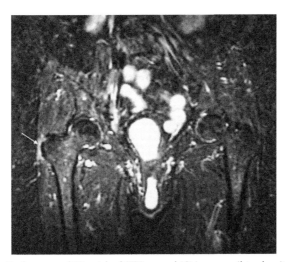

FIGURE 2.—On fat saturated T2-weighted STIR coronal (C) images, unilateral peritrochanteric high T2 signal is seen (arrows). (Reprinted from European Journal of Radiology, Haliloglu N, Inceoglu D, Sahin G. Assessment of peritrochanteric high T2 signal depending on the age and gender of the patients. *Eur J Radiol.* 2010;75:64-66, with permission from Elsevier.)

an early state of subsequent tendinosis. We are including this article to call attention to the need for a high level of suspicion that chronic trochanteric bursitis may in fact be a degenerative attachment of the abductors.

B. F. Morrey, MD

Analysis of the microbial load in instruments used in orthopedic surgeries
Pinto FMG, de Souza RQ, da Silva CB, et al (Univ of São Paulo, Brazil; Dept of Hosp Infection Control of Irmandade Santa Casa de Misericordia de São Paulo, Brazil)
Am J Infect Control 38:229-233, 2010

Background.—Because of advances in technology, the number of orthopedic surgeries, mainly hip and knee replacement surgeries, has increased, with a total of 150,000 prosthetic surgeries estimated per year in the United States and 400,000 worldwide.

Methods.—We used an exploratory cross-sectional study, with a quantitative approach to determine the microbial load in instruments used in orthopedic surgeries, quantifying and identifying the microbial growth genus and species, according to the surgical potential of contamination that characterizes the challenge faced by the Material and Sterilization Center at the Institute of Orthopedics and Traumatology of Hospital das Clinicas of the School of Medicine of the University of Sao Paulo, Brazil. The orthopedic surgical instruments were immersed, after their use, in sterilized distilled water, sonicated in an ultrasonic washer, and posteriorly agitated. Subsequently, the wash was filtrated through a 0.45-μm membrane and incubated in aerobic and anaerobic mediums and in medium for fungi and yeasts.

Results.—In clean surgeries, 47% of the instruments were contaminated; in contaminated surgeries, 70%; and, in infected surgeries, 80%. Regardless of the contamination potential of the surgeries, the highest quantitative incidence of microorganism recovery was located in the 1 to 100 colony-forming unit range, and 13 samples presented a microbial growth potential >300 colony-forming units. Regardless of the contamination potential of the surgeries, there was a convergence in the incidence of negative-coagulase *Staphylococcus* growth (28%, clean surgeries; 32%, contaminated surgeries; and 29%, infected surgeries) and *Staphylococcus aureus* (28%, contaminated surgeries; and 43%, infected surgeries).

Conclusion.—Most of the microorganisms recovered from the analyzed instruments (78%) were vegetative bacteria that presented their death curve at around 80°C, characterizing a low challenge considering the processes of cleaning and sterilization currently employed by the Material and Sterilization Center. Fewer microorganisms were recovered from instruments used in clean surgeries in comparison with those used in contaminated and infected surgeries.

▶ There are few studies of this nature in the orthopedic literature. How often do we consider the tissue cultures taken later in the case as more (or less) valid, because of the issue of contamination, than those taken earlier? Even if we are sensitive to this issue, I suspect few of us routinely consider the possibility of instrument contamination. It should come as no surprise that colonies can be isolated from instruments at the end of a case. That the counts would be higher in the contaminated and frankly infected procedure than a clean one is also intuitive. This work quantifies the expected differences. Of final note is that the counts are typically not of such a magnitude nor of a virulence as to cause clinical infection. Nonetheless, it does provide food for thought.

B. F. Morrey, MD

A Prospective, Randomized Clinical Trial Comparing an Antibiotic-Impregnated Bioabsorbable Bone Substitute With Standard Antibiotic-Impregnated Cement Beads in the Treatment of Chronic Osteomyelitis and Infected Nonunion
McKee MD, Li-Bland EA, Wild LM, et al (St Michael's Hosp and the Univ of Toronto, Ontario, Canada)
J Orthop Trauma 24:483-490, 2010

Objectives.—We sought to compare the effectiveness of an antibiotic-impregnated bioabsorbable bone substitute (BBS, tobramycin-impregnated medical-grade calcium sulfate) with antibiotic-impregnated polymethyl-methacrylate (PMMA) cement beads after surgical débridement in patients with chronic nonhematogenous osteomyelitis and/or infected nonunion.
Design.—A prospective, randomized clinical trial.
Setting.—A university-affiliated teaching hospital.
Patients/Participants.—Thirty patients requiring surgical treatment for chronic long bone infection or infected nonunion were included: BBS (15 patients, mean age 44.1 years) PMMA (15 patients, mean age 45.6 years).
Intervention.—Patients were randomized to receive either BBS or PMMA to the bone void created by surgical débridement.
Main Outcome Measurements.—Eradication of infection, new bone growth, rate of union, repeat operative procedures complications.
Results.—Patients were followed for a mean 38 months (range, 24—60 months). One patient was lost to follow-up in each group. In the BBS group, infection was eradicated in 86% (12 of 14) of patients. Seven of eight patients achieved union of their nonunion, and five patients underwent seven further surgical procedures. In the PMMA group, infection was eradicated in 86% (12 of 14) of patients. Six of eight patients achieved union of their nonunion, and nine patients required 15 further surgical procedures. There were more reoperations in the PMMA group (15 versus seven, $P = 0.04$), and these procedures tended to be of greater magnitude.
Conclusions.—The results of this preliminary study suggest that, in the treatment of chronic osteomyelitis and infected nonunion, the use of an

antibiotic-impregnated BBS is equivalent to standard surgical therapy in eradicating infection and that it may reduce the number of subsequent surgical procedures. A larger, definitive study on this topic is required.

▶ The topic of treating musculoskeletal infection is as old as our specialty, but it is getting renewed interest with the recent military actions. There have been numerous efforts through the years to develop a biodegradable carrier for the antibiotic because the removal of polymethylmethacrylate spacers requires another procedure and is expensive.

Nonetheless, it is the standard of care. Hence, an effective bioabsorbable option is very attractive. After years of investigation, we may be getting close to a clinically useful product.

B. F. Morrey, MD

Increased cancer risks among arthroplasty patients: 30 year follow-up of the Swedish Knee Arthroplasty Register
Wagner P, Olsson H, Lidgren L, et al (Lund Univ, Sweden)
Eur J Cancer 47:1061-1071, 2011

Background.—An increasing number of young patients are undergoing knee arthroplasties. Thus, the long-term risks of having a knee prosthesis must be evaluated. This study focuses on the potential carcinogenic effects of the prosthesis; it is a long-term follow-up of all patients in Sweden between 1975 and 2006.

Methods.—The incidence of cancer in a total population of operated individuals was compared to the overall national cancer incidence in Sweden by means of standardised incidence ratios. Analysis of cancer latency period was performed to identify potential aetiological factors.

Results.—For male and female patients with rheumatoid arthritis (RA) or osteoarthritis (OA), the overall cancer risks were elevated, ranging from 1.10 (95% confidence interval (CI): 1.03–1.18) for men with OA to 1.26 (1.23–1.29) for men with RA. The greatest increases in risk were observed for the leukaemia subtypes, myelodysplastic syndromes (MDS) and essential thrombocytosis (ET), ranging from 3.31 (1.24–8.83) for ET in men with OA to 7.38 (1.85–29.51) for ET in women with RA. Increases in risk were also observed for breast cancer, prostate cancer and melanoma. The latency analysis revealed elevated risks late in the study period for both solid and haematopoietic cancers. However, only increases in MDS and possibly prostate cancer and melanoma rates appeared to be connected to the operation.

Conclusion.—This study showed that OA and RA arthroplasty patients have a significantly higher risk of cancer than the general population. Elevated risks of MDS and possibly prostate cancer and melanoma indicated a potential connection to exposure to metals in the implant. The

TABLE 4.—Latency Analysis for Women and Men with OA. SIRs were Calculated for Each 5-Year Interval After the First Operation

Site	Interval	Women Obs.	Women Exp.	Women SIR	Women 95% CI	Men Obs.	Men Exp.	Men SIR	Men 95% CI
All	0−5	3316	2742	1.21	(1.17−1.25)	2676	2355	1.14	(1.09−1.18)
	5−10	2155	1614	1.34	(1.28−1.39)	1576	1271	1.24	(1.18−1.30)
	10−15	877	671	1.31	(1.22−1.40)	607	480	1.27	(1.17−1.37)
	15−20	215	188	1.14	(1.00−1.31)	130	115	1.13	(0.95−1.34)
	20−25	54	48	1.14	(0.87−1.48)	27	31	0.87	(0.60−1.27)
	25−30	8	8.3	0.96	(0.48−1.92)	6	5.7	1.05	(0.47−2.34)
Leukaemia	0−5	54	30	1.82	(1.40−2.38)	44	22	1.97	(1.46−2.64)
	5−10	34	18	1.86	(1.33−2.61)	19	12	1.56	(1.00−2.44)
	10−15	11	7.9	1.4	(0.77−2.52)	14	4.6	3.05	(1.80−5.14)
	15−20	1	2.2	0.45	(0.06−3.17)	2	1.1	1.81	(0.45−7.25)
	20−25	2	0.6	3.49	(0.87−13.9)	0	0.3	0	−
	25−30	0	0.1	0	−	0	0.1	0	−
MDS	0−5	17	3.7	4.64	(2.88−7.46)	15	3.3	4.58	(2.76−7.60)
	5−10	9	2.4	3.74	(1.95−7.19)	8	2	4.06	(2.03−8.11)
	10−15	7	1	6.79	(3.24−14.25)	3	0.8	3.91	(1.26−12.11)
	15−20	1	0.3	3.34	(0.47−23.73)	0	0.2	0	−
	20−25	1	0.1	12.61	(1.78−89.49)	0	0.1	0	−
	25−30	0	0.01	0	−	0	0.01	0	−
ET	0−5	8	1.13	7.1	(3.55−14.17)	3	0.7	4.34	(1.40−13.44)
	5−10	3	0.8	3.9	(1.26−12.08)	1	0.3	2.97	(0.42−21.07)
	10−15	2	0.4	4.79	(1.20−19.16)	0	0.1	0	−
	15−20	0	0.1	0	−	0	0.03	0	−
	20−25	0	0.03	0	−	0	0.01	0	−
	25−30	0	0.01	0	−	0	0	0	−
Malignant	0−5	135	75	1.8	(1.52−2.13)	112	61	1.84	(1.53−2.21)
melanoma	5−10	74	44	1.68	(1.33−2.10)	55	32	1.71	(1.31−2.23)
	10−15	32	19	1.7	(1.20−2.40)	23	12	1.86	(1.23−2.79)
	15−20	2	5.3	0.37	(0.09−1.50)	3	3	1.01	(0.33−3.13)
	20−25	1	1.4	0.71	(0.10−5.04)	1	0.8	1.21	(0.17−8.58)
	25−30	1	0.3	3.83	(0.54−27.19)	1	0.2	5.92	(0.83−42.00)
Prostate	0−5	0	0	0	−	950	813	1.17	(1.10−1.25)
	5−10	0	0	0	−	489	437	1.12	(1.03−1.22)
	10−15	0	0	0	−	199	161	1.23	(1.07−1.42)
	15−20	0	0	0	−	28	38	0.74	(0.51−1.07)
	20−25	0	0	0	−	9	10	0.87	(0.45−1.68)
	25−30	0	0	0	−	3	1.8	1.67	(0.54−5.17)
Breast	0−5	779	623	1.25	(1.17−1.34)	5	3.6	1.38	(0.57−3.32)
	5−10	433	342	1.27	(1.15−1.39)	1	2.1	0.49	(0.07−3.45)
	10−15	176	138	1.27	(1.10−1.48)	2	0.8	2.4	(0.60−9.60)
	15−20	48	38.4	1.25	(0.94−1.66)	0	0.2	0	−
	20−25	5	9.8	0.51	(0.21−1.23)	0	0.06	0	−
	25−30	2	1.7	1.16	(0.29−4.64)	0	0.01	0	−

MDS − myelodysplastic syndrome and ET − essential thrombocytemia.

observed excessive incidence of ET was likely associated with the inflammatory disease (Tables 4 and 5).

▶ This important article represents a clear advantage of registry data. Only with large numbers can such an important question be asked, and answered! The timeliness of this work cannot be overstated. To date, most studies failed to show a relationship between malignancy and arthroplasty. This study offers a different conclusion. The reader is referred to the data for both osteoarthritis

TABLE 5.—Latency Analysis for Women and Men with RA. SIRs were Calculated for Each 5-Year Interval After the First Operation

Site	Interval	Women Obs.	Exp.	SIR	95% CI	Men Obs.	Exp.	SIR	95% CI
All	0–5	357	339	1.05	(0.94–1.17)	158	148	1.07	(0.91–1.25)
	5–10	249	247	1.01	(0.89–1.14)	138	103	1.34	(1.13–1.58)
	10–15	184	141	1.3	(1.13–1.51)	78	55	1.43	(1.15–1.79)
	15–20	76	65	1.16	(0.93–1.46)	24	21	1.12	(0.75–1.68)
	20–25	31	25	1.25	(0.88–1.78)	7	7.2	0.97	(0.46–2.03)
	25–30	8	5.2	1.55	(0.78–3.11)	0	1.4	0	–
Leukaemia	0–5	4	3.6	1.1	(0.41–2.93)	2	1.5	1.3	(0.33–5.21)
	5–10	5	2.7	1.88	(0.78–4.51)	2	1	1.93	(0.48–7.71)
	10–15	4	1.5	2.66	(1.00–7.09)	1	0.5	1.9	(0.27–13.50)
	15–20	1	0.7	1.41	(0.20–10.03)	0	0.2	0	–
	20–25	1	0.3	3.72	(0.52–26.40)	0	0.1	0	–
	25–30	0	0.1	0	–	0	0.01	0	–
MDS	0–5	0	0.3	0	–	0	0.2	0	–
	5–10	1	0.3	3.97	(0.55–28.17)	0	0.1	0	–
	10–15	2	0.2	12.3	(3.08–49.18)	0	0.1	0	–
	15–20	0	0.1	0	–	0	0.03	0	–
	20–25	1	0.04	24.5	(3.45–173.6)	0	0.01	0	–
	25–30	0	0.01	0	–	0	0	0	–
ET	0–5	0	0.1	0	–	0	0.04	0	–
	5–10	1	0.1	12.36	(1.74–87.73)	0	0.03	0	–
	10–15	1	0.1	18.33	(2.58–130.1)	0	0.02	0	–
	15–20	0	0.03	0	–	0	0.01	0	–
	20–25	0	0.01	0	–	0	0	0	–
	25–30	0	0.0	0	–	0	0	0	–
Malignant	0–5	19	9.2	2.08	(1.32–3.25)	3	3.8	0.8	(0.26–2.48)
melanoma	5–10	12	6.7	1.79	(1.02–3.15)	2	2.6	0.76	(0.19–3.05)
	10–15	2	3.9	0.51	(0.13–2.05)	4	1.4	2.86	(1.07–7.62)
	15–20	4	1.9	2.14	(0.80–5.71)	2	0.6	3.53	(0.88–14.11)
	20–25	2	0.8	2.68	(0.67–10.71)	0	0.2	0	–
	25–30	0	0.2	0	–	0	0.04	0	–
Prostate	0–5	0	0.0	0	–	45	45	1	(0.75–1.34)
	5–10	0	0.0	0	–	35	33	1.06	(0.76–1.48)
	10–15	0	0.0	0	–	19	18	1.05	(0.67–1.65)
	15–20	0	0.0	0	–	7	7.2	0.97	(0.46–2.04)
	20–25	0	0.0	0	–	1	2.5	0.4	(0.06–2.81)
	25–30	0	0.0	0	–	0	0.5	0	–
Breast	0–5	83	83	1	(0.80–1.24)	0	0.2	0	–
	5–10	44	58	0.76	(0.56–1.01)	0	0.2	0	–
	10–15	35	33	1.07	(0.77–1.49)	0	0.1	0	–
	15–20	16	15.0	1.06	(0.65–1.74)	0	0.03	0	–
	20–25	4	5.8	0.69	(0.26–1.84)	0	0.01	0	–
	25–30	0	1.2	0	–	0	0	0	–

MDS – myelodysplastic syndrome and ET – essential thrombocytemia.

(Table 4) and rheumatoid arthritis (Table 5). An increased incidence in certain, especially haematopoietic, malignancies is noted for both diagnoses. Of interest, the authors implicate exposure to the metallic component as the most likely etiology. These observations, especially the delay to presentation, are extremely relevant today with the proliferation of the metal-on-metal bearing implant.

B. F. Morrey, MD

Are Dropped Osteoarticular Bone Fragments Safely Reimplantable in Vivo?

Bruce B, Sheibani-Rad S, Appleyard D, et al (Rhode Island Hosp, Providence; McLaren Regional Med Ctr/Michigan State Univ, Flint; et al)
J Bone Joint Surg Am 93:430-438, 2011

Background.—There are limited data detailing the appropriate management of nondisposable autologous osteoarticular fragments that have been contaminated by the operating room floor. The goal of the present study was to perform a comprehensive, three-phase investigation to establish an appropriate intraoperative algorithm for the management of the acutely contaminated, but nondisposable, autologous osteoarticular bone fragment.

Methods.—Phase I of the study was performed to quantify the rate of contamination and microbial profile of human osteoarticular fragments that were dropped onto the operating room floor (n = 162). Phase II was performed to assess the feasibility and optimal means of decontaminating 340 similar fragments that underwent controlled contamination with bacteria that were identified in Phase I; decontamination was performed with use of cleansing agents that are routinely available in an operating room. Phase III was performed to assess the effect of each decontamination process on fragment chondrocyte viability through histologic evaluation.

Results.—The contamination rate in Phase I was 70%. Coagulase-negative Staphylococcus was the most commonly cultured organism. In Phase II, varying exposure time to the chemical agents did not make a significant difference in decontamination rates. Mechanical scrubbing was superior to mechanical saline solution lavage (zero of fifty-six cultures compared with twenty of fifty-six cultures were positive for coagulase-negative Staphylococcus; p < 0.001). As a whole, bactericidal agents were found to be more effective decontaminating agents than normal saline solution. Povidone-iodine and 4% chlorhexidine gluconate were the most effective decontaminating agents, with none of the twenty-eight specimens that were decontaminated with each agent demonstrating positive growth on culture. Phase III demonstrated that the groups that were treated with normal saline solution and povidone-iodine retained the greatest number of live cells and the least number of dead cells. Mechanical scrubbing significantly decreased chondrocyte viability as compared with a normal saline solution wash (p < 0.05).

Conclusions.—The majority of osteochondral fragments that contact the operating room floor produce positive bacterial cultures. Five minutes of cleansing with a 10% povidone-iodine solution followed by a normal saline solution rinse appears to provide the optimal balance between effective decontamination and cellular toxicity for dropped autologous bone in the operative setting.

▶ This is a well-designed and well-executed study. Dropping a critical known disposable item on the operating room and floor can be a disaster. We will ultimately be faced with this problem at some time in our career. The authors have provided us with good information as to how to proceed in such a situation. Cell viability is particularly important in this situation. Isopropyl alcohol and chlorhexidine are particularly toxic solutions. The use of povidone-iodine solution is not only effective in the decontaminating the graft, but it is also the least detrimental solution to cellular viability. Dropping a unique one-of-a-kind critical allograft is a constant source of anxiety for surgeons performing allograft reconstructions. This method of decontamination could be applied to the situation if there are no alternate options.

C. P. Beauchamp, MD

2 Basic Science

Introduction

As with other medical disciplines, the most significant basic investigations regarding the musculoskeletal system relate to the genetic control of the disease processes. This expresses itself as the host variation that is observed in these processes as well as in response to treatment. There is relatively little genetic research being conducted in the musculoskeletal arena. A greater area of interest, of course, relates to growth factors in their various forms, including augmentation and potentiation of the osseous healing process. These areas have been covered in this YEAR BOOK edition. In addition, we have focused attention on clinically related basic investigations, particularly relating to insight and understanding regarding complications and untoward reactions. It is hoped that this section will provide the orthopedic surgeon some awareness of the direction and spectrum of basic investigations being conducted in the musculoskeletal arena, as well as some practical applications of relevant findings.

Bernard F. Morrey, MD

Perivascular Lymphocytic Infiltration Is Not Limited to Metal-on-Metal Bearings

Ng VY, Lombardi AV Jr, Berend KR, et al (The Ohio State Univ, Columbus; Joint Implant Surgeons, Inc, New Albany, OH)

Clin Orthop Relat Res 469:523-529, 2011

Background.—Perivascular lymphocytic infiltration (PVLI) suggests an adaptive immune response. Metal hypersensitivity after THA is presumed associated with idiopathic pain and aseptic loosening, but its incidence and relationship to metallic wear leading to revision are unclear as are its presence and relevance in non-metal-on-metal arthroplasty.

Questions/Purposes.—We compared (1) incidence and severity of PVLI in failed hip metal-on-metal (MoM) to non-MoM implants and TKA; (2) PVLI in MoM and non-MoM hip arthroplasty based on reason for revision; and (3) PVLI grade to diffuse lymphocytic infiltration (DLI) and tissue reaction to metal particles.

Patients and Methods.—We retrospectively examined incidence and severity of PVLI, DLI, and tissue reaction in periprosthetic tissue from 215 THA and 242 TKA revisions including 32 MoM hips.

Results.—Perivascular lymphocytic infiltration was present in more TKAs (40%) than overall hip arthroplasties (24%) without difference in severity. Compared to non-MoM hips, MoM bearings were more commonly associated with PVLI (59% versus 18%) and demonstrated increased severity (41% versus 3% greater than mild). Histologically, PVLI correlated (r = 0.51) with DLI, but not tissue reaction. In THA, PVLI was most commonly associated with idiopathic pain (70%) and aseptic loosening (54%) in MoM, and infection in all hip revisions (53%).

Conclusions.—Perivascular lymphocytic infiltration is more extensive in revisions of MoM and in aseptic loosening, idiopathic pain, or infection but is also present in TKA, non-MoM, and different reasons for revision. It correlates with other signs of metal hypersensitivity, but not with histologic measures of metal particulate load.

Level of Evidence.—Level III, diagnostic study. See the Guidelines for Authors for a complete description of levels of evidence.

▶ This study addresses the ever-growing concern about hypersensitivity to metal ions elaborated from the implant-bearing surface. By studying both hip and knee replacements, and metal on metal as well as metal on polyethylene bearings, a focused perspective is possible. Sure enough, the perivascular infiltrate is greater in the metal on metal devices (Figs 1 and 2 in the original article) and is correlated with pain, loosening, and infection. That the response is also present to a lesser extent in the knee and polyethylene bearing is not surprising and implies that the response is dose dependent. Once again, the metal bearing exhibits a potential for an adverse reaction that is not present with the polyethylene-bearing surface.

B. F. Morrey, MD

Lymphocyte Proliferation Responses in Patients with Pseudotumors following Metal-on-Metal Hip Resurfacing Arthroplasty

Kwon Y-M, Thomas P, Summer B, et al (Univ of Oxford, UK; der Ludwig-Maximilians-Universität, München, Germany)
J Orthop Res 28:444-450, 2010

Locally destructive soft tissue pseudotumor has been reported in patients following metal-on-metal hip resurfacing arthroplasty (MoMHRA). A delayed hypersensitivity reaction type IV to nickel (Ni), chromium (Cr), or cobalt (Co) has been suggested to play a role in its aetiology. The aim of this study was to investigate the incidence and level of metal-induced systemic hypersensitivity in patients with MoMHRA, both with and without pseudotumor by measuring lymphocyte proliferation responses to metals. A total of 92 patients were investigated: (1)MoMHRA patients

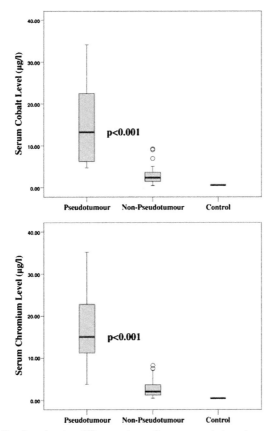

FIGURE 2.—Boxplots showing differences in median serum cobalt and serum chromium level measurements. (Reprinted from Kwon Y-M, Thomas P, Summer B, et al. Lymphocyte proliferation responses in patients with pseudotumors following metal-on-metal hip resurfacing arthroplasty. *J Orthop Res*. 2010;28:444-450, with permission from Orthopaedic Research Society.)

with pseudotumors (nine female, one male); (2)MoMHRA patients without pseudotumors (30 female, 30 male); and (3) age-matched control subjects without metal implants (9 female, 13 male). The venous blood samples were collected for serum Ni, Co, and Cr ion level measurements and lymphocyte transformation tests (LTT). A higher incidence and level of enhanced lymphocyte reactivity only to Ni was found in patients with MoMHRA compared to the patients without MoM implants, reflecting exposure and immune reactivity. However, lymphocyte reactivity to Co, Cr, and Ni did not significantly differ in patients with pseudotumors compared to those patients without pseudotumors. This suggests that systemic hypersensitivity type IV reactions, as measured by lymphocyte proliferation response to these metals, may not be the dominant biological

TABLE 2.—Incidence of Positive Metal Reactivity (SI ≥2.0) within Each Patient Group

Patient Groups	Subgroups	Nickel	Cobalt	Chromium
Pseudotumor	Overall	8/10 (80%)	0%	0%
	Male	1/1 (100%)	0%	0%
	Female	7/9 (78%)	0%	0%
	Male Bilateral	1/1 (100%)	0%	0%
	Female Bilateral	5/7 (71%)	0%	0%
Non-pseudotumor	Overall	29/60 (45%)	1/60 (2%)	3/60 (5%)
	Male	12/30 (40%)	1/30 (3%)	2/30 (7%)
	Female	15/30 (50%)	0/30 (0%)	1/30 (3%)
	Male Bilateral	3/10 (30%)	0/10 (0%)	1/10 (10%)
	Female Bilateral	6/8 (75%)	0/8 (0%)	0/8 (0%)
Control	Overall	3/22 (13%)	0%	0%
	Male	2/13 (15%)	0%	0%
	Female	1/9 (11%)	0%	0%

reaction involved in the occurrence of the soft tissue pseudotumors (Fig 2, Table 2).

▶ This is an important article, as it addresses one of the major and growing clinical concerns in orthopedics today: adverse reaction to the components of metal-on-metal articulations. The uncommon but potentially devastating impact of a hypersensitivity reaction to the metal ions is becoming increasingly recognized. This study is predicated on the observation that these reactions are lymphocytic mediated. The study design uses an adequate size and varied patient characteristics to allow reasonable conclusions. That some, but not all, patients developed the classic pseudotumor allows the important finding shown in Fig 2. Specifically, both cobalt and chromium concentrations are elevated in these patients. Overall, however, nickel appears in the greatest concentration and in the broadest spectrum of patient samples (Table 2). While it seems this study may introduce as many questions as it answers, it does highlight this concern.

B. F. Morrey, MD

Mechanical Loading Increased BMP-2 Expression which Promoted Osteogenic Differentiation of Tendon-Derived Stem Cells
Rui YF, Lui PPY, Ni M, et al (The Chinese Univ of Hong Kong, Hong Kong SAR, China)
J Orthop Res 29:390-396, 2011

This study aimed to investigate the effect of repetitive tensile loading on the expression of BMP-2 and the effect of BMP-2 on the osteogenic differentiation of tendon-derived stem cells (TDSCs) in vitro. Repetitive stretching was applied to TDSCs isolated from rat patellar tendon at 0%, 4%, and 8%, 0.5 Hz. The expression of BMP-2 was detected by Western blotting and qPCR. To study the osteogenic effects of BMP-2 on TDSCs, BMP-2 was added to the TDSC monolayer for the detection of ALP activity and calcium nodule formation in a separate experiment. TDSCs adhered, proliferated, and aligned along the direction of externally applied tensile force while they were randomly oriented in the control group. Western blotting showed increased expression of BMP-2 in 4% and 8% stretching groups but not in the control group. Up-regulation of *BMP-2* mRNA was also observed in the 4% stretching group. BMP-2 increased the osteogenic differentiation of TDSCs as indicated by higher ALP cytochemical staining, ALP activity, and calcium nodule formation. Repetitive tensile loading increased the expression of BMP-2 and addition of BMP-2 enhanced osteogenic differentiation of TDSCs. Activation of BMP-2 expression in TDSCs during tendon overuse might provide a possible explanation of ectopic calcification in calcifying tendinopathy.

▶ This elegant study helps understand the link between mechanical and genetically controlled physiologic responses. That tensile loading stimulates various responses in various tissues is well known. The observation and findings reported herein are relevant not only in the manner suggested by the authors, but also, generically, in providing a basis for rehabilitation of healing tissues.

B. F. Morrey, MD

Novel Nanostructured Scaffolds as Therapeutic Replacement Options for Rotator Cuff Disease

Taylor ED, Nair LS, Nukavarapu SP, et al (Univ of Virginia, Charlottesville; Univ of Connecticut Health Ctr, Farmington)
J Bone Joint Surg Am 92:170-179, 2010

Background.—About 300,000 rotator cuff surgical procedures are done annually in the United States. Rotator cuff injuries cause significant shoulder pain and dysfunction. Active people are highly susceptible to these injuries, especially as they age. Surgical repair involves reapproximating the tendon edge to an anatomic footprint using an open, mini-open, or arthroscopic approach, depending on the tear's size, shape, and chronicity. Open techniques produce larger dissection and take longer; the arthroscopic technique involves a small working area, a longer learning curve, and a greater chance of recurrent lesions. Synthetic augmentation devices to support torn rotator cuff healing are available, but few truly mimic the biomechanical behavior of a natural rotator cuff tendon. A tissue-engineered approach combining biological, chemical, and engineering principles to design a suitable bioresorbable rotator cuff scaffold was investigated in a rodent model.

Methods.—Through electrospinning a biodegradable polymeric solution was used to create resorbable polymer scaffolds from poly(85 lactic acid-*co*-15 glycolic acid) (PLAGA). Patellar tendon cells were obtained from adult New Zealand White rabbits, cultured, trypsinized, and seeded on nanofiber matrices, which were then irradiated with ultraviolet light to reduce contamination. Scanning electron microscopy (SEM) was used to analyze the cellular network development and adhesion properties. MTS assays were used to quantify cell proliferation, and LIVE/DEAD assay evaluated cell viability on the matrices and cell number increases over time. A biomechanical testing machine was used to determine the Young modulus of the matrices; suture strength was also analyzed. Forty-eight Sprague-Dawley rats underwent operative procedures, with the supraspinatus exposed, superficial musculature elevated, and the coracoacromial arch reflected. The supraspinatus tendon was separated longitudinally from other tissues and detached from the greater tuberosity. Repair involved primary reapproximation, with the cut end secured directly to bone using a modified Kessler stitch technique. For augmentation, a scaffold sample was sutured over the primary repair site. The coracoacromial arch, superficial shoulder muscles, and skin were repaired, then animals were allowed free movement in their cages until sacrifice 4 or 8 weeks after surgery for biomechanical evaluation.

Results.—With time the cellular network on the matrices increased. MTS assay found a significant increase in the measured absorbance from the scaffold, indicating cellular activity and proliferation. LIVE/DEAD assay found qualitative evidence of increased surface area of viable cells with time. The cellular network increased the mechanical properties of the cell-seeded scaffold throughout the period of cellular proliferation. Cell-seeded matrices had a higher Young modulus than cell-free scaffolds. Using maximal load to failure as a measure of suture strength, the amount of load needed to produce failure declined insignificantly over time. Suture pullout from the scaffold was the mode of construct breakdown in 14 of the 15 samples tested. No wound complications or premature deaths occurred. All animals had full use of the operated upper extremity and could reach overhead for feeding. Animals with augmentation had a significantly higher Young modulus than those having primary supraspinatus repair only.

Conclusions.—The bioresorbable nanostructured scaffold developed as an augmentation device for regenerating a torn rotator cuff produced biomechanical properties comparable to those with currently available alternative extracellular matrices. The scaffold approach has promise as a potential replacement option for surgical repair of torn rotator cuffs.

▶ Tissue engineering to address voids of the musculoskeletal system is of great scientific interest and shows great clinical promise as well. Much focus has been on osseous deficiencies; hence, the application of the technology to deficiencies of soft tissue is of value. Massive rotator cuff tears remain an unsolved issue. The use of nanotechnology is very attractive in general and appears to be quite applicable in this setting (Fig 3A-C in the original article). The key, as always when dealing biological regeneration, is the strength of the reconstructive tissue. This is an attractive direction.

B. F. Morrey, MD

Ibuprofen Upregulates Expressions of Matrix Metalloproteinase-1, -8, -9, and -13 without Affecting Expressions of Types I and III Collagen in Tendon Cells

Tsai W-C, Hsu C-C, Chang H-N, et al (Chang Gung Univ, Taoyuan County, Taiwan)
J Orthop Res 28:487-491, 2010

Nonsteroidal antiinflammatory drugs are widely used to treat sports-related tendon injuries or tendinopathy. This study was designed to investigate the effect of ibuprofen on expressions of types I and III collagen, as well as collagen-degrading enzymes including matrix metalloproteinase (MMP)-1, -2, -8, -9, and -13. Rat Achilles tendon cells were treated with ibuprofen and then underwent MTT[3-(4,5-Dimethylthiazol-2-yl)-2,5-diphenyltetrazolium bromide] assay. Reverse transcription-polymerase chain reaction was used to evaluate mRNA expressions of types I and III collagen, MMP-1, -2, -8, -9, and -13. Protein expressions of types I and III collagen, MMP-1, -8, and -13 were determined by Western blot analysis. Gelatin zymography was used to evaluate the enzymatic activities of MMP-2 and MMP-9. The results revealed that ibuprofen upregulated expressions of MMP-1, -8, -9, and -13, both at mRNA and protein levels. There was no effect of ibuprofen on mRNA and protein expressions of types I and III collagen. Gelatin zymography revealed that the enzymatic activity of MMP-9 was upregulated after ibuprofen treatment. In conclusion, ibuprofen upregulates the expressions of collagenases including MMP-1, -8, -9, and -13 without affecting the expressions of types I and III collagen. These findings suggest a molecular mechanism potentially accounting for the inhibition of tendon healing by ibuprofen.

▶ The usefulness of this study is simple. In spite of the details that are of less concern to the orthopedic surgeon, it does reinforce the relationship of nonsteroidal anti-inflammatory drugs on tissue healing. While we may be less aware of an adverse impact of such management in our clinical practice, there are clear interactions that are occurring at a molecular level. In our laboratory, we are investigating the concept of individual host variation as accounting for the varied, and lack of, clinical relevance to such well-documented interactions. This is an area of great potential relevance and deserves close monitoring by the clinician.

B. F. Morrey, MD

Autologous Chondrocyte Implantation Using the Original Periosteum-Cover Technique Versus Matrix-Associated Autologous Chondrocyte Implantation: A Randomized Clinical Trial

Zeifang F, Oberle D, Nierhoff C, et al (Orthopädische Universitätsklinik Heidelberg, Germany)

Am J Sports Med 38:924-933, 2010

Background.—Autologous chondrocyte implantation (ACI) is frequently used to treat symptomatic defects of the articular cartilage.

Purpose.—To test whether matrix-associated autologous chondrocyte implantation or the original periosteal flap technique provides superior outcomes in terms of clinical efficacy and safety.

Study Design.—Randomized controlled trial; Level of evidence, 2.

Methods.—Twenty-one patients (mean age, 29.3 ± 9.1 years) with symptomatic isolated full-thickness cartilage defects (mean 4.1 ± 09 cm^2) at the femoral condyle were randomized to matrix-associated autologous chondrocyte implantation or the original periosteal flap technique. The primary outcome parameter was the postoperative change in knee function as assessed by the International Knee Documentation Committee (IKDC) score at 12 months after ACI. In addition, the IKDC score was assessed at 3, 6, 12, and 24 months after surgery. Secondary outcome parameters were postoperative changes in health related quality of life (Short Form-36 Health Survey), knee functionality (Lysholm and Gillquist score), and physical activity (Tegner Activity Score) at 3, 6, 12, and 24 months after ACI. Magnetic resonance imaging was performed to evaluate the cartilage 6, 12, and 24 months after ACI and rated using the Magnetic Resonance Observation of Cartilage Repair Tissue score. Adverse events were recorded to assess safety.

Results.—The primary outcome parameter showed improvement of patients 1 year after autologous chondrocyte implantation, but there was no difference between the periosteal flap technique and matrix-associated ACI ($P = .5573$); 2 years after ACI, a similar result was found ($P = .4994$). The study groups did not show differences in the Short Form-36 categories and in knee functionality as assessed by Tegner Activity Score 12 months ($P = .4063$) and 24 months ($P = .1043$) after ACI. There was a significant difference in the Lysholm and Gillquist score at 12 months ($P = .0449$) and 24 months ($P = .0487$) favoring the periosteal flap technique group. At 6 months after surgery, a significantly lower Magnetic Resonance Observation of Cartilage Repair score was obtained in the matrix-associated ACI group ($P = .0123$), corresponding to more normal magnetic resonance imaging diagnostic findings. Twelve and 24 months after ACI, the differences between the 2 groups were not significant (12 months, $P = .2065$; 24 months, $P = .6926$). Adverse events were related to knee problems such as transplant delamination, development of an osseous spur, osteochondral dissection, and transplant hypertrophy. Systemic (allergic, toxic, or autoimmune) reactions did not occur.

Conclusion.—There was no difference in the efficacy between the original and the advanced ACI technique 12 and 24 months after surgery regarding International Knee Documentation Committee, Tegner Activity Score, and Short Form-36; however, with respect to the Lysholm and Gillquist score, better efficacy was observed in the periosteal flap technique group.

▶ There are several reasons to review this interesting article. First, as a prospective randomized study, it does bring the rigor of the scientific process to its conclusions. Second, it is a relevant topic and a relevant question. That no differences were found between the 2 techniques with the tools used to study outcome, in my mind, probably reflects the lack of sophistication of our methods more than there truly being no difference. That the periosteal flap technique appears to provide a marginally better outcome is also in keeping with my interpretation of prior literature on this subject. Importantly, we are improving our ability to treat localized cartilage lesions. In the end, the technique that is the least expensive and easiest to accomplish will win the day.

B. F. Morrey, MD

Development of simulated arthroscopic skills: A randomized trial of virtual-reality training of 21 orthopedic surgeons
Andersen C, Winding TN, Vesterby MS (Silkeborg Regional Hosp, Denmark)
Acta Orthop 82:90-95, 2011

Background and Purpose.—Previous studies have shown that there is a correlation between arthroscopic experience and performance on a virtual-reality (VR) unit. We analyzed the development inexperienced surgeons went through during VR training of shoulder arthroscopy.

Methods.—14 inexperienced surgeons from Silkeborg Regional Hospital were randomized into an intervention group and a control group. 7 experienced surgeons constituted another control group. All were tested twice on insightMIST—an advanced arthroscopic VR trainer—within a period of 6−15 days. The intervention group also received a 5-hour training program on the VR unit.

Results.—The average time for the arthroscopy in the intervention group was reduced from 720 (SD 239) seconds to 223 (SD 114) seconds (p = 0.03 compared to the inexperienced control group). Distance travelled by the camera was reduced from 367 (SD 151) cm to 84 (SD 44) cm in the intervention group (p = 0.02 compared to the inexperienced control group). Depth of collisions was also significantly reduced, whereas distance travelled by the probe and number of collisions were improved in the intervention group, although not statistically significantly.

Interpretation.—VR training is a possible way for young and inexperienced surgeons to achieve basic navigation skills necessary to perform

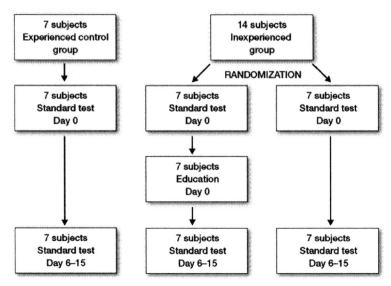

FIGURE 3.—Flow chart of the experiment. (Reprinted from Andersen C, Winding TN, Vesterby MS. Development of simulated arthroscopic skills: a randomized trial of virtual-reality training of 21 orthopedic surgeons. *Acta Orthop.* 2011;82:90-95, with permission from Taylor and Francis Group.)

arthroscopic surgery. Further studies regarding the transferability of the skills acquired on the VR unit to the operating theater are desirable (Fig 3).

▶ This study caught my eye, as it was the topic of discussion just this week. The comment was made that arthroscopic simulation was of little value and no substitute for true clinical experience. While none would argue the point that simulation isn't perfect, when considered from a risk-benefit patient perspective, the issue does deserve critical assessment. This is just what this study does. The study is well designed and well executed (Fig 3). Hence, the findings are legitimate. Simulated arthroscopic education is effective, at least at the shoulder. There is little reason to feel that this is no less true for the knee or other joints. With time, the simulation techniques and models will continue to improve. I believe that the orthopedic community can be confident that surgeons and patients alike will benefit.

B. F. Morrey, MD

Experimental Knee Pain Reduces Muscle Strength
Henriksen M, Rosager S, Aaboe J, et al (Frederiksberg Hosp, Denmark; et al)
J Pain 12:460-467, 2011

Pain is the principal symptom in knee pathologies and reduced muscle strength is a common observation among knee patients. However, the relationship between knee joint pain and muscle strength remains to be

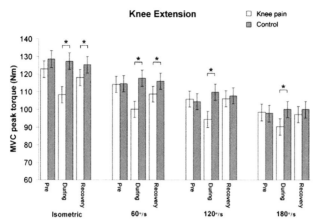

FIGURE 2.—Average (± SE) knee extension maximal voluntary contraction (MVC) peak torque data recorded isometrically, and isokinetically, at 60 degrees/second, 120 degrees/second, and 180 degrees/second, before, during, and after experimental pain by injections of painful hypertonic saline (open bars) into the infrapatellar fat pad or a control injection of nonpainful isotonic saline (grey bars). *$P < .001$. (Reprinted from Henriksen M, Rosager S, Aaboe J, et al. Experimental knee pain reduces muscle strength. *J Pain*. 2011;12:460-467, with permission from the American Pain Society.)

clarified. This study aimed at investigating the changes in knee muscle strength following experimental knee pain in healthy volunteers, and if these changes were associated with the pain intensities. In a crossover study, 18 healthy subjects were tested on 2 different days. Using an isokinetic dynamometer, maximal muscle strength in knee extension and flexion was measured at angular velocities 0, 60, 120, and 180 degrees/second, before, during, and after experimental pain induced by injections of hypertonic saline into the infrapatellar fat pad. On a separate day, isotonic saline injections were used as control condition. The pain intensity was assessed on a 0- to 100-mm visual analogue scale. Knee pain reduced the muscle strength by 5 to 15% compared to the control conditions ($P < .001$) in both knee extension and flexion at all angular velocities. The reduction in muscle strength was positively correlated to the pain intensity. Experimental knee pain significantly reduced knee extension and flexion muscle strength indicating a generalized muscle inhibition augmented by higher pain intensities.

Perspective.—This study showed that knee joint pain has a significant impact on muscle function. The findings provide evidence of a direct inhibition of muscle function by joint pain, implying that rehabilitative strengthening exercises may be antagonized by joint pain (Fig 2).

▶ This interesting and straightforward study documents what we have all recognized clinically—reflex inhibition from pain. The quantification of up to 15% strength reduction is of value as well (Fig 2). The importance of including the study is that it is a nice example of evidence-based medicine.

B. F. Morrey, MD

Influence of icing on muscle regeneration after crush injury to skeletal muscles in rats

Takagi R, Fujita N, Arakawa T, et al (Kobe Univ Graduate School of Health Sciences, Japan; et al)
J Appl Physiol 110:382-388, 2011

The influence of icing on muscle regeneration after crush injury was examined in the rat extensor digitorum longus. After the injury, animals were randomly divided into nonicing and icing groups. In the latter, ice packs were applied for 20 min. Due to the icing, degeneration of the necrotic muscle fibers and differentiation of satellite cells at early stages of regeneration were retarded by ∼1 day. In the icing group, the ratio of regenerating fibers showing central nucleus at 14 days after the injury was higher, and cross-sectional area of the muscle fibers at 28 days was evidently smaller than in the nonicing group. Besides, the ratio of collagen fibers area at 14 and 28 days after the injury in the icing group was higher than in the nonicing group. These findings suggest that icing applied soon after the injury not only considerably retarded muscle regeneration but also induced impairment of muscle regeneration along with excessive collagen deposition. Macrophages were immunohistochemically demonstrated at the injury site during degeneration and early stages of regeneration. Due to icing, chronological changes in the number of macrophages and immunohistochemical expression of transforming growth factor (TGF)-β1 and IGF-I were also retarded by 1 to 2 days. Since it has been said that macrophages play important roles not only for degeneration, but also for muscle regeneration, the influence of icing on macrophage activities might be closely related to a delay in muscle regeneration, impairment of muscle regeneration, and redundant collagen synthesis.

▶ This is an elegant study that addresses one of the most common issues in muscle trauma management. How should the initial injury be handled? The application of ice is universally accepted and taught as a standard of care. Although the experimental setting is not directly applicable, this study does call to question not only whether ice is a value but even whether it may be detrimental. The study methodology is thorough and sophisticated and demonstrates, ultimately, a retardation in the healing process. One could still argue that, even if retarded, the quality of the healing is greater with the intervention of early icing, but there are no data to indicate that this is true. I find it interesting and sobering when a traditional value and practice is challenged with science. Stay tuned.

B. F. Morrey, MD

3 Trauma and Amputation

Introduction

Although the transition to the new on-line method of screening manuscripts for inclusion and commentary has decreased the number of selections in the trauma and amputation chapter, the quality has not suffered. This year's crop contains high-quality systematic reviews and controlled trials. Of particular interest to the orthopedic community are several well-done investigations published with the purpose of gaining a better understanding of femoral fractures associated with bisphosphonate therapy for osteoporosis. This crop of articles leads us to conclude that the risk of these subtrochanteric and diaphyseal fractures is far lower when compared with the benefit of these drugs in preventing a hip fracture. We also note that their widespread use should continue with consideration of a "drug holiday" for patients who have been taking the drug for longer than 5-7 years. Further progress in the production of level 1 and level 2 evidence for trauma and amputation topics, along with higher-quality cohort studies, has again been observed this year.

Marc F. Swiontkowski, MD

General Topics

Atypical Fractures as a Potential Complication of Long-term Bisphosphonate Therapy

Sellmeyer DE (Johns Hopkins School of Medicine, Baltimore, MD)
JAMA 304:1480-1484, 2010

The development of bisphosphonate therapy represented an important advance in the treatment of low bone mass and osteoporosis, conditions that affect more than half of individuals older than 50 years. Currently available bisphosphonates have been shown to reduce spine, nonspine, and hip fractures in individuals at increased risk of fracture. Case reports and limited clinical series over the past 5 years have raised concern that prolonged bisphosphonate therapy may suppress bone remodeling to the extent that normal bone repair is impaired, resulting in increased fracture risk. Fractures potentially resulting from suppressed bone turnover have been described as "atypical," affecting sites such as the subtrochanteric femur that are infrequently affected by osteoporotic fractures. A prodrome of thigh pain, lack of trauma prior to the fracture, and specific radiological characteristics have also been reported. Data are limited on the prevalence of, risk factors for, and treatment of this potential problem. Current strategies include fracture risk assessment, targeting bisphosphonate therapy appropriately to individuals at increased risk of fracture, considering a 12-month interruption in therapy after 5 years in patients who are clinically stable, and considering teriparatide treatment in individuals who experience an atypical fracture while receiving bisphosphonate therapy.

▶ The association between long-term bisphosphonate therapy for osteoporosis and femoral fractures, particularly in the subtrochanteric and shaft, has become public knowledge this year. Many patients now present to their primary care physicians and orthopedic surgeons with questions regarding risk. Although retrospective analyses of the controlled trials that brought a wide range of bisphosphonates to Food and Drug Administration approval have not confirmed increased risk, case series continue to be published that advance the concern. These analyses are underpowered to definitively identify the association or lack thereof. In the meantime, this case discussion provides useful summary information of the current status of knowledge on the subject. A 1-year drug holiday for every 5 years on therapy is the recommendation. Dual-energy X-ray absorptiometry scans should be regularly preformed to inform these decisions.

M. F. Swiontkowski, MD

Bisphosphonates and Fractures of the Subtrochanteric or Diaphyseal Femur

Black DM, for the Fracture Intervention Trial and HORIZON Pivotal Fracture Trial Steering Committees (Univ of California at San Francisco; et al)
N Engl J Med 362:1761-1771, 2010

Background.—A number of recent case reports and series have identified a subgroup of atypical fractures of the femoral shaft associated with bisphosphonate use. A population-based study did not support this association. Such a relationship has not been examined in randomized trials.

Methods.—We performed secondary analyses using the results of three large, randomized bisphosphonate trials: the Fracture Intervention Trial (FIT), the FIT Long-Term Extension (FLEX) trial, and the Health Outcomes and Reduced Incidence with Zoledronic Acid Once Yearly (HORIZON) Pivotal Fracture Trial (PFT). We reviewed fracture records and radiographs (when available) from all hip and femur fractures to identify those below the lesser trochanter and above the distal metaphyseal flare (subtrochanteric and diaphyseal femur fractures) and to assess

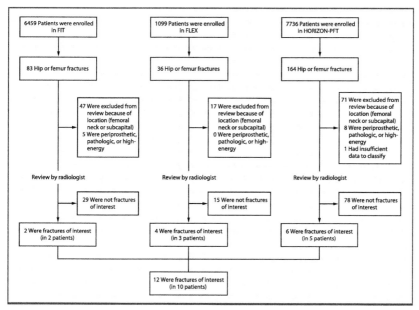

FIGURE 1.—Process for Review of Hip and Femur Fractures from Three Clinical Trials. FIT denotes fracture intervention trial, FLEX FIT long-term extension (ClinicalTrials.gov number, NCT00398931), and HORIZON-PFT health outcomes and reduced incidence with zoledronic acid once yearly pivotal fracture trial (NCT00049829). (Reprinted from Black DM, for the Fracture Intervention Trial and HORIZON Pivotal Fracture Trial Steering Committees. Bisphosphonates and fractures of the subtrochanteric or diaphyseal femur. *N Engl J Med.* 2010;362:1761-1771. Copyright © [2010] Massachusetts Medical Society. All rights reserved.)

atypical features. We calculated the relative hazards for subtrochanteric and diaphyseal fractures for each study.

Results.—We reviewed 284 records for hip or femur fractures among 14,195 women in these trials. A total of 12 fractures in 10 patients were classified as occurring in the subtrochanteric or diaphyseal femur, a combined rate of 2.3 per 10,000 patient-years. As compared with placebo, the relative hazard was 1.03 (95% confidence interval [CI], 0.06 to 16.46) for alendronate use in the FIT trial, 1.50 (95% CI, 0.25 to 9.00) for zoledronic acid use in the HORIZON-PFT trial, and 1.33 (95% CI, 0.12 to 14.67) for continued alendronate use in the FLEX trial. Although increases in risk were not significant, confidence intervals were wide.

Conclusions.—The occurrence of fracture of the subtrochanteric or diaphyseal femur was very rare, even among women who had been treated with bisphosphonates for as long as 10 years. There was no significant increase in risk associated with bisphosphonate use, but the study was underpowered for definitive conclusions (Fig 1, Tables 1 and 2).

▶ Increasing concern in the orthopedic community regarding the incidence of proximal femur stress fractures of the proximal and femoral shaft in patients who

TABLE 1.—Review of Fracture Location in Three Randomized Trials of Bisphosphonates*

Variable	Fracture Intervention Trial (FIT) Alendronate (N = 3236)		Placebo (N = 3223)		Relative Hazard (95% CI)	P Value	HORIZON Pivotal Fracture Trial Zoledronic Acid (N = 3875)	
	no. (%)	per 10,000 patient-yr	no. (%)	per 10,000 patient-yr			no. (%)	per 10,000 patient-yr
Fractures reviewed	15		15				35	
Results of review								
Intertrochanteric	12 (0.4)	9.8	12 (0.4)	9.8	1.00 (0.45–2.22)	0.99	22 (0.6)	20.5
Intertrochanteric and subtrochanteric	1 (<0.1)	0.8	1 (<0.1)	0.8	1.00 (0.06–15.93)	0.99	5 (0.1)	4.7
Subtrochanteric or diaphyseal femur	1 (<0.1)	0.8	1 (<0.1)	0.8	1.03 (0.06–16.46)	0.98	3 (0.1)	2.8
Distal metaphysis	1 (<0.1)	0.8	1 (<0.1)	0.8	1.00 (0.06–15.95)	0.99	1 (<0.1)	0.9
Femoral neck[†]	16 (0.5)	13.1	31 (1.0)	25.5	0.51 (0.28–0.94)	0.03	21 (0.5)	19.6

During the HORIZON-PFT study, an additional category of subcapital fractures was used. In the table, such fractures were combined into the category of femoral-neck fractures.
*High-trauma fractures were excluded according to the original study protocols. CI denotes confidence interval, and NA not applicable.
[†]Data regarding fractures of the femoral neck are based on classification during original studies but were not reviewed as part of this analysis.

have been on prolonged diphosphonate therapy for osteoporosis is the current situation. This well-performed investigation looked at the incidence and location of potentially related fractures in the controlled phase 3 trials, which were the basis of Food and Drug Administration approval for these drugs. Although the pooled studies were underpowered to definitively answer the question, the research indicated no increased risk for stress fracture among the subjects of the trials, some of whom were on therapy for as long as 10 years. This clinical problem will be a subject of active discussion and investigation for at least the next several years.

M. F. Swiontkowski, MD

HORIZON Pivotal Fracture Trial Placebo (N = 3861)				FIT Long-Term Extension (FLEX)					
				Alendronate/ Alendronate (N = 662)		Alendronate/ Placebo (N = 437)			
no. (%)	per 10,000 patient-yr	Relative Hazard (95% CI)	P Value	no. (%)	per 10,000 patient-yr	no. (%)	per 10,000 patient-yr	Relative Hazard (95% CI)	P Value
47				11		6			
Results of review									
39 (1.0)	36.3	0.57 (0.34−0.95)	0.03	10 (1.5)	31.6	5 (1.1)	23.7	1.34 (0.46−3.91)	0.60
4 (0.1)	3.7	1.26 (0.34−4.68)	0.73	0	NA	0	NA	NA	NA
2 (0.1)	1.9	1.50 (0.25−9.00)	0.65	2 (0.3)	6.3	1 (0.2)	4.7	1.33 (0.12−14.67)	0.82
3 (0.1)	2.8	0.34 (0.03−3.23)	0.34	0	NA	0	NA	NA	NA
45 (1.2)	41.9	0.47 (0.28−0.79)	0.004	10 (1.5)	31.5	7 (1.6)	33.2	0.95 (0.36−2.49)	0.91

TABLE 2.—Characteristics of 10 Patients with 12 Fractures of the Subtrochanteric or Diaphyseal Femur*

Patient No.	Study	Study Medication	Age	Days from Randomization to Fracture	Compliance†	Level of Trauma‡	Associated Medications before or during Study	Bone Metabolism Marker (Reference Range)§	Other Comments
1	FIT	Placebo	75 yr	962	>75%	Fall from step, stair, or curb	None	CTX, 0.408 ng/ml (0.110–0.628); P1NP, 43.2 ng/ml (16.3–78.2); BSAP, 14.5 ng/ml (5.1–15.3)	
2	FIT	Alendronate	69 yr	1682	>75%	Unknown	None	CTX, 0.067 ng/ml (0.110–0.628); P1NP, 9.4 ng/ml (16.3–78.2); BSAP, 7.5 ng/ml (5.1–15.3)	
3	HORIZON	Zoledronic acid	65 yr	454	100%	Minimal	Raloxifene (before and during study)	NA	Hip pain reported as adverse event at previous visit; transverse fracture on radiography
4	HORIZON	Placebo	78 yr	1051	100%	Fall from step, stair, or curb	None	NA	Hip pain reported as adverse event at previous visit
5	HORIZON	Zoledronic acid	65 yr	732	100%	Minimal	None	NA	Spiral fracture on radiography
6	HORIZON	Placebo	72 yr	321	100%	Fall from step, stair, or curb	Injected calcitonin (before and during study)	NA	
7 Two fractures	HORIZON	Zoledronic acid	71 yr	934	100%	Minimal	Bisphosphonate (>4 yr) and HRT (both before study)	NA	Bone pain reported as adverse event at previous visit; simultaneous fractures of both femurs

8	First fracture	FLEX	Alendronate/ alendronate	79 yr	1250	Stopped study medication 3 yr before fracture	Minimal	6 yr alendronate (in FIT before FLEX)	NTX, 14.0 pmol/μmol (9.2–51.8); BSAP, 12.0 ng/ml (5.1–15.3)
	Second fracture				1369		Minimal trauma other than fall		
9		FLEX	Alendronate/ placebo	80 yr	1257	Stopped study medication 3 yr before fracture	Minimal	6 yr alendronate (in FIT before FLEX)	NTX, 54.0 pmol/μmol (9.2–51.8); BSAP, 9.5 ng/ml (5.1–15.3)
10		FLEX	Alendronate/ alendronate	83 yr	1006	>75%	Minimal	5 yr alendronate (in FIT before FLEX)	NTX, 11.0 pmol/μmol (9.2–51.8); BSAP, 5.5 ng/ml (5.1–15.3)

*NA denotes not available.

†The level of compliance was assessed on the basis of the pill count in the FIT and FLEX trials; in the HORIZON trial, all five patients had three infusions of zoledronic acid (100% compliance).

‡The level of trauma was recorded as one of the following categories: minimal (fall from standing height or less); fall from a step, stair, or curb; fall from more than standing height (≥20 in.); minimal trauma other than fall; moderate or severe trauma other than fall; and pathologic fracture.

§Listed are patients' most recent measurements of biochemical markers of bone metabolism before fracture. Markers of bone metabolism that were used in the FIT and FLEX trials included serum C-terminal telopeptide of type 1 collagen (CTX), serum procollagen type 1 N-propeptide (P1NP), serum bone-specific alkaline phosphatase (BSAP), and serum N-terminal telopeptide of type 1 collagen (NTX). In the HORIZON trial, markers were assessed only in a sample of subjects. None of the five subjects with subtrochanteric or diaphyseal femur fractures were in this sample.

East Practice Management Guidelines Work Group: Update to Practice Management Guidelines for Prophylactic Antibiotic Use in Open Fractures
Hoff WS, Bonadies JA, Cachecho R, et al (St Luke's Hosp, Bethlehem, PA; Hosp of St Raphael, New Haven, CT; Crozer Chester Med Ctr, Upland, PA; et al)
J Trauma 70:751-754, 2011

Based on a review of the literature published subsequent to their original presentation, the recommendations published in the original EAST guidelines remain valid. Antibiotics are an important adjunct to the management of open fractures and should be initiated as soon as possible. Gram-positive coverage is recommended for type I and type II fractures. Broader antimicrobial coverage is recommended for type III fractures.

Despite the potential clinical and resource advantages of fluoroquinolones, current research does not support their use as single-agent therapy, and studies suggest these agents may impair fracture healing. When required, aminoglycosides may be prescribed in a once-daily regimen.

▶ This is an updated literature review performed as a meta-analysis regarding antibiotic therapy for open fractures. The information displayed as level I and level II (listed as Fig 1 and Fig 2 in the original article) should be reviewed by all orthopedic surgeons treating patients with fractures so as to stay current with evidence-based recommendations.

M. F. Swiontkowski, MD

The Relationship Between Time to Surgical Débridement and Incidence of Infection After Open High-Energy Lower Extremity Trauma
Pollak AN, the LEAP Study Group (Univ of Maryland School of Medicine, Baltimore; et al)
J Bone Joint Surg Am 92:7-15, 2010

Background.—Urgent débridement of open fractures has been considered to be of paramount importance for the prevention of infection. The purpose of the present study was to evaluate the relationship between the timing of the initial treatment of open fractures and the development of subsequent infection as well as to assess contributing factors.

Methods.—Three hundred and fifteen patients with severe high-energy lower extremity injuries were evaluated at eight level-I trauma centers. Treatment included aggressive débridement, antibiotic administration, fracture stabilization, and timely soft-tissue coverage. The times from injury to admission and operative débridement as well as a wide range of other patient, injury, and treatment-related characteristics that have been postulated to affect the risk of infection within the first three months after injury were studied, and differences between groups were calculated. In addition, multivariate logistic regression models were used to control

TABLE 1.—Time to Treatment and Risk of Infection

	N	From Injury to Admission	From Admission to Débridement	From Injury to Débridement	From Débridement to Soft-Tissue Coverage
			Time* (*hr*)		
All infections					
Present	84	$5.2 \pm 6.5^\dagger$	6.5 ± 6.3	11.6 ± 9.3	117.8 ± 89.6
Absent	223	3.5 ± 5.2	8.0 ± 9.6	11.5 ± 10.6	131.1 ± 121.8
Major infections					
Present	50	$6.2 \pm 7.5^\dagger$	7.3 ± 7.4	13.5 ± 10.6	106.3 ± 79.8
Absent	257	3.5 ± 5.1	7.7 ± 9.1	11.2 ± 10.1	137.2 ± 118.4

*The values are given as the mean and the standard deviation.
$^\dagger P < 0.01$, t test.

TABLE 2.—Time from Injury to Débridement and Risk of Infection*

Time from Injury to Débridement	N	Percentage with Infection	Percentage with Major Infection
<5 hr	93	28.0	15.1
5 to 10 hr	86	29.1	14.0
>10 hr	128	25.8	18.8

*No significant differences were detected at the $p < 0.05$ level.

for the effects of potentially confounding patient, injury, and treatment-related variables.

Results.—Eighty-four patients (27%) had development of an infection within the first three months after the injury. No significant differences were found between patients who had development of an infection and those who did not when the groups were compared with regard to the time from the injury to the first débridement, the time from admission to the first débridement, or the time from the first débridement to soft-tissue coverage. The time between the injury and admission to the definitive trauma treatment center was an independent predictor of the likelihood of infection.

Conclusions.—The time from the injury to operative débridement is not a significant independent predictor of the risk of infection. Timely admission to a definitive trauma treatment center has a significant beneficial influence on the incidence of infection after open high-energy lower extremity trauma (Tables 1-3).

▶ The investigators used the extensive data collected in the Lower Extremity Assessment Project (LEAP) trial to investigate the influence of time to debridement to the development of deep infection in severe open injuries of the lower extremity. The time-honored rule that all open fractures need to be brought to the operating room for surgical debridement is not based in high-quality clinical research. For ethical reasons, this treatment guideline will likely not be addressed in a randomized clinical trial. This essentially forces the use of advanced statistical

TABLE 3.—Time from Injury to Admission and Risk of Infection

	N	Percentage with Infection	Percentage with Major Infection
Patients admitted directly to trauma center			
≤2 hr	142	20.4	11.3
>2 hr	43	55.8*	30.2*
Patients transferred to trauma center			
1 to 3 hr	53	17.0	13.2
4 to 10 hr	33	27.3	12.1
11 to 24 hr	36	36.1†	27.8†

*The risks of infection and major infection were significantly higher for patients for whom the time at the scene or in transit was prolonged (more than two hours from the time of injury to admission) as compared with those for whom the time from injury to admission was two hours or less (p < 0.01, chi-square test).
†The risks of infection and major infection were significantly higher in the eleven-to-twenty-four-hour group as compared with the one-to-three-hour group (p < 0.05, chi-square test of homogeneity).

techniques on nonrandomized data sets, such as multivariate regression, to control for injury severity and other treatment factors. The LEAP data were collected with great care and precision, and the elements of time to transfer to 1 of 8 level-I centers and the time from admission to surgical debridement were prospectively collected. The conclusion from these analyses is therefore valid to impact local decision making regarding patient care. The time to initial debridement is not related to the risk of deep infection. The time from injury to transfer to the definitive level-I center is an independent predictor of the likelihood of infection. The former can be a factor in local hospital decision making, and the latter will require discussion at the regional trauma system level.

M. F. Swiontkowski, MD

Osteoporosis as a Risk Factor for Distal Radial Fractures: A Case-Control Study

Øyen J, Brudvik C, Gjesdal CG, et al (Univ of Bergen, Norway; Haukeland Univ Hosp, Bergen, Norway)
J Bone Joint Surg Am 93:348-356, 2011

Background.—Distal radial fractures occur earlier in life than hip and spinal fractures and may be the first sign of osteoporosis. The aims of this case-control study were to compare the prevalence of osteopenia and osteoporosis between female and male patients with low-energy distal radial fractures and matched controls and to investigate whether observed differences in bone mineral density between patients and controls could be explained by potential confounders.

Methods.—Six hundred and sixty-four female and eighty-five male patients who sustained a distal radial fracture, and 554 female and fifty-four male controls, were included in the study. All distal radial fractures were radiographically confirmed. Bone mineral density was assessed with use of dual x-ray absorptiometry at the femoral neck, total hip (femoral neck, trochanter, and intertrochanteric area), and lumbar spine (L2-L4). A self-administered questionnaire provided information on health and lifestyle factors.

Results.—The prevalence of osteoporosis was 34% in female patients and 10% in female controls. The corresponding values were 17% in male patients and 13% inmale controls. In the age group of fifty to fifty-nine years, 18% of female patients and 5% of female controls had osteoporosis. In the age group of sixty to sixty-nine years, the corresponding values were 25% and 7%, respectively. In adjusted conditional logistic regression analyses, osteopenia and osteoporosis were significantly associated with distal radial fractures in women. Osteoporosis was significantly associated with distal radial fractures in men.

Conclusions.—The prevalence of osteoporosis in patients with distal radial fractures is high compared with that in control subjects, and osteoporosis is a risk factor for distal radial fractures in both women and men. Thus, patients of both sexes with an age of fifty years or older who have a distal radial fracture should be evaluated with bone densitometry for the possible treatment of osteoporosis (Tables 2 and 3).

▶ This well-done case cohort study evaluates the prevalence of osteoporosis in patients older than 50 years who present with a distal radius fracture from a fall

TABLE 2.—Factors Associated with Distal Radial Fractures in Women on Unadjusted and Adjusted Conditional Logistic Regression Analyses*,†

	Unadjusted OR (95% CI)	P Value	Adjusted‡ OR (95% CI)	P Value
BMD femoral neck§				
Normal	1		1	
Osteopenia	2.7 (1.9 to 3.9)	<0.001	2.7 (1.9 to 3.9)	<0.001
Osteoporosis	7.1 (4.3 to 11.6)	<0.001	6.8 (4.1 to 11.2)	<0.001
BMI				
≥22 kg/m²	1		1	
<22 kg/m²	1.34 (0.9 to 1.9)	0.098	1.0 (0.7 to 1.5)	0.954
Hip fracture in a parent				
No	1		1	
Yes	0.7 (0.5 to 1.1)	0.106	0.7 (0.4 to 1.1)	0.093
Previous low-energy fracture				
No	1		1	
Yes	1.6 (1.1 to 2.3)	0.010	1.5 (1.0 to 2.2)	0.050
Menopause				
≥45 yr	1		1	
<45 yr	1.5 (1.0 to 2.3)	0.042	1.5 (0.9 to 2.4)	0.064
Current smoking				
No	1.0			
Yes	1 (0.7 to 1.4)	1.000		

*The analysis included 664 patients and 554 controls.
†OR = odds ratio, CI = confidence interval, BMD = bone mineral density, BMI = body-mass index.
‡Variables that were included in the adjusted model included osteopenia, osteoporosis, a body-mass index of <22, hip fracture in a parent, previous low-energy fracture, and menopause at an age of less than forty-five years.
§A normal BMD is defined as a T score of −1.0 or greater, osteopenia is defined as a T score of less than −1.0 or more than −2.5, and osteoporosis is defined as a T score of −2.5 or less.

TABLE 3.—Factors Associated with Distal Radial Fractures in Men on Unadjusted and
Adjusted Conditional Logistic Regression Analyses[*,†]

	Unadjusted OR (95% CI)	P Value	Adjusted[‡] OR (95% CI)	P Value
BMD femoral neck[§]				
Normal	1		1	
Osteopenia	3.4 (1.1 to 10.5)	0.032	3.1 (1.0 to 9.8)	0.051
Osteoporosis	8.5 (1.6 to 44.7)	0.011	8.1 (1.4 to 47.4)	0.021
BMI				
≥22 kg/m²	1		1	
<22 kg/m²	2.5 (0.7 to 9.8)	0.183	2.6 (0.5 to 12.3)	0.238
Current smoking				
No	1		1	
Yes	2.6 (0.9 to 6.8)	0.060	1.6 (0.5 to 5.1)	0.386
Hip fracture in a parent				
No	1			
Yes	0.8 (0.1 to 2.3)	0.437		

*The analysis included eighty-five patients and fifty-four controls.
†OR = odds ratio, CI = confidence interval, BMD = bone mineral density, BMI = body-mass index.
‡Variables that were included in the adjusted model included osteopenia, osteoporosis, a body-mass index of <22, and current smoking.
§A normal BMD is defined as a T score of −1.0 or greater, osteopenia is defined as a T score of less than −1.0 or more than −2.5, and osteoporosis is defined as a T score of −2.5 or less.

from a standing height. The findings from a careful cohort match are clear (Tables 2 and 3). The findings are clear for both men and women. Patients presenting with this diagnosis should be evaluated with a dual-energy x-ray absorptiometry scan and treated appropriately. This study leads to the rapidly increasing body of literature that strongly suggests that orthopedic surgeons be involved with appropriate diagnosis of patients presenting with fragility fractures.

M. F. Swiontkowski, MD

Ultrasound-guided reduction of distal radius fractures
Chinnock B, Khaletskiy A, Kuo K, et al (Univ of California, San Francisco)
J Emerg Med 40:308-312, 2011

Background.—Ultrasound (US) may provide the emergency physician with the ability to do real-time assessment of fracture reduction adequacy.
Objectives.—To assess whether US guidance aids in determining the adequacy of distal radius fracture reduction in the emergency department (ED), and to compare the rates of successful reduction with and without US.
Methods.—We conducted a prospective study of patients who underwent US-guided reduction of a distal radius fracture, compared to a historical cohort without US guidance. After performing US-guided reduction, but before post-reduction radiographs, physicians filled out a form stating whether reduction was successful or unsuccessful. Successful radiographic reduction was determined by two orthopedic surgeons based on radiographic

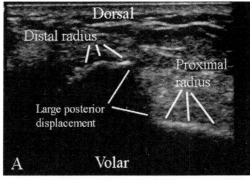
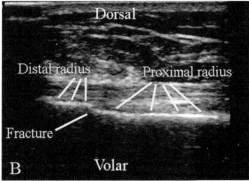

FIGURE 1.—Pre- and post-reduction ultrasound images of a distal radius fracture. The pre-reduction image (A) demonstrates significant dorsal displacement of the distal radius. Post-reduction image (B) demonstrates good alignment with minimal displacement. (Reprinted from Chinnock B, Khaletskiy A, Kuo K, et al. Ultrasound-guided reduction of distal radius fractures. *J Emerg Med.* 2011;40:308-312, Copyright 2011, with permission from Elsevier.)

findings. Main outcome measures were the sensitivity and specificity of US-guided ED physician assessment of successful reduction, and reduction success compared against the historical cohort.

Results.—We enrolled 46 patients in the US-guided group and compared them to 44 patients in the historical cohort. Pre-reduction characteristics were similar in both groups. Physician assessment of reduction success by US had a sensitivity of 94% (95% confidence interval [CI] 88-98%) and specificity of 56% (95% CI 31-71%) for identifying a successful reduction on post-reduction radiographs. The overall success rates of the US-guided and control groups were similar (83% and 80%, respectively).

Conclusions.—Physicians had a high sensitivity in predicting adequate reduction of distal radius fractures using US guidance in the ED. The overall rate of successful fracture reduction was similar with or without US. Further study may determine whether US guidance reduces the time spent in the ED for fracture reduction (Fig 1 and Table 1).

▶ Ultrasound utilization for multiple purposes has become a topic of widespread interest. A partial list of conditions where ultrasound is of help in the

TABLE 1.—Pre-reduction Characteristics of Patients Having Fracture Reduction With and Without US Guidance

Pre-reduction Characteristics	Control Patients (n = 44)	US-guided Patients (n = 46)
Subject characteristics		
Age in years, mean (range)	30 (3–87)	32 (6–77)
Female gender n (%)	21 (48)	20 (43)
Fracture characteristics		
Angulation of distal fragment		
Posterior, n (%)	32 (73)	37 (80)
Anterior, n (%)	6 (13.5)	6 (13)
None, n (%)	6 (13.5)	3 (7)
Angulation > 20°, n (%)*	24 (55)	22 (48)
AP displacement[†]		
None, n (%)	19 (43)	17 (37)
Partial, n (%)	9 (20)	11 (24)
Total, n (%)	16 (37)	18 (39)
Shortening, n (%)[‡]	26 (59)	28 (61)
Intra-articular, n (%)	4 (9)	9 (20)
Comminution, n (%)	6 (17)	9 (20)
Ulna fracture, n (%)	25 (57)	25 (54)
Radioulnar dislocation, n (%)	1	1
Mechanism of injury		
Fall, n (%)	34 (77)	35 (76)
MVA, n (%)	8 (18)	7 (15)
Other, n (%)	2 (5)	4 (9)
Pre-reduction assessment of reduction difficulty		
Difficult, n (%)	17 (39)	21 (47)
Interrater agreement of reduction difficulty (%)	75	85

All p-values non-significant.
*Angulation was measured by drawing lines through the center of the proximal and distal fragments, and measuring the angle at the intersection.
[†]AP displacement was described as "none" if the anterior cortex of the proximal and distal fragments were in contact, "partial" if there was any overlap of the proximal and distal fragments, and "total" if there was no overlap between the proximal and distal fragments.
[‡]Shortening was present if the proximal portion of the distal fragment lay proximal to the distal portion of the proximal bone. MVA = motor vehicle accident; F = female; AP = anteriorposterior.

clinical situation includes foreign body location, evaluation of ligament and tendon integrity, evaluation of joint reduction, and assessment of fracture reduction. This exploratory uncontrolled trial evaluates the utility of ultrasound in judging the quality of reduction of distal radius fracture. It proves to be reproducible and a technology capable of evaluating the quality of reduction but no better than the standard of care (using radiographs). This is not a cost-benefit study, and therein may lie the real benefit in addition to limiting the use of radiographs. The technology is highly technician dependent, and that fact cannot be minimized. Ultrasound will be the subject of numerous investigations in the next 2 to 4 years.

M. F. Swiontkowski, MD

Traumatic and Trauma-Related Amputations: Part I: General Principles and Lower-Extremity Amputations
Tintle SM, Keeling JJ, Shawen SB, et al (Walter Reed Army Med Ctr, Washington, DC; Natl Naval Med Ctr, Bethesda, MD)
J Bone Joint Surg Am 92:2852-2868, 2010

Deliberate attention to the management of soft tissue is imperative when performing an amputation. Identification and proper management of the nerves accompanied by the performance of a stable myodesis and ensuring robust soft-tissue coverage are measures that will improve patient outcomes.

Limb length should be preserved when practicable; however, length preservation at the expense of creating a nonhealing or painful residual limb with poor soft-tissue coverage is contraindicated.

While a large proportion of individuals with a trauma-related amputation remain severely disabled, a chronically painful residual limb is not inevitable and late revision amputations to improve soft-tissue coverage,

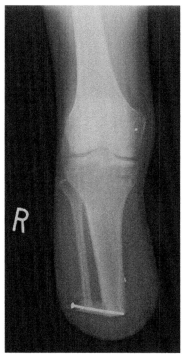
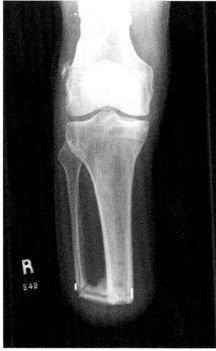

Fig. 7-A   **Fig. 7-B**

FIGURE 7.—Anteroposterior radiographs showing transtibial amputations with a distal bridge synostosis complicated by fracture and implant failure (Fig. 7-A) and with stable, uncomplicated early consolidation of the osteosynthesis sites (Fig. 7-B). (Reprinted from Tintle SM, Keeling JJ, Shawen SB, et al. Traumatic and trauma-related amputations: part I: general principles and lower-extremity amputations. *J Bone Joint Surg Am.* 2010;92:2852-2868, with permission The Journal of Bone and Joint Surgery, Inc.)

mentation procedure

TABLE 1.—Checklist for Successful Performance of Trauma-Related Amputations

Perform an aggressive initial (and subsequent) debridement and irrigation; do not attempt to definitively close the wound at the index procedure
Preserve reconstructive options via appropriate length selection and salvage of all viable tissue at the initial debridement procedure
Salvage functional joint levels; manage proximal fractures via standard techniques
Perform a traction neurectomy for all named nerves and all grossly visible cutaneous nerves well proximal to the end of the residual limb
Identify, isolate, and securely ligate all named vessels
Bevel and smooth all sharp bone ends of the residual limb; respect the periosteum
Perform a stable myodesis under physiologic muscle tension and augment with a secondary myoplasty
Ensure robust and viable distal padding
Maintain close follow-up in the early postoperative period and then pursue a consistent subsequent follow-up plan to identify operative complications and problems early and prevent nonoperative issues from escalating into operative ones

TABLE 2.—Documented Technical Errors in the Operative Care of Trauma-Related Amputations and Subsequent Untoward Results

Technical Error	Resulting Complication(s)
Improper length selection	Length salvage may be inappropriately aggressive with little concern for soft-tissue coverage, leading to a poorly padded residual limb; conversely, length selection may be overly conservative, leading to an unnecessarily shortened residual limb
Failure to perform traction neurectomies	Symptomatic neuromas, which can negatively affect prosthetic wear or require revision surgery
Inappropriate management of bone	Inappropriate handling of the periosteum or failure to smooth bone ends may lead to sharp, symptomatic spurs or edges
Failure to adequately stabilize distal musculature	Decreased residual limb control, retraction of distal padding, or overt subluxation or snapping of distal muscle groups
Failure to achieve a robust distal soft-tissue envelope	Delayed healing, pain, and soft-tissue breakdown
Failure to balance remaining muscular forces on the residual limb	Decreased residual limb control and proximal joint contractures
Inadequate attention to balanced incision closure	Dog ears, or soft-tissue redundancy, producing ulceration or pain
Inadequate short and intermediate-term follow-up	Failure to adequately recognize and treat frequent complications

stabilize the soft tissues (revision myodesis), or remove symptomatic neuromas can dramatically improve patient outcomes.

Psychosocial issues may dramatically affect the outcomes after trauma-related amputations. A multidisciplinary team should be consulted or created to address the multiple complex physical, mental, and psychosocial issues facing patients with a recent amputation (Fig 7 and Tables 1, 2).

▶ This is a comprehensive summary detailing amputation surgery principles to obtain optimum functional and pain outcomes. Summary Tables 1 and 2 are particularly valuable. The summary regarding the potential benefits of the Ertl variation of the below-knee amputation (Fig 7A and B) is accurate and unbiased. Any surgeon who performs the occasional amputation will find value in reviewing this article.

M. F. Swiontkowksi, MD

Femur Fractures

Is Surgery Necessary for Femoral Insufficiency Fractures after Long-term Bisphosphonate Therapy?
Ha Y-C, Cho M-R, Park KH, et al (Chung-Ang Univ College of Medicine, Seoul, South Korea; Daegu Catholic Univ College of Medicine, South Korea; Chung General Hosp, Seongnam, South Korea; et al)
Clin Orthop Relat Res 468:3393-3398, 2010

Background.—Prolonged use of bisphosphonates in patients with osteoporosis reportedly induces femoral insufficiency fractures. However, the natural course of these fractures and how to treat them remain unknown.

Questions/Purposes.—We determined the rates of fracture displacement and subsequent operations of undisplaced insufficiency fractures of the femur in patients treated with prolonged bisphosphonate therapy.

Patients and Methods.—We retrospectively collected and reviewed the clinical course of 11 patients (14 fractures) who had been diagnosed as having an insufficiency fracture of the femur after prolonged use (mean, 4.5 years; range, 3–10 years) of bisphosphonate. All patients were women with a mean age of 68 years (range, 57–82 years). The fracture site was subtrochanteric in six and femoral shaft in eight. The minimum followup was 12 months (mean, 27 months; range, 12–60 months).

Results.—During the followup period, secondary displacement of the fracture occurred in five of the 14 fractures after a mean of 10 months (range, 1–19 months). Three fractures were treated with internal fixation using a compression hip screw and two with intramedullary nailing. Because five additional fractures were treated surgically owing to intractable pain, surgery was performed in 10 of 14 insufficiency fractures during the followup period. All 10 fractures healed during followup. The remaining four patients (four fractures) not undergoing any surgery had persistent pain.

Conclusions.—Femoral insufficiency fractures after prolonged bisphosphonate therapy seldom healed spontaneously and most patients had surgery either for fracture displacement or persistent pain (Table 1).

▶ The issue of femoral insufficiency fracture related to prolonged bisphosphonate treatment of osteoporosis has received increased attention in the popular media over the last year and has prompted Food and Drug Administration review of the association. Yearlong drug holidays for every 5 years of treatment are now broadly recommended. The issue of how to manage these fatigue fractures is not completely clear at this time. This cohort study adds important

TABLE 1.—Data for 11 Patients With Insufficiency Fractures of the Femur

Patient Number	Age (years)	Side	Fracture Location	Bisphosphonate	Duration of Bisphosphonate Treatment (years)	DXA	Fracture Displacement	Interval* (months)	Surgical Treatment	Followup (months)
1	63	Left	Subtrochanter	Alendronate	4	−1.7	No		Not done	18
2	64	Left	Subtrochanter	Alendronate	5	−1.6	No		IM nailing	24
3	75	Left	Midshaft	Pamidronate	5	−2.9	No		Plate fixation	12
4	75	Right	Midshaft	Alendronate	10	−1.5	Yes	12	IM nailing	12
5	67	Left	Subtrochanter	Pamidronate	3	−2.2	Yes	1	CHS fixation	12
	78	Left	Midshaft				No		Plate fixation	18
6	65	Left	Subtrochanter	Alendronate	4	−2.7	No		IM nailing	48
	65	Right	Subtrochanter				Yes	19	CHS fixation	48
7	60	Left	Subtrochanter	Alendronate	4	−1.7	No		IM nailing	36
	60	Right	Subtrochanter				Yes	3	CHS fixation	36
8	57	Right	Midshaft	Alendronate	3	−1.9	No		Not done	24
9	68	Right	Midshaft	Alendronate	5	−3.8	No		Not done	36
10	82	Right	Midshaft	Alendronate	4	−4.8	Yes	15	IM nailing	60
11	73	Left	Midshaft	Alendronate	4	−2.9	No		Not done	12

DXA = dual-energy xray absorptiometry (lowest T-score of total femur or lumbar area); IM = intramedullary; CHS = compression hip screw.
*Time between the diagnosis of insufficiency fracture and fracture displacement.

information as the orthopedic surgery community tries to resolve the issue and develop a standard treatment approach. Of the 14 patients in this cohort, 10 eventually had surgical stabilization, 5 for intractable pain and 5 when the fractures displaced. Fortunately, all 10 healed. The question of whether or not parathyroid hormone therapy may be required for some of these fractures to get them to heal is not addressed. Patients who develop these fatigue fractures will generally benefit from stabilization to assure healing and prevent displacement.

M. F. Swiontkowski, MD

Femoral Insufficiency Fractures Associated with Prolonged Bisphosphonate Therapy
Isaacs JD, Shidiak L, Harris IA, et al (The St George and Sutherland Hosp Orthopaedic Depts, Sydney, New South Wales, Australia; The Univ of New South Wales, Sydney, Australia)
Clin Orthop Relat Res 468:3384-3392, 2010

Background.—Emerging evidence has linked the long-term use of bisphosphonates with femoral insufficiency fractures. It has been suggested that the prolonged effect on bone remodeling leads to the accumulation of microfractures and weakening of bone.

Questions/Purposes.—We investigated the association between bisphosphonate use and femoral insufficiency fractures.

Methods.—We evaluated 100 patients with low-energy femoral shaft fractures before and after bisphosphonates became available for use. Twenty-one consecutive patients who presented between January 1995 and February 1997 were compared with 79 consecutive patients who presented between January 2007 and February 2009. The radiographs of all 100 patients were examined for evidence of preexisting insufficiency fractures. We identified insufficiency fractures by a transverse fracture line on the tension side of the femur with lateral cortical thickening immediately adjacent to the fracture. Relevant details from the history were recorded.

TABLE 2.—Clinical Characteristics of Patients with Low-energy Femoral Fractures

Parameter	Insufficiency Fracture Present (n = 41)	Insufficiency Fracture not Present (n = 59)	p Value*
Mean age (years)	73.7 (72.4−75.0)	75.2 (73.5−77.0)	0.76
Mean ASA score	2.5 (2.3−2.6)	2.4 (2.3−2.6)	0.74
History of bisphosphonate use	41[†]	12	−
Duration of bisphosphonate use (years)	7.1 (6.6−7.6)	3.2 (2.6−3.8)	<0.0001
Bilateral insufficiency fracture	18	−	−
Prodrome of pain	29	−	−
Spontaneous nontraumatic fracture	9	−	−

ASA = American Society of Anesthesiologists score.
[†]40 patients had been taking alendronate, one patient had been taking risedronate.
*p values calculated using Student's t test.

TABLE 3.—Association Between Bisphosphonate Use and Insufficiency Fracture

History of Bisphosphonate Use	Insufficiency Fracture Present	Insufficiency Fracture not Present	Total Number of Patients
Yes	41	12	53
No	0	47	47
Totals	41	59	100

Odds ratio = greater than 1000, p < 0.0001; sensitivity = 100%, specificity = 80%, positive predictive value = 77%, negative predictive value = 100%.

TABLE 4.—Reported Clinical Characteristics of Patients with Femoral Insufficiency Fractures

Study	Femoral Insufficiency Fractures	Bilateral Insufficiency Fractures	Prodrome of Pain	Mean Duration of Bisphosphonate Use (Years)	Mean Age (Years)	Insufficiency Fractures Identified with no History of Bisphosphonate Use
Odvina et al., 2005 [46]	5	2	—	5.6 (3—8)	60.0 (49—68)	—
Goh et al., 2007 [26]	6	3	5	4.2 (2.5—5)	66.9 (55—82)	0
Kwek et al., 2008 [33]	17	9	13	4.4 (2—10)	66.1 (53—82)	0
Lenart et al., 2008 [35]	10	2	—	7.3 (5.5—9)	70.4 (55—83)	3
Neviaser et al., 2008 [45]	19	—	—	6.9	69.5	1
Sayed-Noor and Sjoden, 2008 [56]	1	1	1	7.0	72.0	—
Capeci and Tejwani, 2009 [16]	7	7	4	8.6 (5—13)	61.0 (53—75)	—
Sayed-Noor and Sjoden, 2009 [57]	2	1	2	9.0	66.5	—
Schneider, 2009 [59]	3	—	2	7.3 (6—9)	63.3 (59—66)	—
Aspenberg, 2008 [6]	1	1	1	9.0	57.0	—
Edwards et al., 2010 [23]	1	1	1	6.0	60.0	—
Koh et al., 2010 [30]	16	0	7	4.5 (2—7)	68.0 (53—92)	—
Current study	41	18	29	7.1 (4—11)	73.7 (67—85)	0

*The exact number in the literature is unknown owing to multiple publications from the same patient populations; numbers in parentheses denote ranges; — = data not reported.
Editor's Note: Please refer to original journal article for full references.

Results.—Forty-one patients had an underlying femoral insufficiency fracture, all of whom had been receiving bisphosphonate therapy. Among the 21 patients with low-energy femoral fractures before the availability of bisphosphonates, none had insufficiency fractures. Of the 41 patients with insufficiency fractures, 29 (71%) had prodromal pain and 18 (44%) had bilateral insufficiency fractures. Bisphosphonate use was associated (odds ratio greater than 1000) with insufficiency fracture. The mean duration of bisphosphonate use in patients with insufficiency fractures was longer than in patients without fractures (7.1 versus 3.2 years).

Conclusion.—Long-term bisphosphonate use is associated with insufficiency fractures of the femoral shaft, which commonly present with prodromal thigh pain and may be bilateral. These fractures were not seen before bisphosphonates became available for use (Tables 2-4).

▶ This comparative cohort study addresses the issue of femoral shaft fracture in low-energy trauma and the association with bisphosphonate treatment. The authors compared a cohort before and after bisphosphonate therapy came into widespread use. This study design is at risk for detection bias, especially with regard to identifying evidence of insufficiency fracture in the postfracture radiographs. A panel blinded to associated radiographic patient date/cohort would have been preferred to limit this source of bias. Nevertheless, this cohort study adds to the increasing body of knowledge (Table 4) clarifying this association. The risk-benefit ratio of prescribing bisphosphonates favors the use of this medication to limit fracture risk overall, yet patients and physicians alike need to be aware of the association and rapidly investigate any sign of proximal hip or thigh pain with radiographic imaging.

M. F. Swiontkowski, MD

Cumulative Alendronate Dose and the Long-Term Absolute Risk of Subtrochanteric and Diaphyseal Femur Fractures: A Register-Based National Cohort Analysis

Abrahamsen B, Eiken P, Eastell R (Univ of Southern Denmark, Odense, Denmark; Hillerød Hosp, Denmark; Univ of Sheffield, UK)
J Clin Endocrinol Metab 95:5258-5265, 2010

Context.—Bisphosphonates are the mainstay of anti-osteoporotic treatment and are commonly used for a longer duration than in the placebo-controlled trials. A link to development of atypical subtrochanteric or diaphyseal fragility fractures of the femur has been proposed, and these fractures are currently the subject of a U.S. Food and Drug Administration review.

Objective.—Our objective was to examine the risk of subtrochanteric/diaphyseal femur fractures in long term users of alendronate.

Design.—We conducted an age- and gender-matched cohort study using national healthcare data.

Patients.—Patients were alendronate users, without previous hip fracture, who began treatment between January 1, 1996, and December 31, 2005 (n = 39,567) and untreated controls, (n = 158,268).

Main Outcome Measures.—Subtrochanteric or diaphyseal femur fractures were evaluated.

Results.—Subtrochanteric and diaphyseal fractures occurred at a rate of 13 per 10,000 patient-years in untreated women and 31 per 10,000 patient-years in women receiving alendronate [adjusted hazard ratio (HR) = 1.88; 95% confidence interval (CI) = 1.62−2.17]. Rates for men were six and 31 per 10,000 patient-years, respectively (HR = 3.98; 95% CI = 2.62−6.05). The HR for hip fracture was 1.37 (95% CI = 1.30−1.46)) in women and 2.47 (95% CI = 2.07−2.95) in men. Risks of subtrochanteric/diaphyseal fracture were similar in patients who had received 9 yr of treatment (highest quartile) and patients who had stopped therapy after the equivalent of 3 months of treatment (lowest quartile).

TABLE 1.—Baseline Demographics for Subjects in the Matched Cohort Analysis

	Controls (n = 158,268)	Alendronate (n = 39,567)	P Value
Age (yr)	69.8 ± 11.6	69.8 ± 11.6	Matched
Female (%)	82.8	82.8	Matched
Follow-up (yr)	3.4 ± 2.2	3.4 ± 2.3	<0.001
Medications			
Hormone therapy baseline (any, last 12 months) (%)	8.3	7.4	<0.001
Prednisolone at baseline (any, last 12 months) (%)	3.9%	26.0%	<0.001
Prednisolone (mg in the last 12 months)	60.6 ± 420	791.3 ± 1772	<0.001
Number of comedications	5.2 ± 4.7	8.6 ± 6.1	<0.001
Fracture history (%)			
Any fracture after age 50	16.1	29.7	<0.001
Previous spine fracture	0.6	4.7	<0.001
Previous forearm fracture	6.5	12.1	<0.001
Previous humerus fracture	2.3	5.2	<0.001
Previous hip fracture	0.0	0.0	Exclusion
More than one previous fracture	2.2	6.7	<0.001
Comorbid conditions (%)			
Charlson index, mean	0.5 ± 1.2	0.8 ± 1.5	<0.001
0	81.3	70.7	<0.001
1−3	15.5	23.6	
>3	3.2	5.7	
Cardiac failure	7.0	10.2	<0.001
Malignancy	4.1	5.7	<0.001
Pulmonary disease	3.3	12.5	<0.001
Cerebrovascular disease	3.2	4.0	<0.001
Diabetes, w/o complications	2.9	3.2	<0.001
Diabetes, with complications	0.8	0.8	0.90
Myocardial infarction	2.0	2.6	<0.001
Peripheral vascular disease	1.6	2.6	<0.001
Ulcer disease	1.1	2.4	<0.001
Rheumatic or collagen disorder	1.0	7.5	<0.001
Dementia	0.9	0.9	0.44
Renal failure	0.4	0.4	0.24
Mild liver disease	0.3	1.1	<0.001
Severe liver disease	0.0	0.2	<0.001
Hemiplegia	0.1	0.3	<0.001
Solid metastatic tumor	0.3	0.6	<0.001

Treatment-naive patients without previous hip fracture beginning alendronate in Denmark between January 1, 1996, and December 31, 2005, with 4:1 matched bisphosphonate-unexposed control subjects, matched for age, sex, and index year.

TABLE 2.—Fracture Rates in 39,567 Patients Who Began Alendronate 1996–2005, Compared (1:4) with 158,268 Age- and Sex-Matched Control Subjects from the Background Population

	n	Patient-Years	n	Hip, Rate per 10,000 Patient-Years	n	Subtrochanteric or Diaphyseal, Rate per 10,000 Patient-Years, Total (Subtrochanteric/Diaphyseal)	Subtrochanteric or Diaphyseal Fractures (% of all Proximal Femur Fractures)
Men							
Untreated	27276	95826	469	49	59	6 (4.0/2.6)	10.9
Alendronate	6819	19806	264	133	61	31 (19.2/13.1)	18.9
Women							
Untreated	130992	451333	4446	99	578	13 (7.9/5.7)	11.6
Alendronate	32748	112748	1852	164	351	31 (19.4/13.3)	15.9

Test for difference in proportion of subtrochanteric/diaphyseal fractures between alendronate-exposed and unexposed persons: $\chi^2 = 33.4$; $P < 0.0001$.

Conclusions.—Alendronate-treated patients are at higher risk of hip and subtrochanteric/diaphyseal fracture than matched control subjects. However, large cumulative doses of alendronate were not associated with a greater absolute risk of subtrochanteric/diaphyseal fractures than small cumulative doses, suggesting that these fractures could be due to osteoporosis rather than to alendronate (Tables 1 and 2).

▶ This very well done administrative database study using the Danish health care data set addresses the issue of risk of bisphosphonate use for atypical subtrochanteric hip fracture and the dose-response issue and overall impact on hip fracture prevention. The large data set of nearly 40000 treated subjects and untreated controls (nearly 160000) allows a valid comparison. There are limitations to any administrative data set, as radiographs are not reviewed and there is risk of coding error. However, this study proves the associated risk of bisphosphonate therapy at 13 per 10000 patient-years for the untreated and 31 per 10000 patient-years in women receiving alendronate. There was no therapy duration-associated risk identified, leaving us to conclude that there are potent patient factors involved in the overall risk of this complication of therapy. In fact, the fractures may be associated with degree of osteoporosis— these data are not available in this database. Finally, the use of alendronate was importantly associated with a decrease in overall rate of hip fracture, which is critically important to understand (Fig 2 in the original article).

M. F. Swiontkowski, MD

Immediate Spica Casting of Pediatric Femoral Fractures in the Operating Room Versus the Emergency Department: Comparison of Reduction, Complications, and Hospital Charges

Mansour AA III, Wilmoth JC, Mansour AS, et al (Vanderbilt Univ Med Ctr, Nashville, TN; Ohio State Univ Med Ctr, Columbus; Louisiana State Univ School of Medicine, New Orleans)
J Pediatr Orthop 30:813-817, 2010

Background.—Immediate spica casting for pediatric femur fractures is well described as a standard treatment in the literature. The purpose of this study is to evaluate the application of a spica cast in the emergency department (ED) versus the operating room (OR) with regard to quality of reduction, complications, and hospital charges at an academic institution.

Methods.—An institutional review board-approved retrospective review identified 100 children aged 6 months to 5 years between January 2003 and October 2008 with an isolated femur fracture treated with a hip spica cast. Patients were compared based on the setting of spica cast application.

Results.—There were 79 patients in the ED cohort and 21 patients in the OR cohort. There were no significant differences in age, weight, sex, fracture pattern, prereduction shortening, injury mechanism, duration of spica treatment, time to heal, or length of follow-up between cohorts. There were no significant differences in the rate of loss of reduction requiring

TABLE 1.—Comparison of Demographics, Fracture Characteristics, and Treatment

	ED Cohort	OR Cohort	P
Patient			
Total patients	79	21	
No. male	52 (65.8%)	15 (71.4%)	
Average age at injury (y)	2.4	2.9	0.15
Average weight (kg)	13.7	15.1	0.27
NAT workup	22 (27.9%)	5 (23.8%)	0.71
% of high-energy mechanism*	47 (59.5%)	13 (61.9%)	0.96
Fracture location and shortening			
Proximal 1/3	8 (10.1%)	2 (9.5%)	0.74
Middle 1/3	65 (82.3%)	16 (76.2%)	0.75
Distal 1/3	6 (7.6%)	3 (14.3%)	0.59
Nondisplaced fractures	10 (12.7%)	1 (4.8%)	0.52
Average prereduction fracture shortening (mm)	10	11	0.80
Treatment			
Average time from ED admission to spica application (h)	3.8	11.5	<0.0001
Average length of sedation/anesthesia for spica application (min)	40	51	0.007
Length of stay excluding NAT workup (h)	16.8	30.5	0.0002
Average duration of spica treatment (wk)	5.9	6.2	0.10
Average duration of follow-up (wk)	20.5	15.9	0.82
Average time to healing (wk)	6.6	7.4	0.21
Average initial hospital charges	$5150	$15983	<0.0001

ED indicates emergency department; NAT, nonaccidental trauma; OR, operating room.
*High-energy mechanisms were classified as those not resulting from a twisting injury or a fall from standing height.

TABLE 2.—Comparison of Acceptable Radiographic Reduction With Healed Fracture

	ED Cohort	OR Cohort	P
Age <2 y	n = 27	n = 5	
Varus/valgus angulation (>30 degrees)	0 (0%)	0 (0%)	—
Anterior/posterior angulation (>30 degrees)	2 (7.4%)	1 (20%)	0.96
Shortening (>15 mm)	1 (3.7%)	1 (20%)	0.71
Overall unacceptable reduction*	3 (11.1%)	2 (40%)	0.34
Age 2 to 5 y	n = 52	n = 16	
Varus/valgus angulation (>15 degrees)	6 (11.5%)	1 (6.2%)	0.89
Anterior/posterior angulation (>20 degrees)	4 (7.7%)	0 (0%)	0.59
Shortening (>20 mm)	10 (19.2%)	4 (25%)	0.88
Overall unacceptable reduction*	16 (30.8%)	5 (31.3%)	0.78

ED indicates emergency department; OR, operating room.
*Defined as failing at least 1 of the 3 radiographic parameters for acceptable reduction.

TABLE 3.—Comparison of Complications

	ED Cohort (n = 79)	OR Cohort (n = 21)	P
Major			
Loss of reduction requiring revision casting or internal fixation in OR	5 (6.3%)	1 (4.8%)	0.80
Anesthetic complications	0	0	—
Malunion (according to radiographic criteria)	19 (24.1%)	7 (33.3%)	0.67
Minor			
Skin breakdown	10 (12.7%)	3 (14.3%)	0.87
Subsequent wedging to improve alignment	7 (8.9%)	3 (14.3%)	0.23
Cast soiling requiring cast change	5 (6.3%)	0	—
Cast breakage requiring revision cast	1 (1.3%)	0	—
Overall need for revision casting or internal fixation in OR	11 (13.9%)	1 (4.7%)	0.44
Total number of spica-related complications	47	14	
Overall patients with spicarelated complications	33 (41.8%)	11 (52.4%)	0.62

ED indicates emergency department; OR, operating room.

revision casting or operative treatment (6.3% vs. 4.8%), the need for cast wedging (8.9% vs. 14.3%), or minor skin breakdown (12.7% vs. 14.3%). There were no sedation or anesthetic complications in either group. There were no significant differences in the quality of reduction or the rate of complications between the 2 groups. Spica casting in the OR delayed the time from presentation to cast placement as compared with the ED cohort (11.5 h vs. 3.8 h, P < 0.0001) and lengthened the hospital stay (30.5 h vs. 16.9 h, P = 0.0002). The average hospital charges of spica cast application in the OR was 3 times higher than the cost of casting in the ED ($15,983 vs. $5150, P < 0.0001).

Conclusions.—Immediate spica casting in the ED and OR provide similar results in terms of reduction and complications. With the significantly higher hospital charges for spica casting in the OR, alternative settings should be considered.

Level of Evidence.—III—Retrospective comparative study (Tables 1-3).

▶ Immediate application of a spica cast is widely accepted as the treatment of choice for femur fractures in children younger than 6 years. This retrospective cohort study demonstrates that there is no difference in relevant patient clinical or functional outcome between spica casts placed in the emergency department (ED) and the operating room for femoral fractures in children aged 6 months to 5 years. The study used blinded assessment of the radiographic observers, which strengthens the conclusions. Because of the considerable cost differential, application of spica casts for children with femur fractures in the ED should be a standard practice for any ED/orthopedic service where children's fractures are routinely treated.

M. F. Swiontkowski, MD

Femoral Fractures in Adolescents: A Comparison of Four Methods of Fixation
Ramseier LE, Janicki JA, Weir S, et al (Children's Univ Hosp Zurich, Switzerland; Children's Memorial Hosp, Chicago, IL; The Hosp for Sick Children, Toronto, Ontario Canada)
J Bone Joint Surg Am 92:1122-1129, 2010

Background.—The optimal management of femoral fractures in adolescents is controversial. This study was performed to compare the results and complications of four methods of fixation and to determine the factors related to those complications.

Methods.—We conducted a retrospective cohort study of 194 diaphyseal femoral fractures in 189 children and adolescents treated with elastic stable intramedullary nail fixation, external fixation, rigid intramedullary nail fixation, or plate fixation. After adjustment for age, weight, energy of the injury, polytrauma, fracture level and pattern, and extent of comminution, treatment outcomes were compared in terms of the length of the hospital stay, time to union, and complication rates, including loss of reduction requiring a reoperation, malunion, nonunion, refracture, infection, and the need for a reoperation other than routine hardware removal.

Results.—The mean age of the patients was 13.2 years, and their mean weight was 49.5 kg. There was a loss of reduction of two of 105 fractures treated with elastic nail fixation and ten of thirty-three treated with external fixation (p < 0.001). At the time of final follow-up, five patients (two treated with external fixation and one in each of the other groups) had ≥2.0 cm of shortening. Eight of the 104 patients (105 fractures) treated with elastic nail fixation underwent a reoperation (two each because of loss of reduction, refracture, the need for trimming or advancement of the nail, and delayed union or nonunion). Sixteen patients treated with external fixation required a reoperation (ten because of loss of reduction, one for replacement of a pin complicated by infection, one for

TABLE 1.—Results

	Total (N = 194 Fractures, 189 Patients)	Elastic Nail (N = 105 Fractures, 104 Patients)	External Fixation (N = 33 Fractures, 32 Patients)	Rigid Nail (N = 37 Fractures, 37 Patients)	Plate (N = 19 Fractures, 17 Patients)	P Value
Length of hospital stay *(days)*						0.062
Median	5	5	7	6	6	
Mean (stand. dev.)	7.8 (9.0)	6.8 (10.1)	9 (5.5)	7.3 (4.5)	12.9 (12.7)	
Mean time to union (stand. dev.) *(wk)*	12.01 (7.6)	11.2 (7.6)	16.1* (8.9)	10.1 (4.8)	13.1 (7.0)	0.003 (0.016†)

*The time to union was shown to be significantly longer in the external fixation group in pairwise comparisons with the elastic nail group (Bonferroni adjusted p = 0.005) and the rigid nail group (Bonferroni adjusted p = 0.005).
†Adjusted for other baseline factors in multivariate analysis.

TABLE 2.—Clinically Relevant Loss of Reduction and/or Malunion

	Total (N = 194 Fractures, 189 Patients)	Elastic Nail (N = 105 Fractures, 104 Patients)	External Fixation (N = 33 Fractures, 32 Patients)	Rigid Nail (N = 37 Fractures, 37 Patients)	Plate (N = 19 Fractures, 17 Patients)	P Value
Loss of reduction (resulting in reoperation and/or malunion)	12 (6%)	2 (2%)	10 (30%)*	0	0	<0.001 (0.039†)
Malunion	12 (6%)	7 (7%)	3 (9%)	1 (3%)	1 (5%)	0.73
Limb-length discrepancy of ≥2 cm	5 (3%)	1 (1%)	2 (6%)	1 (3%)	1 (5%)	0.36
Total (loss of reduction + malunion + limb-length discrepancy)	25 (13%)	10 (10%)	11 (33%)‡	2 (5%)	2 (11%)	0.004 (0.01†)

*In the pairwise comparisons, the rate of clinically relevant loss of reduction was significantly higher only in the external fixation group compared with the three other fixation groups (Bonferroni adjusted p < 0.001 in all three comparisons).
†Adjusted for other baseline factors in multivariate analysis.
‡The rate of clinically relevant loss of reduction and/or malunion and/or limb-length discrepancy was shown to be significantly higher in the external fixation group in pairwise comparisons with the elastic nail group (p = 0.002) and the rigid nail group (p = 0.003) but not in the pairwise comparison with the plate group (p = 0.09). (All p values are Bonferroni adjusted for multiple comparisons.) No significant difference was found between the elastic nail group and the rigid nail (p = 0.41) or plate (p = 0.95) group.

débridement of the site of a deep infection, three because of refracture, and one for lengthening). One patient treated with a rigid intramedullary nail required débridement at the site of a deep infection, and one underwent removal of a prominent distal interlocking screw. One fracture treated with plate fixation required refixation following refractures. A multivariate analysis with adjustment for baseline differences showed external fixation to be associated with a 12.41-times (95% confidence interval = 2.26

TABLE 3.—Reoperations

Reason for Reoperation	Total (N = 194 Fractures, 189 Patients)	Elastic Nail (N = 105 Fractures, 104 Patients)	External Fixation (N = 33 Fractures, 32 Patients)	Rigid Nail (N = 37 Fractures, 37 Patients)	Plate (N = 19 Fractures, 17 Patients)	P Value
Loss of reduction*	12 (13)	2	10 (11)	—	—	
Malunion/shortening*	1		1	—	—	
Delayed union*	2	2	—	—	—	
Refracture*	6 (7)	2	3	—	1 (2)	
Infection*	3		2	1	—	
Advancement/trimming nails*	2	2	—	—	—	
All reoperations (no.[%])	28 (14%)	8 (8%)	17 (52%)†	1 (3%)	2 (11%)	0.013†

*Number of patients (number of reoperations).
†Only the external fixation group had a significantly higher reoperation rate than the other groups.

to 68.31) greater risk of loss of reduction and/or malunion than elastic stable intramedullary nail fixation.

Conclusions.—External fixation was associated with the highest rate of complications in our series of adolescents treated for a femoral fracture. Although the other three methods yielded comparable outcomes, we cannot currently recommend one method of fixation for all adolescents with a femoral fracture. The choice of fixation will remain influenced by surgeon preference based on expertise and experience, patient and fracture characteristics, and patient and family preferences (Tables 1-3).

► The debate regarding the optimum management of femoral shaft fractures in the adolescent continues. This is a well-conducted retrospective cohort series using sophisticated statistical techniques to compare the treatment of these fractures by external fixation, flexible nailing, interlocking nails, or plates. The major takeaway point from this research is that external fixation clearly has the highest complication rate. Although patient acceptance (and family acceptance) was not evaluated with this study, it is highly likely that this method would also carry the highest level of patient concern. The other 3 methods of treating these fractures seem more or less equivalent, and therefore the choice should be made with the surgeon's experience, institutional resources, and parental input.

M. F. Swiontkowski, MD

Analysis of Postoperative Knee Sepsis After Retrograde Nail Insertion of Open Femoral Shaft Fractures

O'Toole RV, Riche K, Cannada LK, et al (Univ of Maryland School of Medicine, Baltimore; Brigham & Women's Hosp, Boston, MA; St Louis Univ Hosp, MO; et al)
J Orthop Trauma 24:677-682, 2010

Objectives.—Retrograde nailing of open femoral fractures has presumed increased risk of knee sepsis. Our hypothesis was that the incidence of secondary knee infection after retrograde nailing of open femoral fractures is low.

Design.—Retrospective, multicenter.

Setting.—Four Level I trauma centers.

Patients and Methods.—A retrospective review of prospective trauma registries and fracture databases identified all open femoral fractures treated with retrograde intramedullary nailing from January 1, 2003, through February 15, 2007. Patients with ballistic injuries and those with less than 1 month follow up were excluded. Ninety-three open femoral fractures were identified in 90 patients. We defined a septic knee as a knee with infection that required reoperation with arthrotomy or arthroscopy. Infections at an open fracture site were defined as those treated with local irrigation and débridement and intravenously and/or orally administered antibiotics.

Intervention.—Open femoral shaft fractures treated with a retrograde approach.

Main outcome measurements.—Occurrence of an ipsilateral postoperative septic knee.

Results.—One acute septic knee was identified (1.1%; 95% confidence interval, 0.0%−3.2%) noted at time of repeat irrigation and débridement of a massive degloving wound that left no skin coverage over the knee. We also observed one late knee sepsis 2.5 years after the index procedure occurring after quadricepsplasty. The nail had been removed 1.5 years before surgery, so we did not include that case in our knee sepsis rate. Two additional infections at the open wound site did not involve the knee.

Conclusions.—Previous publications have argued that retrograde nailing of open femoral fractures provides a potential conduit for knee infection. Our data show that risk of a septic knee as a direct result of retrograde nailing of an open femoral fracture is relatively low (1.1%; 95% confidence interval, 0.0%-3.2%). To our knowledge, this is the first case series to document the relative safety associated with retrograde nailing of open femoral fractures (Table 3).

▶ The authors attempt to address the issue of the potential complication of a septic knee after retrograde nailing of open femoral fracture with this retrospective multicenter cohort design. The relative rarity of the injury, open femoral fracture, is evident by the small numbers collected from 4 level I trauma centers. The risk at around 1% seems acceptable, but one is left to question what the

---

TABLE 3.—Details of Acute Treatment*

Initial Treatment	
Retrograde nailing	74% (n = 69)
External fixation	26% (n = 24)
Average days from external fixation to retrograde nailing	6.4 (range, 0–42)
Wound treatment	
Primary closure	89% (n = 83)
Average number of irrigation and débridement procedures	1.53
Irrigant type	
Normal saline	90% (n = 84)
Lactated ringers	4% (n = 4)
Not documented	5% (n = 5)
Irrigant volume at first irrigation and débridement procedure	8.2 L (range, 31–2 L)
(data available for only 64 of 93 fractures)	
Retrograde nail technique	
Reamed	97% (n = 90)†
Approach	
Medial parapatellar	72% (n = 67)
Midline split	15% (n = 14)
Through patella fracture or traumatic wound	2% (n = 2)
Lateral parapatellar	6% (n = 6)
Unknown	40% (n = 4)

*Ninety-three open femoral shaft fractures treated with retrograde nails.
†Two fractures were treated with unreamed nails, and for one fracture, the use of reaming could not be determined.

---

impact of this complication can be on patient pain, function, and long-term reconstruction options. Of course, the question of the risk of a septic hip with antegrade nailing of open femoral fracture is also relevant but not addressed in this study. Surgeons must continue to weigh this relatively low risk when choosing between antegrade and retrograde nailing of femoral shaft fractures.

M. F. Swiontkowski, MD

Early Fracture Fixation

Comparison of RIA and conventional reamed nailing for treatment of femur shaft fractures

Streubel PN, Desai P, Suk M (Univ of Florida – Shands Jacksonville; AO Clinical Investigation and Documentation-Duebendorf, Switzerland)
Injury 41:S51-S56, 2010

Introduction.—The standard of care for femoral diaphysis fractures is sequentially reamed, locked, intramedullary nails. However, in the polytraumatized patient perioperative complications such as fat embolism syndrome (FES) and acute respiratory distress (ARDS) are well chronicled. The reamer irrigator aspirator (RIA)has been theorized to minimize such phenomena.

Methods.—A retrospective study comparing conventional reamed nailing for femur fractures versus those treated with the RIA was conducted. From January 2005 to September 2006, 156 patients treated at our institution with an intramedullary nail met inclusion criteria. There were sixty-six

TABLE 1.—Baseline Characteristics

	Sequential (n = 66)	RIA (n = 90)	P-Value
Demographics			
Age (years)[a]	32.5 (±14)	32.2 (±14)	0.89
Male[b]	50 (76)	71 (79)	0.70
BMI (kg/m²)[b]			
<18.5	2 (4)	1 (1)	0.02
18.5−24.9	24 (42)	28 (42)	
25−29.9	12 (21)	28 (42)	
≥30	19 (33)	10 (15)	
Trauma[b]			
GCS			
13−15	60 (91)	82 (91)	1.00
9−12	1 (2)	2 (2)	
3−8	5 (8)	6 (7)	
ISS			
<18	50 (76)	68 (76)	0.69
18−24	7 (11)	8 (9)	
25−39	8 (12)	14 (16)	
>40	1 (2)	0 (0)	
Head	16 (24)	21 (23)	0.52
Chest	8 (12)	14 (16)	0.64

BMI: Body Mass Index, GCS: Glasgow coma scale, ISS: Injury severity score.
[a]Values are given as means with standard deviations in parentheses.
[b]Values are given as number of patients with percentages in parentheses.

TABLE 2.—Fracture Characteristics[a]

	Sequential (n = 68)	RIA (n = 97)	P-Value
Side			
Right	34 (50)	55 (57)	0.43
Left	34 (50)	42 (43)	
Bilateral	4 (6)	14 (16)	0.13
Location			
Proximal	8 (12)	20 (21)	0.41
Middle	44 (65)	52 (54)	
Distal	15 (22)	23 (24)	
Segmental	1 (1)	2 (2)	
AO/OTA			
32A	29 (43)	38 (39)	0.28
32B	24 (35)	45 (46)	
32C	15 (22)	14 (14)	
Open	17 (25)	22 (23)	0.85
I	8 (12)	9 (9)	0.80
II	6 (9)	7 (7)	
IIIA	3 (4)	3 (3)	
IIIB	0 (0)	2 (2)	
IIIC	0 (0)	1 (1)	

[a]Values are given as number of patients with percentages in parentheses.

patients treated with conventional reaming (group A) and ninety patients treated with the RIA (group B). The main outcome measures included length of hospital stay, rate of ARDS, pneumonia, ventilatory failure, overall pulmonary complications, healing rate and death.

TABLE 4.—Hospital Data

	Sequential (n = 66)	RIA (n = 90)	P-Value
Duration (in days)[a]			
Hospital stay	8.7 (±8.8)	10.4 (±11.3)	0.30
ICU stay	1.8 (±5.2)	2.6 (±7.2)	0.12
Mechanical ventilation	1.5 (±4.5)	2.2 (±6.4)	0.49
Complications[b]			
Pulmonary complications	7 (11)	14 (16)	0.48
Pneumonia	5 (8)	7 (8)	1.00
ARDS/Ventilatory failure	3 (5)	8 (9)	0.36
Death	0 (0)	4 (4)	0.14

ICU: Intensive care unit, ARDS: Acute respiratory distress syndrome.
[a]Values are given as means with standard deviations in parentheses.
[b]Values are given as number of patients with percentages in parentheses.

TABLE 5.—Healing Complications

	Sequential[a] (Max. n = 41)	RIA[a] (Max. n = 53)	P-Value
Healing complications	3 (7)	8 (14)	0,35
Delayed-union	2 (5)	5 (9)	0,70
Non-union	1 (2)	3 (5)	0,63

ICU: Intensive care unit, ARDS: Acute respiratory distress syndrome.
[a]Values are given as number of patients with percentages in parentheses.

Results.—No significant differences were found between groups with regard to patient demographics, injury severity and the incidence of head/chest trauma. In addition, no differences were found in length of hospital stay, length of ICU stay or mechanical ventilation. Overall pulmonary complications occurred in 11% (group A) and 16% (group B) respectively (p = 0.48). No fatalities were found in group A while there were four in group B, 4% (p = 0.14). No significant differences were found in delayed union versus nonunion rate between groups, while overall healing complications were seen in 7% and 14% of patients (p = 0.35) in groups A and B respectively.

Conclusion.—No statistical significance was reached with regard to pulmonary complications, healing rates or death. However, we were unable to demonstrate favorable physiologic lung parameters with RIA use compared to conventional reaming as has been described in previous animal studies. We found a trend toward more healing complications in the RIA group, but this was not statistically significant. Further study is warranted (Tables 1, 2, 4, and 5).

▶ The Reamer Irrigation Aspiration system is designed to remove marrow contents in long bones prior to reaming to limit the marrow debris being sent into the pulmonary vasculature system. Its benefits in this regard have been well documented in animal models. The question remains whether these benefits accrue to patients undergoing femoral nailing. This comparative cohort study fails to confirm these benefits in 156 patients treated with reamer irrigator aspirator (RIA) or conventional sequential reaming. Although not statistically significant, the study raises concerns regarding the impact of RIA on fracture healing.

M. F. Swiontkowski, MD

Femur

Femoral Malrotation After Unreamed Intramedullary Nailing: An Evaluation of Influencing Operative Factors
Hüfner T, Citak M, Suero EM, et al (Hannover Med School, Germany; Hosp for Special Surgery, NY; et al)
J Orthop Trauma 25:224-227, 2011

Objective.—The objective of this study was to determine which clinical factors influence the presence and extent of femoral malrotation during unreamed nail insertion performed without a fracture table.
Design.—Retrospective chart review.
Setting.—Academic trauma center.
Intervention.—Patients were treated statically locked femoral nails inserted without reaming in either a retrograde or antegrade manner without the use of a fracture table between April 1, 2000, and December 31, 2005. All patients received postoperative computed tomography scans. Institutional radiographic threshold for revision surgery was 15° of either internal or external rotation.
Main Outcome Measurements.—Postoperative computed tomography measurements of rotation were compared with the opposite side. Patients were grouped by 1) Orthopaedic Trauma Association fracture classification; 2) closed versus mini open reduction; 3) surgeon experience; 4) antegrade versus retrograde femoral nail; and 5) time of day surgery performed (day shift versus night shift). The following parameters were measured from the chart and x-ray: rotational malalignment, x-ray time, and duration of surgery.
Results.—There were 82 femurs in 82 patients, 59 men and 23 women, with a mean age of 32 years (range, 17–83 years). Eighteen femurs (22%) showed a malrotation of greater than 15°. Seven were internally malrotated (mean, 23°; range 16°–32°), whereas 11 were externally malrotated (mean, 24.2°; range, 16°–39.7°). After clinical examination, only 11 of the 18 patients (61%) underwent revision surgery, six patients for external malrotation (mean, 27.47°; range, 21.9°–39.7°) and five for internal malrotation (mean, 23.6°; range, 16°–32°). Malrotation varied significantly with fracture severity with Type C averaging 19.4° (24 patients), Type B 9° (26 patients), and Type A 6.6° (32 patients). No difference was found between an open and closed technique nor the experience of surgeon or the type of implant. There was a significant difference depending on the time of surgery in which an average malrotation of 15.2° (14 patients) was found on the night shift and an average malrotation of 10.3° (68 patients) was found during the day.

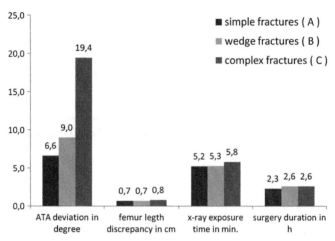

FIGURE 1.—Shown are the analyzed parameters according to the fracture classifications. (Reprinted from Hüfner T, Citak M, Suero EM, et al. Femoral malrotation after unreamed intramedullary nailing: an evaluation of influencing operative factors. *J Orthop Trauma.* 2011;25:224-227, with permission from Lippincott Williams & Wilkins.)

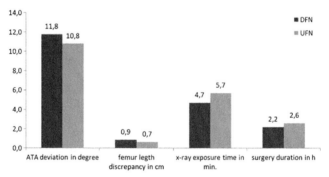

FIGURE 4.—Results for the different implants. (Reprinted from Hüfner T, Citak M, Suero EM, et al. Femoral malrotation after unreamed intramedullary nailing: an evaluation of influencing operative factors. *J Orthop Trauma.* 2011;25:224-227, with permission from Lippincott Williams & Wilkins.)

Conclusion.—Rotational malalignment greater than 15° was found in 22% of femurs treated in this study. Fracture comminution and time of day the surgery was performed had the greatest effect on the severity of malrotation (Figs 1 and 4).

▶ Femur rotation following antegrade or retrograde intramedullary nailing in a large cohort of patients (82) provides valuable insight into this issue. Interestingly, closed versus open reduction and experienced versus junior surgeon did not correlate, which is somewhat surprising, as the major clinical issue seems to be the lack of ability to judge fracture rotational alignment with the C-arm. The fact that there is a higher degree of malrotated femora with late-night surgery speaks to this as a major factor. Twenty-two percent of patients with greater than 15° malrotation confirms that this is not a trivial clinical issue, and approaches to evaluating the rotation of the postreduction femur intraoperatively must be developed.

M. F. Swiontkowski, MD

Functional Outcome After Antegrade Femoral Nailing: A Comparison of Trochanteric Fossa Versus Tip of Greater Trochanter Entry Point
Moein CA, ten Duis H-J, Oey L, et al (Univ Med Centre Groningen, The Netherlands; Univ Med Centre Utrecht, The Netherlands)
J Orthop Trauma 25:196-201, 2011

Objectives.—This study was performed to explore the relationship between entry point-related soft tissue damage in antegrade femoral nailing and the functional outcome in patients with a proximal third femoral shaft fracture.

Design.—Retrospective clinical trial.

Setting.—Level I university trauma center.

Patients.—Seventeen patients with a high femoral shaft fracture treated with an antegrade femoral nail joined the study.

Intervention.—Nine patients with an Unreamed Femoral Nail (UFN; Synthes, Bettlach, Switzerland) inserted at the trochanteric fossa and eight patients with a long Proximal Femoral Nail (PFN; Synthes) inserted at the tip of the greater trochanter.

Main Outcome Measurements.—Pain, gait, nerve, and muscle function along with endurance.

Results.—Five patients with a UFN had a positive Trendelenburg sign and a reinnervated superior gluteal nerve after initial injury of the nerve at operation. None of these findings occurred in the long PFN group ($P = 0.01$). Isokinetic measurements showed diminished abduction as well as external rotator function in the UFN group rather than in the long PFN group. Leg endurance was significantly lower in patients with a UFN.

Conclusions.—Compared with the trochanteric fossa, femoral nailing through the greater trochanter tip may decrease the risk of damage to the superior gluteal nerve and intraoperative damage to the muscular apparatus of the hip region, resulting in some improved muscle function. Therefore, a lateral entry point may be a rational alternative for conventional nailing through the trochanteric fossa (Table 1).

▶ The focus of this investigation is the issue of functional recovery after antegrade femoral nailing, as it relates to starting point. The extensive analyses of function included isokinetic testing, gait analysis, and electromyography. Anatomic evaluation included MRI looking for scarring around the abductors. It does appear that the outcome assessors were not blinded to treatment group. The outcomes favor the trochanteric starting point. One critical element to understand is that all patients were treated with supine position nailing. This editor has long recommended lateral position nailing to minimize injury to the

TABLE 1.—Patient-Reported Outcome in the (A) UFN Group and (B) Long PFN Group

A

Patient Number	Age (years)	Sex	Fracture Type	Trendelenburg (0 = negative, 1 = positive)	EMG Reinnervation (0 = no, 1 = in one or more muscles)	VAS– Pain (0–10)	Pain Interference With Daily Activity (no = 0, slight = 1, moderate = 2, severe = 3)	Walking Distance (0 = infinite)	Reduced Ability Intensive Exercise (no, slight, moderate, severe =1, 2, 3)	Walking Stairs (normal, with some aid, difficult = 0, 1, 2)	Postoperative Change of Profession	HHS
1	18	M	32A	0	0	3	0	0	0	0	No	100
2	27	M	32A	0	1	4	0	0	1	0	No	100
3	46	M	32B	0	0	3	1	0	1	0	No	96
4	38	M	32A	1	0	4	1	0	1	0	No	77
5	45	M	32A	0	0	5	0	0	1	0	No	96
6	49	M	32A	1	1	5	2	<2 km	3	2	Yes	68
7	52	M	32B	1	1	6	2	<2 km	1	0	No	87
8	39	M	32B	1	1	6	3	<2 km	3	2	Yes	35
9	51	M	32B	1	1	4	2	<2 km	3	1	Yes	79
Average (SD)	40.5 (11.5)					4.5 (1.1)						82.0 (18.9)

B

Patient number	Age (years)	Sex	Fracture type	Trendelenburg (0 = negative, 1 = positive)	EMG Reinnervation (0 = no, 1 = in one or more muscles)	VAS– Pain (0–10)	Pain Interference With Daily Activity (no = 0, yes = 1)	Walking Distance (0 = infinite)	Reduced Ability Intensive Exercise (no, slight, moderate, severe =1, 2, 3)	Walking Stairs (normal, with some aid, difficult = 0, 1, 2)	Postoperative Change of Profession	HHS
1	62	M	32A	0	0	5	0	0	1	1	No	95
2	35	M	32A	0	0	5	1	<2 km	3	0	No	89
3	58	M	32B	0	0	4	0	0	1	0	No	69

4	45	M	32A	0	0	3	0	<2 km	3	1	No	80
5	46	M	32A	0	0	4	0	0	3	0	No	78
6	67	M	32A	0	0	3	1	<2 km	3	0	Yes*	69
7	34	M	32B	0	0	2	0	0	1	0	No	95
8	37	M	32A	0	0	1	0	0	0	0	No	95
Average (SD)	48 (12.8)					3.3 (1.2)						89.8 (11.3)

UFN, Unreamed Femoral Nail; PFN, Proximal Femoral Nail; EMG, electromyography; VAS, visual analog scale; HHS, Harris hip score; M, male; SD, standard deviation.

abductor and limit the incision size. The ideal comparison would include patients nailed in the lateral position. This is useful information for clinicians who continue to exclusively use the supine position.

M. F. Swiontkowski, MD

Risk Factors for Femoral Nonunion After Femoral Shaft Fracture

Taitsman LA, Lynch JR, Agel J, et al (Harborview Med Ctr, Seattle, WA)

J Trauma 67:1389-1392, 2009

The purpose of this study was to evaluate risk factors for nonunion after femoral nailing of femoral shaft fractures. A case-control study with two to one matching was conducted. Forty-five patients with 46 femoral nonunions (cases) and 92 patients with healed femoral shaft fractures (controls) were identified from our orthopedic trauma registry. All cases and controls were initially managed with reamed, statically locked femoral nails. The characteristics that were significantly different between the two groups were open fracture, delay to weight bearing, and tobacco use. Fracture classification, gender, direction of nail insertion (antegrade vs. retrograde), and Injury Severity Score were not predictive of nonunion. We conclude that open fracture, tobacco use, and delayed weight bearing are risk factors for femoral nonunion after intramedullary nailing for diaphyseal femur fractures.

▶ Femoral shaft nonunion is a relatively rare complication in uncontrolled cohort studies; the union rate for reamed statically locked nails is in the 98% to 99% range. This study uses a cohort case-control methodology to identify risk factors. In such study designs, the critical issue is the method used to match the cases. Here it was simply a control patient treated with reamed statically locked nail. Matching was not done for fracture pattern; simple patterns are at greater risk for nonunion with nailing in distraction. The risk factors are smoking, open fracture, and delay to weight bearing, likely in part related to multiple injuries. These all make clinical sense as all of these factors impact fracture healing, delaying the invasive remodeling required to heal femoral shaft fractures.

M. F. Swiontkowski, MD

Pelvic and Acetabular Fractures

Outcomes of acetabular fracture fixation with ten years' follow-up

Briffa N, Pearce R, Hill AM, et al (St George's Hosp, Tooting, London, UK)

J Bone Joint Surg [Br] 93-B:229-236, 2011

We report the outcome of 161 of 257 surgically fixed acetabular fractures. The operations were undertaken between 1989 and 1998 and the patients were followed for a minimum of ten years. Anthropometric data, fracture

TABLE 5.—Comparison of Published Results from Other Centres

Author/s	Cases	Mean Follow-up (yrs)	Excellent/Good (%)
Bircher*	161	11.3	73
Madhu et al[10]	237	2.9	76
Deo et al[19]	74	2.6	74
Fica et al[42]	84	5.5	68
Rommens et al[43]	175	2	76
Matta et al[11]	255	6	76
Mayo[44]	163	3.7	75
Ruesch et al[45]	53	1	83
Brueton[9]	26	2	61

Editor's Note: Please refer to original journal article for full references.
*Current study.

TABLE 6.—Relative Frequencies of Fracture Pattern Outcome in 161 Patients

	Outcome			
Fracture Pattern*	Excellent (%)	Good (%)	Fair (%)	Poor (%)
PW	52.17	17.39	4.35	26.09
TV	73.68	26.32	0.00	0.00
PC	14.29	14.29	28.57	42.86
TS	11.11	38.89	33.33	16.67
DC	48.72	33.33	0.00	17.95
TV+PW	28.57	21.43	28.57	21.43
AC	56.25	31.25	0.00	18.75
PC+PW	45.45	27.27	0.00	27.27
AC+PHTV	66.67	33.33	0.00	0.00

*PW, posterior wall; TV, transverse; PC, posterior column; TS, T-shaped; DC, double column; TV + PW, transverse posterior wall; AC, anterior column; PC + PW, posterior column posterior wall; AC + PHTV, anterior column posterior hemitransverse.

pattern, time to surgery, associated injuries, surgical approach, complications and outcome were recorded. Modified Merle D'Aubigné score and Matta radiological scoring systems were used as outcome measures. We observed simple fractures in 108 patients (42%) and associated fractures in 149 (58%).

The result was excellent in 75 patients (47%), good in 41 (25%), fair in 12 (7%) and poor in 33 (20%). Poor prognostic factors included increasing age, delay to surgery, quality of reduction and some fracture patterns. Complications were common in the medium- to longterm and functional outcome was variable. The gold-standard treatment for displaced acetabular fractures remains open reduction and internal fixation performed in dedicated units by specialist surgeons as soon as possible (Tables 5 and 6).

▶ This is a carefully reported cohort study detailing a decade-long follow-up of a large group of over 100 patients with operatively treated acetabular fractures. Seventy-two percent good/excellent results fit well within other long-term reports by skilled surgeons (Table 5). The fracture patterns with the highest risk of poor results remain those with posterior wall and posterior column involvement.

M. F. Swiontkowski, MD

Outcomes of Posterior Wall Fractures of the Acetabulum Treated Nonoperatively After Diagnostic Screening with Dynamic Stress Examination Under Anesthesia
Grimshaw CS, Moed BR (Saint Louis Univ School of Medicine, MO)
J Bone Joint Surg Am 92:2792-2800, 2010

Background.—Dynamic stress fluoroscopy with the patient under general anesthesia has been advocated as a clinical measure of hip stability and congruity in patients with a posterior wall acetabular fracture. The purpose of this study was to establish the predictive value of the dynamic stress fluoroscopic examination for these fractures by evaluating clinical and radiographic outcomes after nonoperative treatment of fractures found to be stable with this examination.

Methods.—Twenty-one consecutive patients with an acute posterior wall fracture of the acetabulum who were shown to have a stable hip joint by dynamic stress fluoroscopy while they were under general anesthesia were treated non-operatively. At the time of follow-up, the patients underwent clinical and/or radiographic evaluation.

Results.—Clinical follow-up was performed for eighteen patients at a minimum of two years after injury, at which time the average modified Merle d'Aubigné score was very good, with no one having less than a good clinical outcome. Fifteen of these eighteen patients had radiographic evaluation at a minimum of two years, and all were found to have a congruent joint with a normal joint space and no evidence of posttraumatic arthritis.

Conclusions.—Hip joint stability determined with dynamic stress fluoroscopy with the patient under general anesthesia after a posterior wall acetabular fracture is predictive of hip joint congruity, an excellent radiographic outcome, and a good-to-excellent early clinical outcome after nonoperative treatment.

▶ This well-done prospective study demonstrates the utility of dynamic stress fluoroscopy in making a decision as to whether or not to stabilize a posterior wall fracture of the acetabulum. The tool is particularly useful when the wall fragment is of small dimensions on the postreduction CT of the pelvis. Operative management of posterior wall fractures does involve risk of complication of a partial list of which includes injury to the sciatic nerve and intra-articular screw placement. This series of patients demonstrated good to excellent longer term radiographic and functional outcome when their hip was determined to be stable using this examination method.

M. F. Swiontkowski, MD

Hip Fracture

External Fixation for Stable and Unstable Intertrochanteric Fractures in Patients Older Than 75 Years of Age: A Prospective Comparative Study
Petsatodis G, Maliogas G, Karikis J, et al (Univ of Thessaloniki, Greece)
J Orthop Trauma 25:218-223, 2011

Objective.—External fixation has been advocated as an alternative treatment method of intertrochanteric fractures in elderly and high-risk patients. However, the efficacy of the technique in all fracture types has not been clearly defined. The null hypothesis of this study was that external fixation showed equal results in either stable or unstable intertrochanteric fractures in patients older than 75 years of age.
Design.—Prospective comparative study.
Setting.—Level I trauma center.
Patients.—Between July 2006 and June 2007, 100 patients older than 75 years of age (mean, 82.3 ± 5.2 years) and American Society of Anesthesiologists 3 or 4 who sustained an isolated intertrochanteric fracture met the inclusion criteria for the study. The patients were followed up at regular intervals until 1 year postoperatively.
Intervention.—All fractures were stabilized with external fixation under epidural anaesthesia. The patients were divided in two groups according to the Orthopaedic Trauma Association classification system for intertrochanteric fractures. Types A1.1, A1.2, A1.3, and A2.1 fractures were considered stable (Group A) and Types A2.2, A2.3, A3.1, A.3.2, and A.3.3 unstable (Group B). Fifty patients were collected in each group.
Main Outcome Measurements.—Operation and hospitalization time, union time, complication rate, Harris hip score, and patients' walking status were evaluated.
Results.—The median operative time was 17 minutes (range, 15–50 minutes) in Group A and 21.5 minutes (range, 15–60 minutes) in Group B ($P < 0.001$). The median hospitalization time was 5 days (range, 2–11 days) in Group A and 7 days (range, 4–17 days) in Group B ($P < 0.001$). The average union time was 11.24 ± 1.66 weeks (range, 9–16 weeks) for Group A and 14.1 ± 1.63 weeks (range, 10–17 weeks) for Group B ($P < 0.001$). The overall complication rate was 8% for the stable fractures and 26% for the unstable fractures ($P = 0.03$). The rate of varus collapse in unstable fractures was 11%. The median Harris hip score was 75 points (range, 28–100) in Group A and 68 points (range, 25–99) in Group B ($P = 0.006$). No difference was found between groups in terms of mortality ($P = 0.913$) or walking status ($P = 0.736$).
Conclusion.—External fixation for the treatment of Orthopaedic Trauma Association Types A2.2, A2.3, A3.1, A.3.2, and A.3.3 intertrochanteric fractures in the elderly was associated with prolonged union time, increased incidence of varus position of the fracture site, and inferior

functional outcome. Therefore, it should be used with caution in the geriatric population with an unstable intertrochanteric fracture.

▶ Throughout the last 3 decades, external fixation for management of proximal femur fractures has been suggested from time to time, with advocates exposing minimal blood loss and acceptable risk of complication. This well-done comparative cohort study should put the concept to rest for all but the most seriously ill patients with stable fracture patterns. The time to union and difficulty maintaining reduction for the 12-week period of time necessary for these fractures to unite are hurdles too large to overcome with any improved frame design that one can anticipate.

M. F. Swiontkowski, MD

The Value of an Organized Fracture Program for the Elderly: Early Results
Kates SL, Mendelson DA, Friedman SM (Univ of Rochester, NY)
J Orthop Trauma 25:233-237, 2011

Objectives.—To describe the early financial results of an organized hip fracture program for older adults.

Design.—Retrospective evaluation of financial data for a 1-year period on a hip fracture program for older adults.

Setting.—University medical center.

Patients.—All 193 adults older than age 60 with a native, nonpathologic hip fracture admitted to the hospital and surgically treated from May 2005 to April 2006 were included as subjects in this study.

Intervention.—The comanaged, protocol-driven fracture management program was used as the specific intervention for treating all patients with hip fractures.

Main Outcome Measure.—The primary outcome was profit or loss resulting from treatment of patients. Key quality measures studied included length of hospital stay, mortality rates, complication rates, and hospital readmission rates.

Results.—With use of an organized program, substantial savings in nearly all areas of expenditure is demonstrated. Adjusting for patient characteristics, costs are demonstrated to be 66.7% of the expected costs nationally. The length of stay, mortality, complication rates, and readmission rates were all noted to be below national averages.

Conclusions.—The improved quality measures suggest that better quality of patient care is associated with reduced costs (Tables 1-3).

▶ This retrospective review of 1-year data for a newly organized hip fracture program in a community hospital confirms the patient and hospital benefits of the program. Substantial cost savings and length of stay decrease accompany the institution of a program like this. Key factors are comanagement of the patients with hospitalists/geriatricians, surgeon collaboration to limit the

TABLE 1.—Patient Characteristics and Costs by Procedure Type

Procedure	Type of Fracture	Age Mean ± SD	Charlson Mean ± SD	LOS Mean ± SD	Total Variable Cost Mean ± SD	Fixed Cost Mean ± SD	Net Profit Mean ± SD
Cannulated screw (n = 22)	Nondisplaced femoral neck	85 ± 6.7	1.7 ± 2.0	4.3 ± 1.8	3666 ± 1408	2625 ± 1427	4859 ± 1907
Hemiarthroplasty (n = 61)	Displaced femoral neck	83 ± 8.6	2.0 ± 1.9	4.6 ± 1.9	5198 ± 4929	3153 ± 2860	4636 ± 2785
SHHS (n = 27)	Stable pertrochanteric	84 ± 6.8	1.5 ± 2.1	3.9 ± 1.1	4401 ± 1146	3121 ± 868	2744 ± 2591
SHS (n = 71)	Stable pertrochanteric	87 ± 12.4	2.2 ± 1.4	4.1 ± 1.9	4223 ± 1550	2784 ± 1020	3413 ± 3091
Blade plate (n = 5)	Unstable pertrochanteric	83 ± 4.3	2.3 ± 1.9	3.8 ± 0.8	4804 ± 1472	3085 ± 559	2314 ± 2934
Nail (n = 7)	Unstable pertrochanteric	89 ± 4.9	1.0 ± 1.8	9.1 ± 9.9	7361 ± 3716	4186 ± 1868	327 ± 5248

SD, standard deviation; LOS, length of stay; SHHS, sliding helical hip screw; SHS, sliding hip screw.

TABLE 2.—Hip Fracture Care Costs by Cost Center

Study dates Category	Hip Fracture Program (N = 193) 2005–2006 Mean ± SD	Median	Comparison 1 (N = 586) 2002–2006 Mean ± SD	Median	Comparison 2 (N = 206) 1996–1999 Mean
Age	85 ± 8	85	74 ± 9		81
Length of stay	4.4 ± 2.6	4	6.3		9.8
Case mix index	2 ± 0.6	1.9			
Net margin	3731 ± 2971	3968			37
Total fixed cost	2988 ± 1127	2605			
Total variable cost	4622 ± 1713	4188			
Non-ICU bed	1582 ± 879	1422			
ICU bed	18 ± 202	0	867 ± 3540	0	
Pharmacy	197 ± 282	122	760 ± 920	532	393
Laboratory	415 ± 287	361	1116 ± 1529	668	471
Radiology	256 ± 252	225	679 ± 1057	305	566
Operating room	953 ± 256	994	3924 ± 1382	3723	837
Preanesthesia	195 ± 51	198			
Cardiology	28 ± 48	15			
Emergency	25 ± 17	23			
Supply	865 ± 573	591	3946 ± 3085	4105	1793
Other	87 ± 82	62	1094 ± 1226	767	
Total cost	7610 ± 2746	6966	17,183 ± 10,252	14,441	10,159

SD, standard deviation; ICU, intensive care unit.

TABLE 3.—Actual Versus Predicted Average Cost in the Geriatric Fracture Center*

Location	Length of Stay Mean ± SD	Costs Mean ± SD	Geriatric Fracture Center Costs Percent of Predicted
Geriatric Fracture Center	4.4 ± 2.6	7610 ± 2746	
Predicted (New York State)	5.9 ± 1.2	11,071 ± 59	68.7
Predicted (United States)	5.2 ± 0.9	11,417 ± 62	66.7

SD, standard deviation.
*Predicted costs adjust for patient characteristics using a national database.

use of more expensive implants, and attention to discharge planning. Most important for patients, the program led to a lower rate of readmission, which would include readmission because of implant failure. This indicates that limiting the use of the more expensive nail implants does not result in a higher incidence of loss of reduction and need for repeat surgery. Another advantage of an organized hip fracture service is that appropriate evaluation and treatment for osteoporosis can more readily be included such that follow-up dual energy x-ray absorptiometry scans with appropriate medical management can be initiated.

M. F. Swiontkowski, MD

Iron Supplementation for Anemia After Hip Fracture Surgery: A Randomized Trial of 300 Patients

Parker MJ (Peterborough District Hosp, UK)
J Bone Joint Surg Am 92:265-269, 2010

Background.—Anemia as a consequence of surgery is often treated with iron therapy. The evidence base for this practice is limited. To determine if oral iron therapy is beneficial for the treatment of anemia after surgery for the treatment of a hip fracture, we undertook a prospective, randomized controlled trial.

Methods.—Three hundred patients with a hemoglobin level of <110 g/L after treatment for a hip fracture were randomized to receive either a twenty-eight-day course of ferrous sulfate therapy or no iron therapy. Hemoglobin levels were measured at six weeks after surgery. The length of the hospital stay and the mortality rate at one year were compared between groups.

Results.—The mean rise in hemoglobin levels six weeks after discharge from the hospital was 21 g/L in the iron group, compared with 18 g/L in the no-iron group (p = 0.07). There was no significant difference between the two groups with regard to the length of hospital stay or the mortality rate. Seventeen percent of the patients who were allocated to iron therapy reported adverse effects of the medication.

Conclusions.—The present study demonstrated that iron therapy had no clinically relevant benefit when used to treat anemia associated with a hip fracture (Tables 2 and 3).

▶ It has been relatively commonly accepted that patients undergoing surgical repair for hip fracture should receive iron therapy in the postoperative period

TABLE 2.—Characteristics of the Patients

	Iron Therapy	No Iron	P Value
No. of patients	150	150	—
Age* *(yr)*	81 (60 to 96)	83 (61 to 104)	0.03
Male *(no. of patients)*	31 (20.7%)	24 (16.0%)	0.37
Resides in own home *(no. of patients)*	134 (89.3%)	124 (82.7%)	0.13
American Society of Anesthesiologists grade[†]	2.6	2.5	0.13
Mobility score[†] *(points)*	6.0	5.5	0.09
Mental test score[†] *(points)*	7.0	7.2	0.54
Intracapsular fracture *(no. of patients)*	63 (42.0%)	73 (47.7%)	0.30
Transfusion (no. of patients)	29 (19.3%)	21 (14.0%)	0.28
No. of units of blood transfused[†]	2.1	2.3	0.29
Managed with arthroplasty *(no. of patients)*	63 (42.0%)	71 (47.3%)	0.42
Managed with intramedullary nail *(no. of patients)*	37 (24.7%)	27 (18.0%)	0.20
Managed with extramedullary fixation *(no. of patients)*	50 (33.3%)	52 (34.7%)	0.90
Hemoglobin level at time of admission[‡] *(g/L)*	126.9 ± 10.8	125.1 ± 10.9	0.15
Hemoglobin level at start of study[†] *(g/L)*	98.6	98.4	0.82

*The values are given as the mean, with the range in parentheses.
[†]The value are given as the mean.
[‡]The values are given as the mean and the standard deviation.

TABLE 3.—Outcome Measures for the Two Groups

	Iron Therapy	No Iron	P Value
Hemoglobin level at six weeks* (g/L)	119.5 ± 11.3	116.7 ± 12.3	0.06
Change in hemoglobin level at six weeks* (g/L)	21.0 ± 13.1	18.1 ± 12.8	0.07
Total hospital stay* (d)	18.8 ± 17.4	21.3 ± 20.6	0.26
Mortality†			
30 days	6 (4.0%)	3 (2.0%)	0.50
90 days	13 (8.7%)	9 (6.0%)	0.51
120 days	16 (10.7%)	12 (8.0%)	0.55
One year	29 (19.3%)	29 (19.3%)	1
Adverse effect of iron therapy (no. of patients)	26 (17.3%)	0	

*The values are given as the mean and the standard deviation.
†The values are given as the number of patients who had died by each time point, with the percentage in parentheses.

to speed recovery of their hemoglobin level to prefracture levels. Nearly all surgeons are aware of the issues with side effects of this treatment as well as issues with patient compliance. This well-done randomized trial has definitively answered the question of the efficacy of this treatment. Supplemental iron in patients with normal dietary intake should no longer be prescribed for patients in the postfracture repair phase.

M. F. Swiontkowski, MD

Intramedullary nailing appears to be superior in pertrochanteric hip fractures with a detached greater trochanter: 311 consecutive patients followed for 1 year

Palm H, Lysén C, Krasheninnikoff M, et al (Hvidovre Univ Hosp, Copenhagen, Denmark)
Acta Orthop 82:166-170, 2011

Background and Purpose.—In recent years, intramedullary nails (INs) for the treatment of pertrochanteric hip fractures have gained prominence relative to conventional, sliding hip screws (SHSs). There is little empirical background for this development, however. A previous series of ours suggested that the use of SHS was not adequate in situations with fragile or fractured lateral femoral walls, where it often led to lack of healing in a maximally telescoped position. We hypothesized that INs would be the superior implant in these specific circumstances.

Methods.—We retrospectively examined 311 consecutive patients treated in our department between 2002 and 2008, with either an IN (n = 158) or an SHS (n = 153) mounted on a 4-hole side-plate, for an AO/OTA type 31A1−2 pertrochanteric fracture with a detached greater trochanter. The status of the lesser trochanter was assessed preoperatively and the integrity of the lateral femoral wall, fracture reduction, and position of the implants were assessed postoperatively. Reoperations due to technical failure were recorded for one year postoperatively.

TABLE 2.—Relationship Between Reoperation Within a Year Postoperatively and Patient Characteristics in the 311 Patients with a Pertrochanteric Fracture with a Detached Greater Trochanter, Operated with Either an Intramedullary Nail or a Sliding Hip Screw

| | | Reoperation Within 1 Year Postoperatively | | | |
| | | Univariate Analysis | | Multivariate Analysis | |
	n (%)	OR (95% CI)	p-Value	OR (95% CI)	p-Value
Age, years[a]	84 (76—90)		1.0	1.0 (1.0—1.1)	0.2
Female sex	240 (77)	0.6 (0.3—1.4)	0.2	0.5 (0.2—1.4)	0.2
Prefracture NMS 0—5	151 (49)	0.7 (0.3—1.5)	0.4	0.5 (0.2—1.4)	0.2
ASA score III—IV	141 (46)	1.1 (0.5—2.5)	0.8	1.2 (0.5—3.0)	0.7
Detached lesser trochanter	217 (70)	0.9 (0.4—2.1)	0.8	1.6 (0.6—4.0)	0.4
Tip-apex distance, mm[a]	20 (15—26)		0.09	1.1 (0.9—1.1)	0.07
Fracture reduction, mm[a]	8 (3—12)		0.02	1.1 (1.0—1.1)	0.01
Sliding hip screw	153 (49)	4.3 (1.7—11)	0.001	5.3 (1.8—15)	0.002

ASA: American Society of Anaesthesiologists; NMS: new mobility score.
Values are presented as number of patients (percentage) and analyzed using the chi-square test.
[a]Except for continuous data, presented as median (interquartiles) and analyzed using the Mann-Whitney test.

Results.—Multivariate logistic regression analysis showed that the groups were similar regarding demographic and biomechanical parameters. The lateral femoral wall was more frequently fractured during SHS implantation (42 patients) than in the IN group (9 patients) (p < 0.001). 6 (4%) of the 158 patients operated with IN had to be reoperated, as compared to 22 (14%) in the SHS group of 153 patients (p = 0.001).

Interpretation.—IN had a lower reoperation rate than SHS in these pertrochanteric hip fractures with a detached greater trochanter. IN left more lateral femoral walls intact (Table 2).

▶ This retrospective comparative cohort study comparing the results of intramedullary nail (IN) hip screws with those of sliding hip screws confirms once again the usefulness of IN screws in situations of fractured greater trochanter and lateral wall of the proximal femur. The fracture of the greater trochanter is most often associated with a fractured lateral wall or compromised very thin lateral wall. This explains the association with patient age and female sex (Table 2). The use of the IN screw in this setting results in lower reoperation rates with complete failure of reduction/fixation. The problem with these devices (IN hip screws) is that they are overused in stable fracture patterns, with associated increase in cost and complications of the use of these devices in that setting. This situation has been extensively studied and reported. The orthopedic community needs to restrict the use of these devices to the unstable fracture patterns detailed in this review.

M. F. Swiontkowski, MD

Foot and Ankle Fractures

Long-term outcome after 1822 operatively treated ankle fractures: A systematic review of the literature

Stufkens SAS, van den Bekerom MPJ, Kerkhoffs GMMJ, et al (Academic Med Ctr, The Netherlands; et al)
Injury 42:119-127, 2011

The aim of this literature review is to systematically gather the highest level of available evidence on the long-term outcome after operatively treated ankle fractures in the English, German and Dutch literature. A search term with Boolean operators was constructed. The search was limited to humans and adults and the major databases were searched from 1966 to 2008 to identify studies relating to functional outcome, subjective outcome and radiographic evaluation at least 4 years after an operatively treated ankle fracture. Of the 42 initially relevant papers, 18 met our inclusion criteria. A total of 1822 fractures were identified. The mean sample-size weighted follow-up was 5.1 years. The initial number of patients that were included in the studies was 2724, which results in a long-term follow-up success rate of 66.9%. Regarding the fracture reduction we found 4 papers reporting on 106 fractures. Of the fractures that were classified according to Danis—Weber, 736 were eligible for correlation with the long-term outcome. In 442 fractures a comparison was possible between supination-external rotation stage 2 and 4 of the Lauge-Hansen classification. Only one study reported on the influence of initial cartilage lesions on the outcome. Regarding the involvement of the posterior malleolus, two studies reported on the long-term outcome. None of the studies addressed the influence of hindfoot varus or valgus on the long-term outcome after ankle fracture. Only 79.3% of the optimally reduced fractures show good to excellent long-term outcome. The Weber A type fractures do not show a better long-term outcome

TABLE 7.—Odd-ratio on Good to Excellent Outcome

Reduction	OR	95% CI	
Optimal versus poor	11.20	(3.65; 34.15)	*
Fair versus poor	6.08	(1.99; 18.59)	*
Optimal versus fair	1.84	(0.60; 5.62)	
Fracture type Weber			
Type A versus type C	2.01	(1.13; 3.57)	*
Type B versus type C	2.17	(1.22; 3.86)	*
Type B versus type A	1.08	(0.61; 1.92)	
Fracture type Lauge-Hansen			
SER-2 versus SER-4	2.93	(1.40; 5.90)	*
Cartilage lesions			
Without versus with	5.00	(0.82; 30.46)	

$*p = 0.05$.

than Weber B type fractures. Recommendations for future research were formulated (Table 7).

▶ This well-done meta-analysis evaluates the impact of fracture location, fracture reduction, and associated cartilage damage on long-term functional outcome following ankle fracture. Eighteen of 42 relevant articles met the criteria for inclusion, which is a commentary in and of itself on the quality of the published literature on the subject. The instruments used to evaluate patient function at the weighted follow-up of 5.1 years were varied. The follow-up percentage of the original patient-pooled cohort was nearly 67%.

The take-home message is that the quality of reduction does impact the long-term functional outcome, as does the presence of cartilage injury. The location of the fracture does, as well, with Weber C level fractures having a worse outcome than B and A level fractures. The literature is overall lacking, and the orthopedic community will benefit by larger well-done long-term functional cohort studies.

M. F. Swiontkowski, MD

Outcomes of Ankle Fractures in Patients with Uncomplicated Versus Complicated Diabetes
Wukich DK, Joseph A, Ryan M, et al (UPMC Comprehensive Foot and Ankle Ctr, Jane St, Pittsburgh, PA)
Foot Ankle Int 32:120-130, 2011

Background.—Patients with diabetes who sustain an ankle fracture are at increased risk for complications including higher rates of in hospital mortality, in-hospital postoperative complications, length of stay and non-routine discharges. The purpose of this study was to retrospectively compare the complications associated with operatively treated ankle fractures in a group of patients with uncomplicated diabetes versus a group of patients with complicated diabetes. Complicated diabetes was defined as diabetes associated with end organ damage such as peripheral neuropathy, nephropathy and/or PAD. Uncomplicated diabetes was defined as diabetes without any of these associated conditions. Our hypothesis was that patients with uncomplicated diabetes would experience fewer complications than those patients with complicated diabetes.

Materials and Methods.—We compared the complication rates of ankle fracture repair in 46 patients with complicated diabetes and 59 patients with uncomplicated diabetes and calculated odds ratios (OR) for significant findings.

Results.—At a mean followup of 21.4 months we found that patients with complicated diabetes had 3.8 times increased risk of overall complications 3.4 times increased risk of a non-infectious complication (malunion, nonunion or Charcot arthropathy) and 5 times higher likelihood of needing revision surgery/arthrodesis when compared to patients with

TABLE 2.—Comparison of Patients with Complicated and Complicated Diabetes Mellitus

	Complicated $n=46$	Diabetes Status Uncomplicated $n=59$	Odds Ratio (95% CI)	p Value
Overall Complications (%)	50.0	22.8	3.8 (1.6–8.9)	0.003
Total Infections (%)	30.4	17.5		0.13
Superficial Infections (%)	28.3	17.5		0.20
Deep Infections (%)	17.4	5.3		0.06
Total Non Infectious (%) (Nonunion, Malunion and/or Charcot Arthropathy)	28.9	11.9	3.4 (1.2–9.2)	0.02
Amputation (%)	8.7	3.4		0.26
Revision Surgery (%)	26.7	6.8	5.0 (1.4–16.8)	0.009

TABLE 3.—Impact of Diabetic Neuropathy on Complication Rate

	With Neuropathy ($n=35$) v. Without Neuropathy ($n=70$)
Any Complication	[OR = 4.7, 95% CI (1.2–9.2), $p=0.001$]
Overall Infection	[$p=0.06$]
Superficial Infection	[$p=0.12$]
Deep Infection	[OR = 6.4, 95% CI (1.6–26.1), $p=0.009$]
Aggregate Noninfectious Complication (Nonunion, Malunion and/or Charcot Arthropathy)	[OR = 3.5, 95% CI (1.3–9.4), $p=0.01$]
Amputation	[$p=0.10$]
Revision Surgery	[OR = 4.4, 95% CI (1.5–13.6), $p=0.009$]

OR, Odds Ratio; CI, Confidence Interval. Significant findings in **bold**.

uncomplicated diabetes. Open ankle fractures in this diabetic population were associated with a three times higher rate of complications and 3.7 times higher rate of infection.

Conclusion.—Patients with complicated diabetes have an increased risk of complications after ankle fracture surgery compared to patients with uncomplicated diabetes. Careful preoperative evaluation of the neurovascular status is mandatory, since many patients with diabetes do not recognize that they have neuropathy and/or peripheral artery disease (Tables 2 and 3).

▶ This retrospective cohort study examines the relationship between diabetic disease severity and complications following ankle fracture. The definition of diabetes associated with end organ disease as being complicated diabetes makes clinical sense. The findings are not surprising. With a 3.8 times higher risk of overall complications and 3.4 times higher risk of nonunion and malunion/Charcot arthropathy, there is reason for careful counseling of patients with these comorbidities as to the risk of fracture complication. Open fracture is particularly of note with a 3.7 times higher risk of infection for individuals with complicated diabetes. This study is of course subject to detection bias and inclusion bias; however, the magnitude of differences in the outcomes warrants attention. The information is of most use in counseling patients early in the management of their fracture as to what the future may hold for their lower extremity.

M. F. Swiontkowski, MD

Shock Wave Therapy Compared with Intramedullary Screw Fixation for Nonunion of Proximal Fifth Metatarsal Metaphyseal-Diaphyseal Fractures
Furia JP, Juliano PJ, Wade AM, et al (SUN Orthopaedics and Sports Medicine, Lewisburg, PA; Penn State Milton S. Hershey Med Ctr, PA; et al)
J Bone Joint Surg Am 92:846-854, 2010

Background.—The current "gold standard" for treatment of chronic fracture nonunion in the metaphyseal-diaphyseal region of the fifth metatarsal is intramedullary screw fixation. Complications with this procedure, however, are not uncommon. Shock wave therapy can be an effective treatment for fracture nonunions. The purpose of this study was to evaluate the safety and efficacy of shock wave therapy as a treatment of these nonunions.

Methods.—Twenty-three patients with a fracture nonunion in the metaphyseal-diaphyseal region of the fifth metatarsal received high-energy shock wave therapy (2000 to 4000 shocks; energy flux density per pulse, 0.35 mJ/mm^2), and twenty other patients with the same type of fracture nonunion were treated with intramedullary screw fixation. The numbers of fractures that were healed at three and six months after treatment in each group were determined, and treatment complications were recorded.

Results.—Twenty of the twenty-three nonunions in the shock wave group and eighteen of the twenty nonunions in the screw fixation group were healed at three months after treatment. One of the three nonunions that had not healed by three months in the shock wave group was healed by six months. There was one complication in the shock wave group (post-treatment petechiae) and eleven complications in the screw-fixation group (one refracture, one case of cellulitis, and nine cases of symptomatic hardware).

Conclusions.—Both intramedullary screw fixation and shock wave therapy are effective treatments for fracture nonunion in the metaphyseal-diaphyseal region of the fifth metatarsal. Screw fixation is more often associated with complications that frequently result in additional surgery.

▶ Intramedullary screw fixation is generally accepted as the treatment of choice for fresh fractures and nonunion of the proximal metaphyseal-diaphyseal junction of the fifth metatarsal. Shock wave therapy has been shown to be effective in placebo-controlled trials for treatment of fracture nonunion. This comparative cohort study has demonstrated that both are relatively effective in gaining radiographic and clinical union of proximal fifth metatarsal nonunions within 3 months after intervention in approximately 90% of cases. Inclusion bias is always a concern in these types of nonrandomized designs, and one would expect that the nonunions perceived to be more difficult to heal would be in the invasive surgical cohort. Because both techniques require an anesthetic intervention, this condition would be ideal for shared decision making with the patient. The patient can choose between the 2 techniques, weighing the risk of an open procedure with potential for infection and need for hardware removal against the less-invasive technique. Of course, the technology for shock wave therapy, with its considerable financial investment, must be available to the patient.

M. F. Swiontkowski, MD

Outcomes of Suture Button Repair of the Distal Tibiofibular Syndesmosis

DeGroot H, Al-Omari AA, El Ghazaly SA (Newton Wellesley Hosp, MA; Jordan Univ of Science and Technology, Ramtha; Ain Shams Univ, Cairo, Egypt)
Foot Ankle Int 32:250-256, 2011

Background.—Recently, a suture button device has been advocated as a simple and effective method of repairing the syndesmosis. Proponents of the device have cited earlier weightbearing and elimination of the need for device removal as potential advantages over metallic screws. However, the available reports generally have short followup. With longer followup, some concerns about the suture button device have surfaced.

Materials and Methods.—We reviewed the clinical and radiographic results of 24 patients with acute injuries to the distal tibiofibular syndesmosis who were treated with suture button fixation. Average followup was 20 months. The primary outcomes measure was the AOFAS ankle hindfoot score. Secondary outcomes measures included a calibrated measurement of the tibiofibular clear space and tibiofibular overlap.

Results.—The average AOFAS score was 94 points. Syndesmotic parameters returned to normal after surgery and remained normal throughout the followup period. One in four patients required removal of the suture endobutton device due to local irritation or lack of motion. Osteolysis of the bone and subsidence of the device into the bone was observed in four patients. Three patients developed heterotopic ossification within the syndesmotic ligament, one mild, one moderate, and one who had a nearly complete syndesmotic fusion.

Conclusion.—The suture button device is an effective way to repair the syndesmosis. In our series, the reduction of the syndesmosis was maintained throughout the followup period. However, reoperation for device removal was more common than anticipated. Osteolysis of the bone near the implant and subsidence of the device may occur.

▶ Use of the suture button technique has been widely adopted over the last 3 to 5 years, and long-term studies evaluating the efficacy are lacking. This is a longer-term cohort study that confirms that syndesmotic reduction can be maintained over the early time frame following syndesmotic injury (average follow-up, 20 months). The fact that osteolysis around the device occurs is not surprising or of concern. The fibula rotates with ankle dorsiflexion and plantar flexion, and internal fixation devices will break or resorption occurs in the bone around the implant; this is true for screws as well. A randomized controlled trial, adequately powered and likely multicenter, comparing the suture endobutton device with screw fixation is heavily anticipated.

M. F. Swiontkowski, MD

A Systematic Review on the Treatment of Acute Ankle Sprain: Brace versus Other Functional Treatment Types
Kemler E, van de Port I, Backx F, et al (Univ Med Centre Utrecht, the Netherlands; et al)
Sports Med 41:185-197, 2011

Ankle injuries, especially ankle sprains, are a common problem in sports and medical care. Ankle sprains result in pain and absenteeism from work and/or sports participation, and can lead to physical restrictions such as ankle instability. Nowadays, treatment of ankle injury basically consists of taping the ankle. The purpose of this review is to evaluate the effectiveness of ankle braces as a treatment for acute ankle sprains compared with other types of functional treatments such as ankle tape and elastic bandages.

A computerized literature search was conducted using PubMed, EMBASE, CINAHL and the Cochrane Clinical Trial Register. This review includes randomized controlled trials in English, German and Dutch, published between 1990 and April 2009 that compared ankle braces as a treatment for lateral ankle sprains with other functional treatments. The inclusion criteria for this systematic review were (i) individuals (sports participants as well as non-sports participants) with an acute injury of the ankle (acute ankle sprains); (ii) use of an ankle brace as primary treatment for acute ankle sprains; (iii) control interventions including any other type of functional treatment (e.g. Tubigrip™, elastic wrap or ankle tape); and (iv) one of the following reported outcome measures: re-injuries, symptoms (pain, swelling, instability), functional outcomes and/or time to resumption of sports, daily activities and/or work. Eight studies met all inclusion criteria. Differences in outcome measures, intervention types and patient characteristics precluded pooling of the results, so best evidence syntheses were conducted. A few individual studies reported positive outcomes after treatment with an ankle brace compared with other functional methods, but our best evidence syntheses only demonstrated a better treatment result in terms of functional outcome. Other studies have suggested that ankle brace treatment is a more cost-effective method, so the use of braces after acute ankle sprains should be considered. Further research should focus on economic evaluation and on different types of

TABLE 3.—Characteristics of Trials Included

Study (Year)	Sample Size (n); Sex	Age (y) [Range]	Participants	Follow-up	Injury Severity	Sports-related Injuries	Treatment (n)	Control (n)	Relevant Outcomes with Significant Results
Twellaar et al.[64] (1993)	116; M 77, F 39	Mean 32	83% SP in the tape group and 73% SP in the brace group	Long term 1.8–2.8 y	All ankle injuries	Percentage of sports injuries NR	Confection brace (53)	Adhesive, non-elastic tape (63)	Functional stability; swelling; blisters; pain – investigating ankle is painful in brace group: 20% vs 47% in tape group; p < 0.05
Neumann et al.[59] (1994)	80; NR	SRO: mean 25.2 [16–46]; EB: mean 23.2 [11–50]	Percentage of SP not reported	Short term (3, 10 d, 3, 6 wk, 4 mo); intermediate term (12 mo)	Grade III	Percentage of sports injuries NR	SRO (31)	EB (33)	Questionnaire with 88-point scale
Dettori et al.[63] (1994)	64; M 60, F 4	Mean 24.2–25.9	All were military personnel	Short term (5 wk)	Moderate and severe injuries	All injuries occurred during military activities	AB (24)	Elastic wrap (22); cast (18)	Number of days before return to full duty; ankle swelling; pain
Leanderson and Wredmark[62] (1995)	73; M 48, F 25	Mean 28 [15–55]	SP + NSP	Short term (24 h, 3–5 d, 2, 4, 10 wk)	Grades II and III	48% sports injuries	ASB (39)	CB (34)	Karlsson's scoring scale Recording sick leave: ASB 5.3 (0–26 days) vs CB 9.1 (0–21 days); p < 0.05; clinical examination with regard to localized tenderness, degree of swelling and range of plantar flexion-dorsiflexion of the ankle
Karlsson et al.[61] (1996)	86; 57 M, 29 F	Mean 22 [16–38]	SP	Long term (12–24 mo, mean 18 mo)	Grades II and III	Percentage of sports injuries NR	Functional treatment, with specially designed compression pads, weightbearing and range-ofmotion training (45)	Conservative treatment with elastic wrapping, partial weight bearing and crutches (39)	Karlsson's scoring scale Return to sports activities – functional treatment with compression pads: 9.6 ± 4.8 d vs 19.2 ± 9.5 days for conventional treatment with elastic wrapping (p < 0.05); reported d of sick leave – functional treatment with compression pads: 5.6 ± 4.2 d vs 10.2 ± 6.8 d for conventional treatment with elastic wrapping (p < 0.05)

Study	Participants (n; sex)	Age	Sport participation	Follow-up	Injury severity/type	Sports injuries	Intervention	Comparator(s)	Outcomes
Boyce et al.[60] (2005)	50, 12 default, 3 excluded (1 lateral malleolus, 1 wrong clinical appointment given and 1 foot injury; ESB M 11, AB M 10	>16 [16–58]	SP + NSP	Short term (10 d, 1 mo)	Moderate or severe	38% sports injuries	AB (18)	ESB (17)	Karlsson's scoring scale: (i) after 10 d: ESB mean = 35 vs AB mean = 50; 95% CI 1.7, 27.7; $p = 0.028$; (ii) after 1 mo: ESB mean = 55 vs AB mean = 68; 95% CI 1.4, 24.8; $p = 0.029$; pain score; ankle girth difference
Beynnon et al.[58] (2006)	212; NR	[16–61]	SP + NSP	Short term, intermediate term (6 mo)	First-time grade I, grade II and grade III	Grade I: 34% sports injuries; grade II: 39% sports injuries; grade III: 71% sports injuries	AB (NR)	Elastic wrap (not reported); AB with wrap (NR); cast (NR)	Number of d required to return to: no pain during weight bearing, full capability in normal daily activities, full capability at work or school, full capability in usual athletic or recreational physical activity; Karlsson's scale; re-injuries
Lamb et al.[65] (2009)	584; M 337, F 247	Mean 30	SP NR	Intermediate term (3 and 9 mo)	Severe ankle sprains	Percentage of sports injuries NR	Tubigrip™ (140)	Below-knee cast (119); Bledsoe boot (148); AB (148)	FAOS including; assessments of pain, symptoms, activities of daily living, sport and quality of life

AB = Aircast® brace; ASB = Air-stirrup® brace; CB = compression bandage; EB = elastic bandage; ESB = elastic support bandage; F = female; FAOS = foot and ankle outcome score; M = male; NR = not reported; NSP = non-sports participants; SP = sports participants; SRO = semi-rigid orthosis.
Editor's Note: Please refer to original journal article for full references.

ankle brace, to examine the strengths and weaknesses of ankle braces for the treatment of acute ankle sprains (Table 3).

▶ Ankle sprain is one of the most common injuries addressed by orthopedic caregivers. Return-to-function questions have dominated prior studies on interventional strategies. This well-done meta-analysis used strict quality criteria to include randomized controlled trials in the data pool to be analyzed. Ankle bracing appears to offer better functional results. More research into cost-effectiveness of this strategy is necessary.

M. F. Swiontkowski, MD

Tibia Fractures

Timing of Definitive Fixation of Severe Tibial Plateau Fractures With Compartment Syndrome Does Not Have an Effect on the Rate of Infection

Zura RD, for the Southeastern Fracture Consortium Foundation (Duke Univ Med Ctr, Durham, NC; et al)
J Trauma 69:1523-1526, 2010

Background.—Tibial plateau fractures with associated compartment syndrome are severe injuries with elevated infection rates. The objective of this article was to analyze whether there is an association between infection and the timing of definitive fracture fixation in relation to fasciotomy closure or coverage.

Methods.—Eighty-one tibial plateau fractures, complicated by compartment syndrome, were treated with four-compartment fasciotomies and definitive fracture fixation before, at, or after fasciotomy closure or coverage.

Results.—Thirty extremities were treated with definitive fixation before fasciotomy closure. Seven (23%) of these extremities developed an infection. Twenty-six extremities were treated with definitive internal fixation at the time of fasciotomy closure of which three (12%) developed an infection. Twenty-five extremities were treated definitively after fasciotomy closure of which four (16%) developed an infection. There was no significant difference in the rate of infection among the groups ($p = 0.5012$).

Conclusions.—This study demonstrated no statistical difference in the rate of infection when tibial plateau fractures with four-compartment fasciotomies were treated with open reduction and internal fixation before fasciotomy closure, at fasciotomy closure, or after fasciotomy closure. Based on the data presented herein, it seems that definitive fracture treatment can be determined by the condition of patient and by surgeon preference and experience without exposing the patient to the additional risk of infection.

▶ This collaborative cohort study focuses on a rather specific clinical question: Does the timing of fasciotomy closure impact the infection risk of patients with combined tibial plateau fracture requiring open reduction internal fixation and compartmental syndrome? The definition of infection was standardized prior to chart review and the cohorts examined for significant confounding variables. This will likely be the definitive work on this clinical question for some time to come, as this is a relatively rare association and is indicative of high-energy trauma to the limb. This makes consideration of a randomization protocol difficult because of the rarity of the association. The take-home message is that with association of injuries, infection is common and the timing of closure of the fasciotomy wounds does not increase or decrease the risk. The timing of the fasciotomy itself, as it relates to tissue necrosis, is probably the larger impact variable.

M. F. Swiontkowski, MD

Upper Extremity

Effect of Calcium Phosphate Bone Cement Augmentation on Volar Plate Fixation of Unstable Distal Radial Fractures in the Elderly

Kim JK, Koh YD, Kook SH (Ewha Womans Univ, Yangcheon-gu, Seoul, South Korea)

J Bone Joint Surg Am 93:609-614, 2011

Background.—Calcium phosphate bone cement increases the stability of implant-bone constructs in patients with an osteoporotic fracture. The purpose of this randomized study was to determine whether augmentation of volar locking plate fixation with calcium phosphate bone cement has any benefit over volar locking plate fixation alone in patients older than sixty-five years of age who have an unstable distal radial fracture.

Methods.—Forty-eight patients (fifty unstable distal radial fractures) were recruited for this study. The mean patient age was seventy-three years. Surgical procedures were randomized between volar locking plate fixation alone (Group 1) and volar locking plate fixation with injection of calcium phosphate bone cement (Group 2). The patients were assessed clinically at three and twelve months postoperatively. Clinical assessments included determinations of grip strength, wrist motion, wrist pain, modified Mayo wrist scores, and Disabilities of the Arm, Shoulder and Hand (DASH) scores. Radiographic evaluations were performed immediately postoperatively and at one year following surgery. The adequacy of the reduction was assessed by measuring radial inclination, volar angulation, and ulnar variance.

Results.—The two groups were comparable with regard to age, sex, fracture type, injury mechanism, and bone mineral density. No significant differences were observed between the groups with regard to the clinical outcomes at the three or twelve-month follow-up examination. No significant intergroup differences in radiographic outcomes were observed immediately after surgery or at the one-year follow-up visit. Furthermore, no complication-related differences were observed, and there were no nonunions.

Conclusions.—Augmentation of metaphyseal defects with calcium phosphate bone cement after volar locking plate fixation offered no benefit

TABLE 2.—Clinical Outcomes*

	3 Months Postop.				12 Months Postop.			
	Group 1		Group 2		Group 1		Group 2	
	Mean and Stand. Dev.	% of Contralat. Side	Mean and Stand. Dev.	% of Contralat. Side	Mean and Stand. Dev.	% of Contralat. Side	Mean and Stand. Dev.	% of Contralat. Side
Range of motion (deg)								
Flexion	51 ± 10	80	53 ± 15	82	61 ± 13	86	61 ± 14	86
Extension	54 ± 11	85	53 ± 10	84	60 ± 15	85	60 ± 15	85
Supination	84 ± 7	95	83 ± 9	84	85 ± 9	95	85 ± 8	97
Pronation	86 ± 5	96	85 ± 6	95	86 ± 5	96	86 ± 6	95
Grip strength *(kg)*	17 ± 9	67	18 ± 10	69	22 ± 13	82	22 ± 15	83
VAS score *(points)*	3.2 ± 2		3.0 ± 2		1.2 ± 2		1.0 ± 2	
MMWS *(points)*	69 ± 11		71 ± 13		80 ± 11		81 ± 13	
DASH score *(points)*	24 ± 15		23 ± 12		10 ± 8		10 ± 7	

*There was no significant difference between groups for any outcome measure.

over volar locking plate fixation alone in elderly patients with an unstable distal radial fracture (Table 2).

▶ Locked plate fixation of distal radius fractures has evolved as the standard treatment for displaced distal radius fractures in adults, including those with intra-articular extension. Because large numbers of these fractures occur in elderly women, there has been a concern on the issue of diminished bone quality related to osteoporosis. This well-done controlled trial documents the results with carefully obtained clinical and radiographic outcomes (Fig 1 in the original article, Table 2). Routine use of calcium phosphate cements offers no benefit to patients by either measure and should not be routinely used. The use of this adjunct should be restricted to extreme cases of communition with markedly diminished bone quality.

M. F. Swiontkowski, MD

Medial and Lateral Pin Versus Lateral-Entry Pin Fixation for Type 3 Supracondylar Fractures in Children: A Prospective, Surgeon-Randomized Study

Gaston RG, Cates TB, Devito D, et al (OrthoCarolina, Charlotte, NC; Emory Univ, Atlanta, GA; et al)
J Pediatr Orthop 30:799-806, 2010

Background.—The purpose of this study is to compare the efficacy of medial and lateral (crossed pin) and lateral-entry pin techniques for Gartland Type 3 supracondylar humerus fractures in children.

Methods.—Six pediatric orthopaedists were divided into the 2 treatment groups (medial and lateral pins or lateral only pins) based on pre-study

TABLE 3.—Results for the Change in Baumann's Angle

Absolute Change of Baumann's Angle	N	Median (25th, 75th Percentile)	P*
Treatment			0.54
Crossed	57	2.9 (1.5, 5.2)	
Lateral	47	3.7 (1.6, 6.1)	
Sex			0.0062
Male	53	4.5(2.2, 6.2)	
Female	51	2.3 (1, 4.3)	
Side			0.39
Right	55	3.6 (1.4, 7)	
Left	49	3.0 (1.8, 4.8)	
Dominant			0.527[†]
Yes	43	3.2 (0.8, 6.1)	0.912[‡]
No	44	2.8 (1.6, 5.0)	
Unknown	17	3.7 (2.3, 5.4)	
Neurovascular injury recovered			0.0852
Intact	78	3.7 (1.8, 5.4)	
Out	26	2.1 (0.8, 4.9)	
Postoperative immobilization			0.77[†]
Cast	58	3.1 (1.8, 5.6)	
Bivalved	34	3.65 (1.6, 5.5)	
Univalved	7	2.0 (0.3, 5.1)	
Splint	5	3.1 (1.6, 3.9)	
Reduction			0.7425
Closed	96	2.9 (1.6, 4.9)	
Open	8	3.5 (1.6, 5.4)	
Delay (d)			0.35
1	45	3.0 (1.1, 6.2)	
<1	55	3.4 (2.0, 5.2)	
Initial displacement			0.028[†]
Posterior	28	4.6 (2.6, 7.7)	
Posterior cortex	29	2.9(1.6, 4.4)	
Posterior-medial	32	2.7 (1.4, 4.4)	

*Wilcoxon Rank-sum test.
[†]Kruskal-Wallis Test.
[‡]Wilcoxon Rank-sum test, comparing the "yes" and "no" groups.

pinning technique preferences. Patients were randomized into 1 of the 2 pinning technique treatment groups based on which attending was on call at the time of patient presentation. One hundred and four patients met inclusion criteria. Forty-seven patients underwent lateral-entry pinning and 57 underwent crossed pinning. The 2 groups were similar with respect to age, sex, preoperative neurovascular injury, direction of fracture displacement, and timing of surgery. Outcome parameters measured included radiographic maintenance of reduction, iatrogenic neurovascular complications, and rate of infection. All radiographic measurements, and interobserver reliability, were determined by a 3 physician panel.

Results.—The results of the interobserver reliability data showed a strong correlation and this data allowed 95% confidence that a change in Baumann's angle of more than 6 degrees and humerocapitellar angle of more than 10 degrees was significant. The lateral-entry patients experienced a median absolute change of Baumann's angle of 3.7 degrees with 12 patients having greater than 6 degrees loss of reduction; whereas those in

TABLE 4.—Results for the Change in HC Angle

Absolute Change of Baumann's Angle	N	Median (25th, 75th Percentile)	P*
Treatment			0.76
Crossed	57	5.1 (2.4, 10.3)	
Lateral	47	4.8 (2.4, 10)	
Sex			0.81
Male	53	5.3 (2.4, 9.8)	
Female	51	4.6 (2.4, 13.2)	
Side			0.29
Right	55	4.7 (2.3, 8.9)	
Left	49	6.4 (2.5, 12.2)	
Dominant			0.39[†]
Yes	43	4.7 (2, 8.9)	0.46[‡]
No	44	5.8 (2.4, 12.9)	
Unknown	17	5.3 (3.5, 10.5)	
Neurovascular injury recovered			0.61
Intact	78	4.9 (2.5, 10.5)	
Out	26	5.05 (1.9, 9.9)	
Postoperative immobilization			0.25[†]
Cast	58	4.9 (3.1, 12.6)	
Bivalved	34	5.3 (2, 10)	
Univalved	7	2.3 (1, 4.5)	
Splint	5	5 (2, 7.4)	
Reduction			0.77
Closed	96	5.0 (2.5, 10.2)	
Open	8	4.9 (1.6, 11.75)	
Delay (d)			0.92
1	45	5.2 (3.1, 8.1)	
<1	55	4.8 (2.3, 12.2)	
Initial displacement			0.897[†]
Posterior	28	5 (2.4, 10.1)	
Posterior cortex	29	3.8 (2, 10.4)	
Posterior-medial	32	4.7 (2.5, 9.2)	

HC indicates humerocapitellar.
*Wilcoxon Rank-sum test.
[†]Kruskal-Wallis Test.
[‡]Wilcoxon Rank-sum test, comparing the "yes" and "no" groups.

the medial and lateral-pin group saw a median change of 2.9 degrees with 10 patients having greater than 6 degrees loss of reduction. In terms of the humerocapitellar angle, the lateral-entry patients experienced a median absolute change of 4.8 degrees with 11 patients having greater than 10 degrees loss of reduction; whereas those in the medial and lateral-pin groups saw a median change of 5.1 degrees with 17 patients having greater than 10 degrees loss of reduction. There was no significant difference in infection rate between the 2 groups but 2 cases of iatrogenic neurovascular injury occurred in patients who had a medial pin placed.

Conclusions.—We found no statistical difference in the radiographic outcomes between lateral-entry and medial and lateral-pin techniques for the management of Type 3 supracondylar fractures in children when evaluated in this prospective and surgeon-randomized trial, but 2 cases of iatrogenic injury to the ulnar nerve occurred with medially placed pins.

Level of Evidence.—Level 2 (Table 3 and 4).

▶ Crossed pin versus lateral-only pin fixation for displaced supracondylar humeral fractures in children has been an issue of debate for more than 2 decades. This surgeon-randomized trial is well conducted and identifies no clinical or radiographic outcome differences with the 2 fixation approaches. The fact that 2 neurovascular complications were related to medial pin fixation and no neurovascular complications occurred with lateral-only pin fixation is the major issue of concern. If surgeons continue to use cross pin fixation as a preference, small incisions with dissection down to the medial epicondyle, particularly where elbow swelling is severe, is advisable to avoid these complications.

M. F. Swiontkowski, MD

A Prospective Study on the Effectiveness of Cotton Versus Waterproof Cast Padding in Maintaining the Reduction of Pediatric Distal Forearm Fractures
Robert CE, Jiang JJ, Khoury JG (Univ of Alabama at Birmingham)
J Pediatr Orthop 31:144-149, 2011

Background.—Distal forearm fractures, one of the most common fractures seen in the pediatric population, are regularly treated by closed reduction and casting. Our study investigates the effectiveness of Gore-Tex-lined casting in maintaining the reduction of 100% displaced distal forearm fractures compared with traditional cotton-lined casts.

Methods.—We screened all patients from February 2007 to July 2009 who presented to Childrens Hospital in Birmingham, AL with a distal radius fracture. Only patients with 100% displaced distal radius fractures were eligible to be assigned to either the cotton-lined or Gore-Tex-lined cast groups. Power analysis was performed to identify an adequate patient sample size. The mean maximum change between initial post-reduction x-rays and follow-up x-rays for anterior-posterior (AP) angulation, AP displacement, lateral angulation, and lateral displacement of the radius were calculated for both cotton and Gore-Tex groups. The rate of subsequent intervention and/or unacceptable results for each group was also analyzed.

Results.—Seven hundred and twenty-two patients were treated with distal radius fractures at our hospital with 59 patients eligible for inclusion in our study. Thirty-six of our patients were treated with cotton-lined casts, and 23 patients were treated with Gore-Tex-lined cast. The mean maximum change in AP angulation, AP displacement, lateral angulation, and lateral displacement of the radius after initial reduction was 9.2 degrees, 6.9%, 13.9 degrees, and 13.6%, respectively, for the cotton-lined cast group and 7.7 degrees, 6.1%, 14.6 degrees, and 9.6%, respectively, for the Gore-Tex-lined cast group. There were no statistical differences between the means of the 4 measurements ($P = 0.33$, 0.69, 0.73, and 0.10, respectively). There were also no significant differences between groups for final AP and lateral angulation and displacement. Subgroup analysis showed no significant differences in all measurements between cotton and Gore-Tex groups.

Conclusion.—Gore-Tex and cotton-lined casts are equally effective in their ability to maintain the reduction of 100% displaced distal forearm fractures. Thus, Gore-Tex-lined casts can be offered to pediatric patients immediately after closed reduction of distal radius fractures of any severity.

Level of Evidence.—Therapeutic level II.

▶ This investigation addresses a practical question: does the use of Gore-Tex cast liners put children with 100% displaced distal forearm fractures at increased risk for repeat manipulation? There are experimental design issues with this protocol; randomization would have been the ideal way to minimize the risk of bias. Potential sources of bias with this comparative cohort design include detection bias and inclusion bias. Nevertheless, with these important caveats, the answer to the question seems to be "no" within the limits of these data.

M. F. Swiontkowski, MD

The Effects of Surgical Delay on the Outcome of Pediatric Supracondylar Humeral Fractures

Bales JG, Spencer HT, Wong MA, et al (Univ of California, Los Angeles; Los Angeles Orthopaedic Med Ctr, CA)
J Pediatr Orthop 30:785-791, 2010

Background.—Occasionally, the treatment of a pediatric supracondylar humeral fracture is delayed owing to lack of an available treating physician, necessitating transfer of the child, or delay in availability of an operating room. The purpose of this study is to prospectively evaluate whether delayed pinning of these fractures affects the outcome or number of complications.

Methods.—We reviewed information that was prospectively collected on 145 pediatric supracondylar humeral fractures that were treated by closed reduction and percutaneous pinning, with a minimum follow-up of 8 weeks. To determine the effect of delayed treatment, we compared a group of fractures that was treated within the first 21 hours after their presentation to our urgent care center (Group A) with a group that was treated after more than 21 hours (Group B). We compared the following variables: need for open reduction, length of surgery, length of hospitalization, the presence of neurologic complications, vascular complications including compartment syndrome, pin tract infection, loss of fixation, final carrying angle, range of motion, and outcome.

Results.—Overall, the mean time from presentation to surgery for both groups was 52 hours. This interval was greater for Gartland type II

TABLE 2.—Confidence Intervals (95%) for the Difference Between Group A and Group B

	All 95% CI of the Difference				Type II 95% CI of the Difference				Type III 95% CI of the Difference			
	Mean Difference		SE	P	Mean Difference		SE	P	Mean Difference		SE	P
Length of surgery (min)	5.0	−2.0 to 12.2	3.6	0.08	3.1	−7.8 to 14.1	5.5	0.3	2.8	−9.0 to 14.6	5.8	0.3
Length of hospital stay (d)	−0.3	−0.5 to −0.07	0.1	0.004	−0.2	−0.6 to 0.2	0.2	0.1	−0.6	−0.8 to −0.3	0.1	<0.00001
Carrying angle (degrees)	−0.6	−1.7 to 0.5	0.6	0.1	−0.3	−2.0 to 1.4	0.9	0.4	−0.5	−1.9 to 1.3	0.8	0.3
Baumann angle (degrees)	−1.9	−4.7 to 0.9	1.4	0.09	−2.5	−6.7 to 1.6	2.1	0.1	−1.4	−5.9 to 3.0	2.2	0.3
Relative arc of motion (%)	1.0	−1.0 to 3.1	1.1	0.2	0.4	−2.8 to 3.6	1.6	0.4	1.9	−1.3 to 5.1	1.6	0.1
Avascular necrosis (%)	0.3	−0.8 to 1.4	0.5	0.7	2.2	2.1 to 2.3	0.1	0.8	3.4	−0.6 to 7.4	2.0	0.6
Pin-site granuloma (%)	−0.6	−1.6 to 0.4	0.5	0.6	−5.0	−9.4 to −0.6	2.3	0.4	—	—	—	—
Unsatisfactory outcome (%)	1.7	−0.8 to 4.2	1.3	0.4	2.7	−2.2 to 7.6	2.5	0.6	3.4	−0.6 to 7.4	2.0	0.6

fractures (65 h) than for Gartland type III fractures (19 h) ($P = 0.00001$). There was no need for an open reduction in either group. There were no significant differences between the groups regarding iatrogenic nerve injuries, vascular complications, compartment syndromes, surgical time, final carrying angle, range of motion, and outcome.

Conclusions.—The results of this prospective study found that a delay in pinning closed supracondylar humeral fractures in children did not lead to a higher incidence of open reduction or a greater number of complications. Although the urgency of treating any child with a supracondylar fracture should be individualized, our study suggests that most of these injuries can be managed safely in a delayed fashion without compromising the clinical outcome. We recommend careful monitoring of any patient with type 3 injury whose treatment is delayed.

Level of Evidence.—II (Table 2).

▶ The issue of the urgency of reduction and pinning of displaced type 3 supracondylar humerus fractures in children is one of many active debates. This well-done retrospective cohort study examines the impact of delay to reduction and pinning on complications, choosing 21 hours as the cutoff for early versus late surgery. Twenty-one hours falls well within the time frame required for all centers to identify a surgeon with the skill to manage a patient with such a fracture. The only significant outcome difference was in length of stay with no difference in complications, including neurovascular compromise. The authors appropriately point out that the decision regarding earlier versus later surgery must be individualized to the patient and the center where the treatment will occur.

M. F. Swiontkowski, MD

The effect of haematoma aspiration on intra-articular pressure and pain relief following Mason I radial head fractures
Ditsios KT, Stavridis SI, Christodoulou AG (1st Orthopaedic Dept of Aristotle Univ, Exohi, Thessaloniki, Greece)
Injury 42:362-365, 2011

Background.—The aspiration of the accompanying haematoma by Mason type I radial head fractures is advocated by several authors to achieve an analgesic effect. The purpose of this study was to investigate the effect of haematoma aspiration on intra-articular pressure and on pain relief after Mason I radial head fractures.

Materials and Methods.—A total of 16 patients (10 men and six women, age 23–47 years) with an isolated Mason I radial head fracture were subjected to haematoma paracentesis. Initially, intra-articular pressure was measured by using the Stryker Intra-Compartmental Pressure Monitor System. After haematoma aspiration, a new pressure measurement without moving the needle was performed. Pain before and after

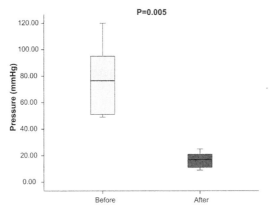

FIGURE 1.—Box-plot of elbow intraarticular pressure before and after aspiration (Wilcoxon signed ranks test $p = 0.005$). Elbow intraarticular pressure decreased significantly after aspiration ($p = 0.005$). (Reprinted from Ditsios KT, Stavridis SI, Christodoulou AG. The effect of haematoma aspiration on intra-articular pressure and pain relief following Mason I radial head fractures. *Injury.* 2011;42:362-365, Copyright (2011), with permission from Elsevier.)

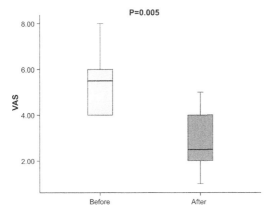

FIGURE 2.—Boxplot of VAS score for pain before and after aspiration (Wilcoxon signed ranks test $p = 0.005$). VAS score for pain decreased significantly after aspiration ($p = 0.005$). (Reprinted from Ditsios KT, Stavridis SI, Christodoulou AG. The effect of haematoma aspiration on intra-articular pressure and pain relief following Mason I radial head fractures. *Injury.* 2011;42:362-365, Copyright (2011), with permission from Elsevier.)

haematoma aspiration was evaluated by using an analogue 10-point pain scale.

Results.—Intra-articular elbow pressure prior to haematoma aspiration varied from 49 to 120 mmHg (median, 76.5 mmHg), while following aspiration, it ranged from 9 to 25 mmHg (median, 17 mmHg). The median quantity of the aspired blood was 2.75 ml (range, 0.5−8.5 ml). Patients reported a decrease in the visual analogue score (VAS) for pain from 5.5 (4−8) before to 2.5 (1−4) after aspiration. Decrease for both pressure and pain was statistically significant ($p = 0.005$).

Conclusion.—The formation of an intra-articular haematoma in the elbow joint following an undisplaced Mason I radial head fracture leads to a pronounced increase of the intra-articular pressure accompanied by intense pain for the patient. The aspiration of the haematoma results in an acute pressure decrease and an immediate patient relief (Figs 1 and 2).

▶ Most orthopedic surgeons have been taught to consider aspirating the elbow hematoma following Mason type I and type II radial head fracture to improve pain and function. This well-done prospective investigation confirms the value of this maneuver to achieve those goals. Surgeons should routinely recommend this treatment for patients with these fractures.

M. F. Swiontkowski, MD

Comminuted fractures of the radial head and neck: is fixation to the shaft necessary?
Neumann M, Nyffeler R, Beck M (Univ of Bern, Switzerland)
J Bone Joint Surg [Br] 93-B:223-228, 2011

Mason type III fractures of the radial head are treated by open reduction and internal fixation, resection or prosthetic joint replacement. When internal fixation is performed, fixation of the radial head to the shaft is difficult and implant-related complications are common. Furthermore, problems of devascularisation of the radial head can result from fixation of the plate to the radial neck.

In a small retrospective study, the treatment of Mason type III fractures with fixation of the radial neck in 13 cases (group 2) was compared with 12 cases where no fixation was performed (group 1). The mean clinical and radiological follow-up was four years (1 to 9). The Broberg-Morrey index showed excellent results in both groups. Degenerative radiological changes were seen more frequently in group 2, and removal of the implant was necessary in seven of 13 cases.

Post-operative evaluation of these two different techniques revealed similar ranges of movement and functional scores. We propose that anatomical reconstruction of the radial head without metalwork fixation to the neck is preferable, and the outcome is the same as that achieved with the conventional technique. In addition degenerative changes of the elbow joint may develop less frequently, and implant removal is not necessary (Tables 1 and 2).

▶ The authors report on the functional outcomes of radial head and neck fractures (Mason type III) treated with fixation of just the articular surface compared with fixation of the surface and to the neck of the radius. It is a small retrospective series, but this is because of the relative rarity of the injury. Additionally, traditional teaching has been that fixation to the neck/shaft is required to allow early active range of motion (ROM), essential to a good

TABLE 1.—Distribution of Fracture Patterns of Mason Type III Fractures According to the Ikeda Sub-Classification[11] and Listing of the Associated Injuries. More than One Associated Injury is Possible in One Elbow

	Group 1	Group 2
Fracture pattern		
IIIA	3	6
IIIB	6	2
IIIC	3	5
Associated injuries		
Lateral collateral ligament	2	6
Medial collateral ligament	0	3
Medial + lateral collateral ligament	0	0
Elbow dislocation	1	6
Fractures at the elbow (coronoid/olecranon fracture)	4	7
Lesion of DRUJ*	1	0

Editor's Note: Please refer to original journal article for full references.
*DRUJ, distal radioulnar joint.

TABLE 2.—Mean (Range) of the Post-Operative Ranges of Movement in the Two Groups. Statistical Comparison by Unpaired *t*-Test

	Group 1	Group 2	p-Value
Flexion	136 (110 to 150)	133 (110 to 150)	0.4759
Extension deficit	8.5 (0 to 30)	14 (0 to 30)	0.1593
Pronation	65 (40 to 90)	64 (30 to 90)	0.9084
Supination	69 (30 to 90)	66 (0 to 90)	0.7260

functional result. The comparative cohorts are similar (Table 1), and the ROM outcomes quite similar (Table 2). This is a thought-provoking series despite the issues with inclusion bias, surgical experience variable, etc. It should influence the development of an adequately powered multicenter controlled trial.

M. F. Swiontkowski, MD

Comparison of Plates versus Intramedullary Nails for Fixation of Displaced Midshaft Clavicular Fractures

Liu H-H, Chang C-H, Chia W-T, et al (Kaohsiung Veterans General Hosp, Taiwan, Republic of China; Hsin Chu General Hosp, Taiwan, Republic of China)
J Trauma 69:E82-E87, 2010

Background.—We compare the use of plate and screws versus intramedullary nails in the operative management of patients with displaced mid-clavicular fractures.

Methods.—Between March 2006 and June 2007, we performed a retrospective comparison of a demographically balanced sample of 110 patients (aged 16–65 years) who had received either plates or nails for completely displaced midshaft clavicular fractures.

Results.—We selected 59 plate-fixed and 51 nail-fixed patients. There was no significant difference between the groups with respect to age, gender, height, dominant arm, fracture angulation, fracture shortening, total fracture displacement, or mechanism of injury. Outcomes were significantly higher in the plate group compared with the nail group for the length of hospital stay (4.6 days ± 2.1 days vs. 5.9 days ± 2.6 days, $p = 0.006$), operative blood loss (67.5 mL ± 36.2 mL vs. 127.9 mL ± 48.8 mL, $p < 0.0001$), and size of surgical wound (11.9 cm ± 4.4 cm vs. 22.3 cm ± 4.5 cm, $p < 0.0001$). There was no significant difference in operative time, time to union, restoration of mobility (forward flexion, abduction, external rotation, and internal rotation), number of nonunions, number of malunions, infection, need for hardware removal, early mechanical failure, time to return to work, and Constant Shoulder and Disabilities of the Arm, Shoulder, and Hand functional scores.

Conclusion.—Our results demonstrate no significant differences in functional outcome and nonunion rates between nails and plates fixation for displaced midshaft clavicular fractures (Tables 1 and 2).

▶ Since the publication of the Canadian Orthopaedic Trauma Society's randomized controlled trial (RCT) on open reduction and internal fixation versus conservative care for markedly displaced clavicle fractures, interest has increased in the operative management of these fractures. There have been concerns regarding plate fixation of these fractures in regard to complication rates. This has brought renewed interest in intramedullary fixation. This retrospective comparative cohort study compares plate fixation with intramedullary fixation. Despite obvious issues with detection bias in such a study design,

TABLE 1.—Comparison of Patient Characteristics: Demographic Data, Characteristics of Fractures, and Details

	Nail (n = 51)	Plate (n = 59)	p
Male*	32 (62.8)	29 (49.2)	0.15
Age (yr)†	33.6 ± 13.5	31.7 ± 9.7	0.41
Height (cm)†	163.5 ± 7.7	162.9 ± 7.3	0.66
Dominant arm*	24 (47.1)	26 (44.1)	0.75
Smokers*	14 (27.5)	18 (30.5)	0.72
Fracture angulation (degrees)†	8.2 ± 4.3	9.7 ± 3.3	0.05
Fracture shortening (mm)†	11.7 ± 5.1	10.8 ± 4.0	0.31
Total fracture displacement (mm)†	15.0 ± 5.1	14.7 ± 5.0	0.78
Mechanism‡			0.61
Fall	3 (5.9)	7 (11.9)	
Sports	4 (7.8)	7 (11.9)	
Motor-vehicle/motorcycle crash	40 (78.4)	41 (69.5)	
Cycling	4 (7.8)	4 (6.8)	

Data presented as n (%) or mean ± SD.
*χ^2 test.
†Student's *t* test.
‡Fisher's exact test.

TABLE 2.—Comparison of Outcomes From Fracture Fixation Using Nails vs. Plates

	Nail (n = 51)	Plate (n = 59)	p
Hospital stay (d)*	4.6 ± 2.1	5.9 ± 2.6	0.006†
Blood loss (mL)*	67.4 ± 36.7	127.9 ± 48.8	<0.0001†
Operative time (min)*	72.8 ± 26.3	75.8 ± 23.0	0.52
Length of surgical wound (cm)*	11.9 ± 4.4	22.3 ± 4.5	<0.0001†
Time to union (wk)*	17.4 ± 6.1	16.8 ± 5.3	0.56
Return to work (wk)*	15.1 ± 4.9	15.6 ± 3.8	0.54
Forward flexion (degree)*	167.5 ± 6.5	167.7 ± 6.3	0.83
Abduction (degree)*	168.7 ± 5.8	170.1 ± 5.0	0.16
External rotation (degree)*	73.9 ± 6.0	75.1 ± 5.6	0.30
Internal rotation (degree)*	76.9 ± 6.2	79.1 ± 5.7	0.06
Constant scores*	86.7 ± 5.3	88.0 ± 4.8	0.17
Disabilities of the Arm, Shoulder, and Hand functional scores*	13.5 ± 3.9	12.9 ± 4.1	0.42
Nonunion‡	5 (9.8)	6 (10.2)	1.00
Malunion requiring further treatment§	4 (7.8)	2 (3.4)	0.41
Wound infection/dehiscence§	3 (5.9)	6 (10.2)	0.50
Hardware irritation requiring removal§	4 (7.8)	12 (20.3)	0.10
Early mechanical failure§	4 (7.8)	5 (8.5)	1.00

Data presented as n (%) or mean ± SD.
*Student's t test.
†$p < 0.05$ was considered statistically significance.
‡χ^2 test.
§Fisher's exact test.

no significant differences were identified in functional or clinical outcomes of interest to patients and their treating surgeons. The choice of internal fixation device should be based on surgeon training and experience with patient input. Care must be taken not to transmit the lessons from this and other well-done RCTs to fractures that are minimally displaced and shortened where conservative care should continue to dominate.

M. F. Swiontkowski, MD

Elastic stable intramedullary nailing is best for mid-shaft clavicular fractures without comminution: Results in 60 patients

Smekal V, Irenberger A, Attal RE, et al (Innsbruck Med Univ, Austria)

Injury 42:324-329, 2011

Introduction.—Elastic stable intramedullary nailing (ESIN) of displaced mid-shaft clavicular fractures is a minimally invasive technique which was reported to be an easy procedure with low complication rates, good cosmetic and functional results, restoration of clavicular length and fast return to daily activities. Recent studies, however, also report on higher complication rates and specific problems with the use of this technique. This prospective study compares ESIN with non-operative treatment of displaced mid-shaft clavicular fractures.

Methods.—Between December 2003 and August 2007, 120 patients volunteered to participate. Of these, 112 patients completed the study

(60 in the operative and 52 in the non-operative group). Patients in the non-operative group were treated with a simple shoulder sling. In the operative group, intramedullary stabilisation was performed within 3 days of the trauma. Clavicular shortening was determined after trauma and after osseous consolidation on thorax posteroanterior radiographs as the proportional length difference between the left and right side with the uninjured side serving as a control for clavicular length (100%). Radiographic union was assessed every 4 weeks on 20° cephalad anteroposterior and posterioranterior radiographs of the clavicle. Constant shoulder scores and DASH scores (DASH, disabilities of the arm, shoulder and hand) were assessed at final follow-up after 2 years.

Results.—ESIN led to faster osseous healing and better restoration of clavicular length in simple fractures. We were not able to restore clavicular length in comminuted fractures using ESIN. Functional outcome at a mean follow-up of 24 months (range: 22−27 months) was better in the operative group. Delayed union and non-union accounted for the majority of complications in the non-operative group. In the operative group, telescoping was the main complication, which occurred in complex fractures with severe post-traumatic shortening only.

Conclusion.—We recommend ESIN for all simple displaced mid-shaft clavicular fractures in order to minimise the rate of delayed union, nonunion and symptomatic mal-union. We also recommend ESIN in comminuted fractures with moderate (≤7%) post-traumatic shortening, as they will heal with moderate shortening. In comminuted fractures with severe shortening, however, we recommend plate osteosynthesis in order to provide for stability, clavicular length and endosteal blood supply (Tables 5 and 6).

▶ This randomized trial compared the use of elastic nails with nonoperative treatment in adult patients with displaced fractures of the midshaft clavicle (defined as no contact between the major fragments). Patients in the operative group benefited in terms of improved function as determined by the validated disabilities of the arm, shoulder, and hand upper extremity functional outcome scale. The complications in this group were primarily related to the fact that this

TABLE 5.—Complications

	Operative Group	Non-Operative Group	*p* Value
All Complications	19	20	0.55
Non-union	0	6	0.00*
Delayed union	2	9	
Symptomatic mal-union	0	2	
Transient plexus irritation	0	3	
Telescoping	7	0	
Infection	1	0	
Medial skin irritation	5	0	
Implant failure	2	0	
Refracture	1	0	

*$p < 0.05$.

TABLE 6.—DASH Score and Constant Score at Final follow-up After Two Years (±SD)

	DASH Score			Constant Score		
	Non-Operative Group	Operative Group	*p* Value	Non-Operative Group	Operative Group	*p* Value
All fracture types	3.1±7.4	0.5±1.8	0.03*	95.1±7.0	98.0±3.6	0.02*
15B1 (Simple)	1.1±2.4	0.2±0.6	0.20	97.4±3.3	96.7±4.1	0.63
15B2 (Wedge)	1.9±4.1	0.2±0.5	0.23	97.0±5.3	98.8±2.2	0.37
15B3 (Comminuted)	5.0±10.0	0.9±2.3	0.04*	92.6±8.8	98.5±3.5	0.00*

*$p < 0.05$.

method of stabilization does not maintain the overall length of the clavicle. This would indicate that comminuted fractures may well be best treated by plate fixation where length can be maintained. This controlled trial adds to the increasing body of evidence that operative treatment of displaced fractures of the clavicle (particularly with 2 cm of shortening or gapping) is best managed with operative stabilization, as the functional results are better and the complication rate is acceptable.

M. F. Swiontkowski, MD

Functional bracing of humeral shaft fractures. A review of clinical studies
Papasoulis E, Drosos GI, Ververidis AN, et al (Democritus Univ of Thrace, Alexandroupolis, Greece)
Injury 41:e1-e7, 2010

Functional bracing has been widely accepted as the gold standard for treating humeral shaft fractures conservatively. We conducted a literature review to verify the efficacy of this treatment method. Sixteen case series and two comparative studies fulfilled the criteria set. Analysis of these clinical studies showed that humeral shaft fractures when treated with functional bracing heal in an average of 10.7 weeks. Union rate is high (94.5%). Statistical analysis showed that proximal third fractures and AO type A fractures have a higher non-union rate although this is not statistically significant. Residual deformity and joint stiffness are considered the main drawbacks of conservative treatment. Angulation—usually varus—rarely exceeded 10°, while full shoulder and elbow motion was achieved in 80% and 85% of the patients, respectively. Nevertheless, in the few studies that subjective parameters such as functional scores, pain and quality of life were assessed results were not so promising (Tables 1, 4, and 6).

▶ This fairly well-done structured literature review (differentiated from a meta-analysis here because of the pooling of cohort study data) carefully details the results of functional brace treatment for humerus fractures. Clinically relevant

TABLE 1.—Articles Included in the Study and their Results in Terms of Union

Study	Study Design	Fractures n	Follow-up n (%)	Union n (%)	Non-Union (%)	Delayed Union n (%)	Time of Brace Application in Weeks (Range)	Follow-up Time Mean (Range)
Sarmiento et al.[21]	Retrospective	51	51 (100)	50 (98)	2		8.5 (3–22.5)	– (2–30 months after removal)
Balfour et al.[1]	Prospective	74	42 (57)	41 (97.6)	2.4	1 (2.4)	7.5 (4–15)	– (6 weeks–3 years, stop when full motion)
Ricciardi-Pollini and Falez[16]	Retrospective	14	14 (100)	14 (100)	0	1 (7.1)	– (8–13)	Not specified
Naver and Aalberg[13]	Prospective	20	20 (100)	18 (90)	10		6.5 (4–24)	13.2 months (6–25 months)
Zagorski et al.[31]	Retrospective	233	170 (73)	167 (98.2)	1.8		10.6 (5–20)	28 weeks (5 weeks–4 years)
Leung et al.[11]	Retrospective	29	29 (100)	29 (100)	0		7 (4–18)	– (at least 9 months)
Wallny et al.[30]	Retrospective	79	79 (100)	74 (93.7)	6.3	1 (3.4)	8.7 (4–17)	2.5 years (2–6 years)
Wallny et al.[29]	Comparative/retrospective	44	44 (100)	42 (95.5)	4.5		– (7–10)	27 months (12–48 months)
Sarmiento et al.[23]	Retrospective	922	620 (67)	604 (97.4)	2.6		11.5 (5–22)	Until union
Fjalestad et al.[8]	Retrospective	67	67 (100)	61 (91.1)	8.9		12 (6–25)	30 weeks (10–152 weeks)
Koch et al.[10]	Retrospective	74	67 (91)	58 (86.6)	13.4	1 (1.4)	10 (5–36)	1 year
Toivanen et al.[27]	Retrospective	93	93 (100)	72 (77.4)	22.6		Not specified	Until union
Rosenberg et al.[18]	Prospective	15	15 (100)	15 (100)	0		22 (10–40)	30 months (12–57 months)
Ekholm et al.[7]	Retrospective/ prospective[a]	78	78/50[a] (100/64)[a]	70 (89.7)	10.3		Not specified	26.4 months
Rutgers et al.[19]	Retrospective	52	49 (94)	44 (89.8)	10.2		Not specified	14 months (2–50 months)
Distal third								
Sarmiento et al.[22]	Retrospective	85	72 (85)	69 (95.8)	4.2		10	Not specified
Pehlivan[14]	Prospective	25	21 (84)	21 (100)	0	3 (14.3)	11.8 (8–30)	39 weeks (29–70 weeks)
Jawa et al.[9]	Comparative/retrospective	21	19 (90)	19 (100)	0		9.7 (8–12)	21 months (2–45 months)

Editor's Note: Please refer to original journal article for full references.

[a]Retrospective study on union (78 fractures)—prospective on function and quality of life (50 patients).

TABLE 4.—Evaluation of Final Outcome

Study	Patients n	Score Used	Excellent %	Good %	Moderate %	Poor %	Other Parameters—Scores
16	14	Their own criteria	85.7				80% no restriction of activity (Grade V)
13	20	Hunter	80	10	5	5	95% content with treatment, 65% no pain
30	74	Hannover Shoulder Score	63	17.7	15.2	3.8	95.5% content with treatment, 50% no pain, 45.5% pain with exercise, 4.5% rest pain, score described by Wulker et al.: 90.8 points
29	44						
8	54/61[a]	Modified Wasmer score	45	24		20	69% no pain, 8% rest pain
10	58/48[b]	Their own criteria	51.7	43.1	5.2	0	11.8 weeks pain, 11.3 weeks off work, 17.2% chronic pain
18	15						Oxford Shoulder score: 34 (12–60, 12 = normal), Constant score: significant lower than normal limb, VAS score on pain: 5 (0–10, 0 = no pain)
7	43	Reported by the patients as full recovery	49				SMFA (Short Musculoskeletal Functional Assessment): Dysfunction index 21.0, Bother index 18.8—SF-36 score on quality of life lower than general population
14	21	Modified Hannover Shoulder Score	86	14			

[a] Fifty-four patients evaluated with Wasmer score, 61 for pain.
[b] Fifty-eight patients evaluated with the scoring system, 48 of the monotrauma group evaluated for pain.

TABLE 6.—Statistics of Non-unions with Regard to Fracture Pattern

Fracture Subtype (Number of Articles with Sufficient Data)	Fractures (n)	Non-unions (n)	Non-union Rate (%)	p
Location (8 articles)				
Proximal	170	14	8.2	
Middle	496	30	6.1	
Distal	289	12	4.2	
Total	955	56	5.9	>0.05
AO type (5 articles)				
A	182	28	15.4	
B	73	7	9.6	
C	19	0	0	
Total	274	35	12.8	>0.05
Fracture configuration (6 articles)				
Spiral	94	12	12.8	
Oblique	57	10	17.5	
Transverse	101	9	8.9	
Comminuted + segmental	66	3	4.5	
Total	318	34	10.7	>0.05

outcomes include a high union rate of nearly 95% with a broad range of time to fracture union estimates centered around 10.7 weeks. Proximal third and transverse fractures had the highest percentage of nonunion. Excellent range of motion outcomes for shoulder and elbow routinely occur in greater than 80% of patients. The cohort studies suffer from quality deficits with retrospective reviews, lack of standard time intervals for patient follow-up, high loss to follow-up, and the lack of the use of validated functional outcome instruments. There is much room for improvement in study design as we seek to understand which patients are optimally treated with functional bracing versus other methods. This review should, however, temper the increasing use of operative intervention for humeral shaft fractures, as these results really are quite acceptable and avoid the risk and expense of other forms of treatment.

M. F. Swiontkowski, MD

Locking Intramedullary Nails and Locking Plates in the Treatment of Two-Part Proximal Humeral Surgical Neck Fractures: A Prospective Randomized Trial with a Minimum of Three Years of Follow-up

Zhu Y, Lu Y, Shen J, et al (Beijing Ji Shui Tan Hosp, People's Republic of China)

J Bone Joint Surg Am 93:159-168, 2011

Background.—Locking intramedullary nails and locking plates specially designed for proximal humeral fractures are widely used. The purpose of our study was to compare the outcomes between these two types of implants in patients with a two-part surgical neck fracture. The advantages and shortcomings of each method were analyzed.

TABLE 2.—Clinical Outcomes

	Locking Nail Group	Locking Plate Group	P Value
1-year follow-up			
Forward elevation* (*deg*)	151.6 ± 20.4	155.4 ± 13.6	0.441
External rotation* (*deg*)	44.0 ± 4.5	38.5 ± 3.2	0.321
Internal rotation†	T9 (T2-buttock)	T8 (T4-L2)	0.433
Strength of supraspinatus (affected side/healthy side)* (%)	64.3 ± 18.3	77.4 ± 20.8	0.032
VAS score‡ (*points*)	1.0 (1.0)	0.5 (1.8)	0.042
ASES score* (*points*)	83.6 ± 11.7	90.8 ± 9.7	0.021
Constant-Murley score* (*points*)	88.0 ± 10.4	92.0 ± 6.3	0.096
3-year follow-up			
Forward elevation* (*deg*)	160.8 ± 11.9	157.3 ± 15.1	0.365
External rotation* (*deg*)	47.8 ± 17.3	40.4 ± 17.4	0.133
Internal rotation†	T8 (T2-buttock)	T8 (T2-buttock)	0.636
Strength of supraspinatus (affected side/healthy side)* (%)	70.2 ± 16.0	79.3 ± 20.4	0.106
VAS score‡ (*points*)	0 (1.0)	0 (0.8)	0.624
ASES score* (*points*)	90.0 ± 8.1	94.0 ± 6.3	0.059
Constant-Murley score* (*points*)	93.3 ± 6.7	94.5 ± 5.8	0.489

*The values are given as the mean and standard deviation.
†The values are given as the mean with the range in parentheses.
‡The values are given as the median with the interquartile range in parentheses.

Methods.—A prospective randomized study was performed. Fifty-one consecutive patients with a fresh two-part surgical neck fracture were randomized to be treated with a locking intramedullary nail (n = 25) or a locking plate (n = 26). Clinical and radiographic assessments were conducted at one year and three years after the surgery. A visual analog scale (VAS) was used to assess shoulder pain. The American Shoulder and Elbow Surgeons (ASES) scores and Constant-Murley scores were recorded to evaluate shoulder function.

Results.—Fracture union was achieved in all patients within three months after the surgery. At one year postoperatively, a significant difference (p = 0.024) was found with regard to the complication rate between the locking plate group (31%) and the locking nail group (4%). The average ASES score, median VAS score, and average strength of the supraspinatus were significantly better in the locking plate group (90.8 compared with 83.6 points [p = 0.021], 1.0 compared with 0.5 point [p = 0.042], and 77.4% compared with 64.3% [p = 0.032]). At three years postoperatively, no significant difference could be found in terms of any parameter between the two groups. Significant improvement in the VAS pain scores, ASES scores, and Constant-Murley scores were found between the one-year and three-year follow-up examinations in each group.

Conclusions.—Satisfactory results can be achieved with either implant in the treatment of two-part proximal humeral surgical neck fractures. There was no difference regarding the ASES scores between these two implants at the time of the final, three-year follow-up. The complication rate was lower in the locking intramedullary nail group, while fixation with a locking plate had the advantage of a better one-year outcome.

Level of Evidence.—Therapeutic Level I. See Instructions to Authors for a complete description of levels of evidence (Table 2).

▶ This well-done controlled trial compares 2 methods of surgical stabilization for 2-part proximal humerus fractures. The 3-year follow-up is excellent, and validated outcomes measures were used. The study demonstrates that when excellent reduction of the fracture can be obtained (Figs 2 and 3 in the original article), equivalent good to excellent clinical and functional outcomes can be achieved. There is no difference between the 2 implant approaches, leaving the decision as to which implant strategy to use to be based on the training and experience of the surgeon. With either technique, excellent fracture reduction must be obtained and maintained.

M. F. Swiontkowski, MD

Wrist function recovers more rapidly after volar locked plating than after external fixation but the outcomes are similar after 1 year: A randomized study of 63 patients with a dorsally displaced fracture of the distal radius
Wilcke MKT, Abbaszadegan H, Adolphson PY (Danderyd Hosp, Stockholm, Sweden)
Acta Orthop 82:76-81, 2011

Background and Purpose.—Promising results have been reported after volar locked plating of unstable dorsally displaced distal radius fractures. We investigated whether volar locked plating results in better patient-perceived, objective functional and radiographic outcomes compared to the less invasive external fixation.

Patients and Methods.—63 patients under 70 years of age, with an unstable extra-articular or non-comminuted intra-articular dorsally displaced distal radius fracture, were randomized to volar locked plating (n = 33) or bridging external fixation. Patient-perceived outcome was assessed with the Disability of the Arm, Shoulder, and Hand (DASH) questionnaire and the Patient-Rated Wrist Evaluation (PRWE) questionnaire.

Results.—At 3 and 6 months, the volar plate group had better DASH and PRWE scores but at 12 months the scores were similar. Objective function, measured as grip strength and range of movement, was superior in the volar plate group but the differences diminished and were small at 12 months. Axial length and volar tilt were retained slightly better in the volar plate group.

Interpretation.—Volar plate fixation is more advantageous than external fixation, in the early rehabilitation period (Tables 2 and 3).

▶ This well-done randomized controlled trial compares a bridging external fixator versus a locked plate for the treatment of distal radius fracture with outcome assessment intervals of 3, 6, and 12 months. The investigators used the Disability of the Arm, Shoulder, and Hand questionnaire as the validated

TABLE 2.—Patient-perceived Results Measured by the DASH and PRWE Scores

	Volar plating	External fixation	p-value[a]
DASH			
3 months	9 (6−12)	27 (20−33)	<0.001
6 months	6 (3−9)	14 (9−19)	0.008
12 months	7 (4−11)	11 (6−16)	0.1
PRWE			
3 months	14 (8−20)	31 (23−39)	<0.001
6 months	9 (5−14)	17 (11−22)	0.02
12 months	11 (6−16)	15 (9−21)	0.3

Values are presented as points (95% CI) corrected for baseline values. Higher scores indicate more disability.
[a]Wilcoxon rank-sum test.

TABLE 3.—Objective Physical Measurements (95% CI) Expressed as a Percentage of the Uninjured Side

	Volar plating	External fixation	p-value[a]
3 months			
Grip strength	72 (64−80)	46 (37−55)	<0.001
Extension	84 (78−90)	59 (49−69)	<0.001
Flexion	81 (77−85)	71 (65−77)	0.009
Ulnar deviation	89 (81−97)	74 (63−86)	0.04
Radial deviation	89 (80−98)	75 (55−95)	0.2
Supination	95 (91−98)	76 (68−85)	<0.001
Pronation	98 (96−100)	89 (84−94)	<0.001
6 months			
Grip strength	89 (83−95)	72 (65−78)	<0.001
Extension	92 (86−97)	77 (68−84)	0.001
Flexion	88 (84−91)	83 (78−88)	0.1
Ulnar deviation	99 (92−106)	91 (79−103)	0.2
Radial deviation	103 (92−115)	89 (70−107)	0.2
Supination	98 (95−100)	88 (84−93)	<0.001
Pronation	100 (100−100)	95 (92−99)	0.005
12 months			
Grip strength	94 (86−102)	85 (79−91)	0.08
Extension	94 (90−98)	85 (77−93)	0.04
Flexion	89 (86−92)	83 (77−89)	0.08
Ulnar deviation	96 (87−105)	83 (72−93)	0.05
Radial deviation	97 (88−106)	89 (77−100)	0.3
Supination	99 (97−100)	89 (81−98)	0.02
Pronation	99 (98−100)	92 (86−99)	0.04

[a]Student's t-test.

functional outcome measure and assessed strength and radiographic outcomes. The strength and radiographic measures were not conducted by individuals blinded to treatment group, which would have increased the impact of the study. The fact that the 3- and 6-month outcomes are superior for the locked plating group is not surprising because of the influence of the nonbridging external fixator on ligament, capsule, and tendon function. Similarly, the lack of functional significance between the 2 treatment groups at 1 year, when these tissues have recovered, is not surprising. This trial adds validity to the increasing use of these plates in managing distal radius fractures based on earlier return to near-normal function.

M. F. Swiontkowski, MD

Should unstable extra-articular distal radial fractures be treated with fixed-angle volar-locked plates or percutaneous Kirschner wires? A prospective randomised controlled trial
McFadyen I, Field J, McCann P, et al (Gloucester Royal Hosp, UK; Cheltenham General Hosp, UK)
Injury 42:162-166, 2011

Fractures of the distal radius are commonly treated with cast immobilisation; however, those potentially unstable injuries with dorsal comminution may need operative intervention. This intervention is usually with manipulation and Kirschner wires but advances in locking-plate technology have enabled surgeons to achieve anatomical reconstruction of complex fracture patterns, even in poor-quality osteoporotic bone.

To ascertain if fixed-angle volar-locked plates confer a significant benefit over manipulation and Kirschner-wire stabilisation, we prospectively randomised 56 adult patients with isolated, closed, unilateral, unstable extra-articular fractures into two treatment groups, one fixed with K-wires and the other fixed with a volar locking plate.

Functional outcomes were assessed using Gartland and Werley and Disabilities of the Arm, Shoulder and Hand (DASH) scores. These were statistically better in the plate group at 3 and 6 months. Radiological assessment showed statistically better results at 6 weeks, 3 months and 6 months, post-operatively. In the plate group, there was no significant loss of fracture reduction (Tables 3 and 4).

▶ This 2-center controlled trial compares internal fixation of extra-articular distal radius fractures with Kirschner wires or locked plates. The postoperative immobilization was standardized with 6 weeks in a cast to remove 1 confounding variable. No patients were lost to follow-up—an advantage of prospective trial design. The functional and radiographic outcomes were superior at 3 and 6 months. The radiographic evaluators were independent of the treating physicians, but they were not blinded to treatment group. In the future, digital techniques should be used to eliminate implants from radiographs to limit this

---

TABLE 3.—Functional Outcome; DASH Scores Showing Statistically Better Results in the Plate Group Compared to the K-wire Group

	Plate	K-wire	p-value
3 months mean score	18.26	27.24	0.001
6 months mean score	15.89	21.45	0.017

TABLE 4.—Radiological Outcome; p-Values Showing Statistically Better Results in the Plate Group Compared with the K-wire Group at the Post-op, 6 Weeks, 3 Months and 6 Months Stage

	Radial inclination	Shortening	Dorsal tilt
Post-op	0.738	0.522	0.001
6 weeks	0.057	0.001	0.001
3 months	0.017	0.071	0.001
6 months	0.006	0.040	0.001

potential source of bias. No cost data are provided. Although statistically better, one will need to consider cost-benefit and clinical significance in the overall equation before recommending treatment. On the whole, this well-done randomized controlled trial supports the continued use of locked plates for these extra-articular fractures, as the benefits from them are likely even greater when extensive cast immobilization is not used.

M. F. Swiontkowski, MD

Long-Term Outcomes of Fractures of Both Bones of the Forearm
Bot AGJ, Doornberg JN, Lindenhovius ALC, et al (Academic Med Ctr Amsterdam, The Netherlands; et al)
J Bone Joint Surg Am 93:527-532, 2011

Background.—Previous studies identified limited impairment and disability several years after diaphyseal fractures of both the radius and ulna, although the relationship between impairment and disability was inconsistent. This investigation studied skeletally mature and immature patients more than ten years after injury and addressed the hypotheses that (1) objective measurements of impairment correlate with disability, (2) depression and misinterpretation of nociception correlate with disability, and (3) patients injured when skeletally mature or immature have comparable impairment and disability.

Methods.—Seventy-one patients with diaphyseal fractures of the radius and ulna were evaluated at an average of twenty-one years after injury. Twenty-five of the thirty-five patients who were skeletally immature at the time of injury were treated nonoperatively, and thirty-one of the thirty-six skeletally mature patients were treated operatively. Objective evaluation included radiographs, functional assessment, and grip strength. Validated questionnaires were used to measure arm-specific disability (the Disabilities of the Arm, Shoulder and Hand [DASH] score), misinterpretation of pain (Pain Catastrophizing Scale [PCS]), and depression (the validated Dutch form of the Center for Epidemiologic Studies-Depression scale [CES-D]).

Results.—The average DASH score was 8 points (range, 0 to 54); 97% of patients had excellent or satisfactory results according to the criteria of

TABLE 2.—Range of Motion and Grip Strength at the Time of Final Follow-up*

	Skeletally Immature	Skeletally Mature	P Value
Motion			
Elbow flexion-extension arc *(deg)*	153 (100%)	143 (97%)	0.003
Wrist flexion-extension arc *(deg)*	142 (99%)	123 (89%)	0.001
Pronation-supination arc *(deg)*	169 (96%)	151 (87%)	0.002
Radioulnar deviation arc *(deg)*	59 (94%)	50 (87%)	0.008
Grip strength *(kg)*	32 (98%)	29 (89%)	Not significant

*Values are given as the mean, with the percent of that measured in the uninjured arm in parentheses.

Anderson et al., and 72% reported no pain. Both the forearm rotation and the wrist flexion/extension arc was 91% of that seen on the uninjured side; grip strength was 94%. There were small but significant differences in rotation (151° versus 169°, p = 0.004) and wrist flexion-extension (123° versus 142°, p = 0.002) compared with the results in the uninjured arm. There was no difference in disability between patients who were skeletally mature or immature at the time of injury. Pain, pain catastrophizing (misinterpretation of nociception), and grip strength were the most important predictors of disability.

Conclusions.—An average of twenty-one years after sustaining diaphyseal fractures of both the radius and the ulna, patients who were skeletally immature or mature at the time of fracture have comparable disability. Disability correlates better with subjective and psychosocial aspects of illness, such as pain and pain catastrophizing, than with objective measurements of impairment.

Level of Evidence.—Therapeutic Level IV. See Instructions to Authors for a complete description of levels of evidence (Table 2).

▶ The authors report on the minimum 10-year outcomes of a large group of patients treated for fracture of both bones of the forearm. The immature group was primarily treated with nonoperative methods and the adults with open reduction and internal fixation. The outcomes are generally very good (Table 2) with minor functional and range of motion deficits. The objective measures do not directly correlate with the functional outcomes as assessed by validated scales highlighting the key impact of depression and sensitivity to pain stimuli on functional outcome. The study gives us substance to reassure patients that if treated for such a fracture, the outcomes can be expected to be generally good but not equivalent to the preinjury function.

M. F. Swiontkowski, MD

Complications of K-Wire Fixation in Procedures Involving the Hand and Wrist

Hsu LP, Schwartz EG, Kalainov DM, et al (Northwestern Univ Feinberg School of Medicine, Chicago, IL; Univ of Illinois School of Medicine, Rockford, IL; JFK Med Ctr, Edison, NJ; et al)
J Hand Surg 36A:610-616, 2011

Purpose.—Surgeons often use smooth K-wires for bone stabilization in the hand and wrist. The purposes of this study were to observe the incidence of postoperative complications of K-wire fixation in the hand and wrist and to identify associated risk factors.

Methods.—A total of 189 patients underwent bone and soft tissue procedures in the hand and wrist with insertion of 408 smooth K-wires. All patients were instructed to comply with a uniform pin care protocol and were observed for a minimum of 1 examination after pin removal. Complications were categorized as minor or major, with 3 subcategories for infectious complications. We compared total complications and infectious complications with patient age, comorbidities, soft tissue integrity, pin exposure (external or buried), number of pins inserted, pin location, compliance with pin site care, and empiric antibiotic treatment.

Results.—We found that 39 patients experienced postoperative complications involving 58K-wires (14% of all pins). Most complications were minor, commonly superficial pin track infection (24 pins, 6% of all pins). Major complications occurred less frequently (11 pins, 3% of all pins) and included complications that led to additional surgery (deep infection, malunion, or nonunion) and fractures through the pin track. The development of an infectious complication was associated with 2 factors: pin location in the hand versus the wrist and poor compliance with pin site care. Patient age, medical comorbidities, soft tissue integrity, pin exposure,

TABLE 2.—Categories of K-Wire Complications

Complication	Complication Type	Patients (n)	Pins (n [% of 408 Pins])
Total		39	58 (14%)
Minor		36	52 (12%)
Major		6	11 (3%)
Total infectious		19	26 (6%)
Redness	Minor	3	6 (2%)
Drainage	Minor	2	2 (<1%)
Superficial pin track infection	Minor and infectious	18	24 (6%)
Pin loosening	Minor	11	12 (3%)
Pin migration	Minor	5	9 (2%)
Skin overgrowth	Minor	1	1 (<1%)
Delayed wound healing	Minor	1	1 (<1%)
Infection requiring drainage	Major and infectious	1	2 (<1%)
Nonunion requiring surgery	Major	2	4 (<1%)
Malunion requiring surgery	Major	2	3 (<1%)
Fracture through pin track	Major	1	2 (<1%)
Septic arthritis/osteomyelitis	Major and infectious	0	0 (0%)

number of pins inserted, and empiric antibiotic treatment had no statistically significant relationships to the occurrence of complications.

Conclusions.—Complications with smooth K-wire fixation in the hand and wrist are relatively uncommon. Most complications involve minor, superficial pin track infections. Location of pins in the hand as compared with the wrist and poor patient compliance with pin site care may increase the risk of infection (Table 2).

▶ All orthopedic surgeons who treat patients with hand and wrist injuries use Kirschner wires routinely. We all have seen problems with these devices yet rely upon them, as they are unique in their ability to control fracture and joint position. This is a careful analysis of the problems with these devices. As we would predict, most of the complications are minor. Antibiotic protocols do not affect the impact of the complications, which is useful information. As with most complications in orthopedic surgery, patient noncompliance plays a major role. Table 2 is a useful summary of the issues and is worthy of note, as we continue to rely on these implants.

M. F. Swiontkowski, MD

Impact on Outcome

Successful Reconstruction for Complex Malunions and Nonunions of the Tibia and Femur
Buijze GA, Richardson S, Jupiter JB (Harvard Med School, Boston, MA)
J Bone Joint Surg Am 93:485-492, 2011

Background.—Information regarding the long-term outcomes of the treatment of lower-extremity fracture malunion and nonunion is lacking.

Methods.—Twenty-nine secondarily referred patients with complex malunion or nonunion of the tibia or femur, treated by a single surgeon, were followed for a median of twenty years (range, twelve to thirty-five years) after injury. The patients were referred at a median of twenty months (range, 1.5 to 360 months) postinjury and had undergone a median of three prior surgical procedures (range, zero to twenty-eight). At the time of final follow-up, patient-based outcomes, patient satisfaction, and pain were evaluated.

Results.—All twenty-nine patients had healing following treatment of the complex malunion or nonunion of the tibia or femur and were able to bear full weight and walk one block or more. The Lower Extremity Functional Scale (LEFS) outcome tool revealed that twenty patients (69%) experienced moderate-to-severe difficulties in carrying out activities because of their lower-limb disability. The median Short Form-36 (SF-36) score was 67, with a median physical component score of 61 and a median mental component score of 71, indicating substantial impact on physical health status when compared with the norm.

Conclusions.—Reconstruction can be a worthwhile endeavor and should be considered for all patients with complex malunion or nonunion of the tibia or femur.

▶ This retrospective series of a fairly large group of patients with femoral or tibial nonunion treated by a single expert surgeon confirms good clinical outcome with improved function in the vast majority. Patient satisfaction is high in that this cohort of patients had treatment elsewhere over many months prior to referral to this center. Functional impairment and pain issues remain, but both were improved over the preoperative status at a minimum of 12 years and maximum of 35 years of follow-up. This series documents what is possible in the hands of an expert surgeon and should not be construed as to what the occasional nonunion surgeon might be able to achieve with similar patients.

M. F. Swiontkowski, MD

Amputation Surgery: Outcome

Optimized Perioperative Analgesia Reduces Chronic Phantom Limb Pain Intensity, Prevalence, and Frequency: A Prospective, Randomized, Clinical Trial

Karanikolas M, Aretha D, Tsolakis I, et al (Patras Univ School of Medicine, Greece; et al)
Anesthesiology 114:1144-1154, 2011

Background.—Severe preamputation pain is associated with phantom limb pain (PLP) development in limb amputees. We investigated whether optimized perioperative analgesia reduces PLP at 6-month follow-up.

Methods.—A total of 65 patients underwent lower-limb amputation and were assigned to five analgesic regimens: (1) Epi/Epi/Epi patients received perioperative epidural analgesia and epidural anesthesia; (2) PCA/Epi/Epi patients received preoperative intravenous patient-controlled analgesia (PCA), postoperative epidural analgesia, and epidural anesthesia; (3) PCA/Epi/PCA patients received perioperative intravenous PCA and epidural anesthesia; (4) PCA/GA/PCA patients received perioperative intravenous PCA and general anesthesia (GA); (5) controls received conventional analgesia and GA. Epidural analgesia or intravenous PCA started 48 h preoperatively and continued 48 h postoperatively. The results of the visual analog scale and the McGill Pain Questionnaire were recorded perioperatively and at 1 and 6 months.

Results.—At 6 months, median (minimum—maximum) PLP and P values (intervention groups *vs.* control group) for the visual analog scale were as follows: 0 (0—20) for Epi/Epi/Epi ($P = 0.001$), 0 (0—42) for PCA/Epi/Epi ($P = 0.014$), 20 (0—40) for PCA/Epi/PCA ($P = 0.532$), 0 (0—30) for PCA/GA/PCA ($P = 0.008$), and 20 (0—58) for controls. The values for the McGill Pain Questionnaire were as follows: 0 (0—7) for Epi/Epi/Epi ($P < 0.001$), 0 (0—9) for PCA/Epi/Epi ($P = 0.003$), 6 (0—11) for PCA/Epi/PCA ($P = 0.208$), 0 (0—9) for PCA/GA/PCA ($P = 0.003$), and 7 (0—15) for

TABLE 1.—Anesthesia and Analgesia Protocol by Group

Analgesia Group	Preoperative Analgesia	Intraoperative Anesthesia	Postoperative Analgesia
Epi/Epi/Epi	Epi	Epi	Epi
PCA/Epi/Epi	IV PCA	Epi	Epi
PCA/Epi/PCA	IV PCA	Epi	IV PCA
PCA/GA/PCA	IV PCA	GA	IV PCA
Control	IM Me, PO CA, IV Ac, IV Parecoxib	GA	IM Me, PO CA, IV Ac, IV Parecoxib

Ac = acetaminophen; CA = codeine/acetaminophen tablets; Epi = Epidural; GA = general anesthesia; IM = intramuscular; IV = intravenous; Me = meperidine; PCA = patient-controlled analgesia; PO = oral.

controls. At 6 months, PLP was present in 1 of 13 Epi/Epi/Epi, 4 of 13 PCA/Epi/Epi, and 3 of 13 PCA/GA/PCA patients *versus* 9 of 12 control patients ($P = 0.001$, $P = 0.027$, and $P = 0.009$, respectively). Residual limb pain at 6 months was insignificant.

Conclusions.—Optimized epidural analgesia or intravenous PCA, starting 48 h preoperatively and continuing for 48 h postoperatively, decreases PLP at 6 months (Table 1).

▶ Phantom limb pain (PLP) following amputation remains a troubling clinical issue. This well-done 5-arm clinical trial investigates the impact of anesthesia technique on this clinically important outcome. The study confirms that optimum anesthesia technique with patient-controlled analgesia and/or epidural anesthesia minimizes the intensity of postoperative PLP. One issue that limits the impact of the study is that of detection bias. A single observer who may have not been blinded to the treatment group did the postoperative interviews. Nevertheless, this study points to the optimization principle for anesthesia for patients undergoing amputations.

M. F. Swiontkowski, MD

Outcomes Associated with the Internal Fixation of Long-Bone Fractures Proximal to Traumatic Amputations
Gordon WT, O'Brien FP, Strauss JE, et al (Walter Reed Natl Military Med Ctr, Washington, DC)
J Bone Joint Surg Am 92:2312-2318, 2010

Background.—Preservation of optimal residual limb length following a traumatic amputation can be challenging. The purpose of this study was to determine if acceptable results can be achieved by definitive fixation of a long-bone fracture proximal to a traumatic amputation.

Methods.—We identified thirty-seven active-duty military service members who underwent internal fixation of a long-bone fracture proximal to a traumatic amputation. Functional status was assessed with the

TABLE 1.—Injury and Demographic Data on the Thirty-Seven Patients

Characteristic	No.
Median age (range) (*yr*)	23 (20-38)
Sex*	
Male	35 (95)
Female	2 (5)
Method of injury*	
Improvised explosive device	30 (81)
Rocket-propelled grenade	3 (8)
Gunshot wound	1 (3)
Fall from height	1 (3)
Vehicular accident	2 (5)
Major fractures in contralateral lower extremity* (n = 8)	
Femur	1 (13)
Tibial plateau	1 (13)
Tibia and fibula	3 (38)
Tibial plafond	1 (13)
Calcaneus	2 (25)
Method of fixation*	
Intramedullary nail	21 (57)
Cannulated screw fixation	1 (3)
Plate-and-screw fixation	14 (38)
External fixation	1 (3)
ORIF and amputation in same osseous segment* (n = 12)	
Humerus	3 (25)
Femur	2 (17)
Tibia	7 (58)
Fracture site on extremity with amputation*	
Humerus	4 (11)
Femur	22 (59)
Femur and tibia	3 (8)
Tibia	8 (22)
Timing of amputation and ORIF*	
Amputation closure prior to ORIF	6 (16)
ORIF prior to amputation closure	27 (73)
Amputation and ORIF performed during same procedure	4 (11)
Time to definitive surgical procedure[†] (*days*)	
ORIF	12 (2-36)
Amputation closure	19 (6-43)
Time to union[‡] (*mo*)	6 (2-32)
Length of follow-up[‡] (*mo*)	44 (10-170)
Infection*	
No infection	4 (11)
Infection at amputation site	31 (84)
Infection at fracture site and amputation site	2 (5)
Heterotopic ossification*	
Present	28 (76)
Absent	9 (24)
Heterotopic ossification treatment* (n = 28)	
Observation only	17 (61)
Symptomatic ossification requiring excision	11 (39)

*The values are given as the number, with the percentage in parentheses. ORIF = open reduction and internal fixation.
†The values are given as the median number of days after the injury, with the range in parentheses.
‡The values are given as the median, with the range in parentheses.

Tegner activity level scale and prosthesis use. Secondary outcome measures were the development of nonunion, infection, and heterotopic ossification. *Results.*—Twelve patients (32%) underwent amputation and fracture in the same osseous segment. Ten patients (27%) sustained bilateral traumatic

TABLE 2.—Amputation Data

Characteristic	No. of Patients
Unilateral amputations (n = 27)	
Transhumeral	2
Transradial	2
Transfemoral	2
Knee disarticulation	2
Transtibial	19
Bilateral amputations (n = 10)	
Transfemoral	2
Transtibial	3
Knee disarticulation	1
Ipsilateral transtibial and contralateral transfemoral	1
Ipsilateral knee disarticulation and contralateral transfemoral	1
Ipsilateral knee disarticulation and contralateral transtibial	1
Ipsilateral transtibial and contralateral Chopart	1

amputations, and eight (22%) had a major fracture of the contralateral extremity. The median times to fracture fixation and amputation closure were twelve days and nineteen days, respectively, after the injury. The mean Tegner activity score was 3.32 (range, 1 to 6); patients with isolated extremity injuries had significantly higher Tegner scores than those with severe bilateral injuries (3.59 and 2.38, respectively; $p = 0.04$). Thirty-three patients (89%) developed an infection requiring surgical debridement. However, all fractures were treated until union occurred, and amputation level salvage was successful in all instances. Heterotopic ossification developed in twenty-eight patients (76%), with operative excision required in eleven patients (39%).

Conclusions.—High complication rates, but acceptable final results, can be achieved with internal fixation of a fracture proximal to a traumatic amputation to preserve functional joint levels or salvage residual limb length (Tables 1 and 2).

▶ The authors performed a retrospective case review of a cohort of severely injured warriors from the recent ongoing conflicts to evaluate the impact of fracture treatment proximal to an amputation. They document high complication rates as anticipated with these very high-energy combat injuries. Roughly one-third developed heterotopic ossification of significant impact that resection was necessary to improve pain, function, and prosthetic wear. Heterotopic ossification is nearly universal. The take-home message from this cohort study is that fracture stabilization proximal to an amputation in high-energy injuries has an extremely high rate of complications, yet it is worthwhile to preserve limb length and ultimate patient function.

M. F. Swiontkowski, MD

4 Total Hip Arthroplasty

Introduction

As is, of course, well recognized, joint replacement has become the standard orthopedic procedure and is done by the vast majority of orthopedic surgeons. Topics related to hip replacement are widespread, and today many articles describe the successful outcome of various designs. I intentionally avoided such contributions but rather have focused on what I think are timely issues. Hence, several articles discuss the impact of metal-on-metal outcomes, but a greater emphasis is placed on the potential of adverse reaction. The reason for this emphasis is my personal concern that the widespread use of the hard metal-on-metal bearing surfaces will result in an increasing number of significant complications that can only be solved by removing the implant. Since there are viable alternatives to the metal-on-metal implant, I feel it is important to call attention to these potential adverse effects that should temper their selection, particularly when considering these are generally felt to be most suitable for the young patient. In addition to this topic, a broad spectrum of hip replacement complications is addressed, along with outcomes of projections for the future. The literature is replete with the documentation of this as a successful operation. It is hoped that this information will place the current state of hip replacement in a reasonable perspective.

Bernard F. Morrey, MD

A Population-Based Study of Trends in the Use of Total Hip and Total Knee Arthroplasty, 1969-2008
Singh JA, Vessely MB, Harmsen WS, et al (Mayo Clinic, Rochester, MN; et al)
Mayo Clin Proc 85:898-904, 2010

Objective.—To study the rates of use of total hip arthroplasty (THA) and total knee arthroplasty (TKA) during the past 4 decades.

Methods.—The Rochester Epidemiology Project was used to identify all Olmsted County, Minnesota, residents who underwent THA or TKA from January 1, 1969, through December 31, 2008. We used a population-based

TABLE 1.—Use of Total Hip Arthroplasty Among Olmsted County, MN, Residents by Period, 1969-2008

Period	Age-Adjusted Sex-Specific Rates (95% CI) Females	Males	Total Age- and Sex-Adjusted Rates (95% CI)
1969-1972	62.3 (48.3-76.2)	32.4 (20.7-44.2)	50.2 (40.5-59.8)
1973-1976	76.6 (61.7-91.4)	67.4 (50.3-84.5)	73.9 (62.6-85.2)
1977-1980	90.9 (75.1-106.8)	58.3 (42.3-74.4)	75.9 (64.8-87.1)
1981-1984	71.8 (58.4-85.3)	76.7 (59.9-93.6)	74.7 (64.1-85.3)
1985-1988	70.9 (58.0-83.8)	64.5 (49.8-79.3)	68.4 (58.7-78.0)
1989-1992	81.0 (67.7-94.3)	73.2 (58.0-88.4)	77.6 (67.7-87.6)
1993-1996	71.1 (59.1-83.1)	76.1 (62.1-90.1)	73.4 (64.3-82.4)
1997-2000	91.4 (78.6-105.1)	74.6 (61.8-87.4)	84.8 (75.5-94.2)
2001-2004	108.1 (94.4-121.8)	93.8 (79.6-107.9)	102.1 (92.2-111.9)
2005-2008	150.2 (134.6-165.8)	138.9 (122.2-155.6)	145.5 (134.2-156.9)
1969-2008	91.0 (86.6-95.5)	81.6 (76.7-86.5)	87.2 (83.9-90.5)

Adjusted to the 2000 US Census white population; rates given per 100,000 person-years. CI = confidence interval.

TABLE 2.—Use of Total Knee Arthroplasty Among Olmsted County, MN, Residents by Period, 1971-2008

Period	Age-Adjusted Sex-Specific Rates (95% CI) Females	Males	Total Age- and Sex-Adjusted Rates (95% CI)
1971-1976	38.8 (30.1-47.4)	21.8 (14.1-29.6)	31.2 (25.3-37.1)
1977-1980	35.8 (26.0-45.7)	27.8 (16.9-38.6)	32.6 (25.3-40.0)
1981-1984	71.4 (58.1-84.7)	49.2 (35.4-62.9)	62.5 (52.8-72.2)
1985-1988	107.3 (91.4-123.1)	88.8 (70.5-107.1)	99.4 (87.5-111.3)
1989-1992	107.4 (92.1-122.7)	120.2 (100.6-139.8)	113.5 (101.4-125.6)
1993-1996	119.9 (104.3-135.5)	90.9 (74.9-106.9)	107.1 (95.9-118.2)
1997-2000	147.4 (130.7-164.2)	118.5 (101.6-135.5)	134.6 (122.7-146.6)
2001-2004	203.1 (184.1-222.0)	150.5 (132.2-168.8)	178.0 (164.9-191.1)
2005-2008	255.1 (234.6-275.6)	184.4 (164.7-204.2)	220.9 (206.7-235.0)
1971-2008	129.3 (123.9-134.8)	104.0 (98.2-109.8)	117.6 (113.7-121.5)

Adjusted to the US Census 2000 white population; rates given per 100,000 person-years. CI = confidence interval.

approach because few data are available on long-term trends in the use of THA and TKA in the United States. Rates of use were determined by age- and sex-specific person-years at risk. Poisson regression was used to assess temporal trends by sex and age group.

Results.—The age- and sex-adjusted use of THA increased from 50.2 (95% confidence interval [CI], 40.5-59.8) per 100,000 person-years in 1969-1972 to 145.5 (95% CI, 134.2-156.9) in 2005-2008, whereas TKA increased markedly from 31.2 (95% CI, 25.3-37.1) per 100,000 person-years in 1971-1976 to 220.9 (95% CI, 206.7-235.0) in 2005-2008. For both procedures, use was greater among females, and the rate generally increased with age.

Conclusion.—In this community, TKA and THA use rates have increased steadily since the introduction of the procedures and continue to increase for all age groups. On the basis of these population-based data, the probable need for TKA and THA exceeds current federal agency projections (Tables 1 and 2).

▶ As orthopedic surgeons, we are or should be aware of the financial impact of managing hip and knee arthritis in our society. You may be familiar with the projections of the dramatic increase in the expected incidence of hip replacement over the next decade and, even more, the almost meteoric rise in rates of knee replacement. The reason is of course multifactorial: baby boomers, broadening indications, motivation (?), better outcomes, etc. The data contained in this very carefully performed population-based study are compelling, as they quantify the rate change over the last several decades.

For the hip, the increase is approximately 3 for I (Table 1); for the knee, the increased rate is approximately 7-fold (Table 2)! Something is going to have to give for our profession. I think it means we must be more resource utilization conscious, among other things. Will we? Based on past performance, not unless we have to!

B. F. Morrey, MD

Choice of Hospital for Revision Total Hip Replacement
Katz JN, Wright EA, Wright J, et al (Brigham and Women's Hosp, Boston, MA; et al)
J Bone Joint Surg Am 92:2829-2834, 2010

Background.—Little is known about how often patients have revision total hip replacement in the same hospital in which they had the primary procedure.

Methods.—We examined Medicare claims data to identify patients who had primary total hip replacement from July 1995 to June 1996 and subsequently had revision through December 31, 2006. We examined whether the revision was performed in the same or different hospital from the primary procedure, with different hospitals being categorized as being in a lower, a higher, or the same hospital volume stratum. Hospital strata included twenty-five or fewer cases of total hip replacement annually in the Medicare population, twenty-six to fifty cases, fifty-one to 100 cases, and >100 cases. We calculated the number of revisions generated (primary procedures eventuating in revision) by hospitals in each volume stratum and the number of revisions performed in these hospitals.

Results.—Of 4448 revision procedures, 3306 (74%) were performed in hospitals in the same volume stratum as the hospital where the primary procedure was performed. Four hundred twenty-nine revisions (9.6%) were performed in a lower-volume hospital, and 713 (16%) were performed in a higher-volume hospital. Thirty-one (3%) of 960 patients who had revision within one year after the primary total hip replacement had the revision in a lower-volume center, compared with 204 (15%) of 1393 who had revision more than six years after the primary procedure (odds ratio = 4.6; 95% confidence interval, 3.0 to 6.8). The ratio of revisions performed to revisions generated was 1.21 for the highest-volume centers and 0.86 for the lowest-volume centers.

Conclusions.—Of 4448 revisions examined in this study, 429 (<10%) were performed in centers with a lower volume of total hip replacement than the center at which the initial hip replacement was performed, whereas 713 (16%) were performed in higher-volume centers. Higher-volume centers performed 21% more revisions than they generated (531 revisions performed, compared with 438 generated). These data will help to inform health-care policy with regard to the utilization of resources for revision total hip replacement.

▶ The authors explore an interesting and timely question. The use of large Medicare databases is of value but has limitations of lack of detail. However, a question such as posited here can be definitely answered by this methodology. The relevance of this issue is the reality that revision surgeon is not reimbursed at a fair rate, compared with the primary. The practice of adverse selection, sending problem cases to referral centers, is in the best interest of the patient and the referring physician. This study quantifies the extent of this pattern for revision hips. The larger hospitals do 20% more revisions than they generate. The trend will and should continue. Reimbursement should follow the trend, but it won't.

B. F. Morrey, MD

Hospital Economics of Primary THA Decreasing Reimbursement and Increasing Cost, 1990 to 2008

Rana AJ, Iorio R, Healy WL (Lahey Clinic Med Ctr, Burlington, MA)
Clin Orthop Relat Res 469:355-361, 2011

Background.—The introduction of new technology has increased the hospital cost of THA. Considering the impending epidemic of hip osteoarthritis in the United States, the projections of THA prevalence, and national cost-containment initiatives, we are concerned about the decreasing economic feasibility of hospitals providing THA.

Questions/Purposes.—We compared the hospital cost, reimbursement, and profit/loss of THA over the 1990 to 2008 time period.

Methods.—We reviewed the hospital accounting records of 104 patients in 1990 and 269 patients in 2008 who underwent a unilateral primary THA. Hospital revenue, hospital expenses, and hospital profit (loss) for THA were evaluated and compared in 1990, 1995, and 2008.

Results.—From 1990 to 2008, hospital payment for primary THA increased 29% in actual dollars, whereas inflation increased 58%. Lahey Clinic converted a $3848 loss per case on Medicare fee for service, primary THA in 1990 to a $2486 profit per case in 1995 to a $2359 profit per case in 2008. This improvement was associated with a decrease in inflation-adjusted revenue from 1995 to 2008 and implementation of cost control programs that reduced hospital expenses. Reduction of length of stay and implant costs were the most important drivers of expense reduction. In

TABLE 5.—THA Economic Trends From 1990 to 2008

Year	Actual Dollars			Inflation-Adjusted Dollars		
	Revenue	Expense	Profit	Revenue	Expense	Profit
1990 (Medicare only)	$8500	$12,348	−$3848	$14,002	$20,341	−$6339
1995 [6] (Medicare only)	$13,590	$11,104	$2486	$19,199	$15,687	$3512
1996 [7] (All patients)	$13,446	$9600	$3846	$18,451	$13,173	$5278
2004 [10] (All patients)	$12,769	$9855	$2914	$14,554	$11,232	$3321
2007 [11] (All patients)	$14,305	$11,445	$2860	$14,854	$11,884	$2969
2008 (All patients)	$15,789	$11,688	$4101	$15,789	$11,688	$4101
2008 (Medicare FFS patients)	$14,033	$11,674	$2359	$14,033	$11,674	$2359
2008 (managed Medicare patients)	$11,405	$10,755	$650	$11,405	$10,755	$650

FFS = fee for service.
Editor's Note: Please refer to original journal article for full references.

addition, the managed Medicare patient subgroup reported a per case profit of only $650 in 2008.

Conclusions.—If hospital revenue for THA decreases to managed Medicare levels, it will be difficult to make a profit on THA. The use of technologic enhancements for THA add to the cost problem in this era of healthcare reform. Hospitals and surgeons should collaborate to deliver THA at a profit so it will be available to all patients. Government healthcare administrators and health insurance payers should provide adequate reimbursement for hospitals and surgeons to continue delivery of high-quality THAs.

Level of Evidence.—Level III, economic and decision analysis. See Guidelines for Authors for a complete description of levels of evidence (Table 5).

▶ This is truly a sobering analysis. We know that costs are increasing for everything. We know reimbursement is decreasing for everything. This assessment merely quantitates what we know to be true and offers an interpretation that is even more sobering. The current trends are not only not sustainable—they will affect our ability to offer hip replacement in the future unless some dynamic changes occur (Table 5). I would submit that we should not think of ourselves as victims, which we are to some extent. We are clearly also part of the problem. The sooner we act in a cost-effective manner, the better we will be.

B. F. Morrey, MD

Adverse reaction to metal debris following hip resurfacing: The influence of component type, orientation and volumetric wear
Langton DJ, Joyce TJ, Jameson SS, et al (Newcastle Univ and Univ Hosp of North Tees, UK)
J Bone Joint Surg [Br] 93-B:164-171, 2011

We sought to establish the incidence of joint failure secondary to adverse reaction to metal debris (ARMD) following metal-on-metal hip resurfacing in a large, three surgeon, multicentre study involving 4226 hips with a follow-up of 10 to 142 months. Three implants were studied: the Articular Surface Replacement; the Birmingham Hip Resurfacing; and the Conserve Plus. Retrieved implants underwent analysis using a coordinate measuring machine to determine volumetric wear. There were 58 failures associated with ARMD. The median chromium and cobalt concentrations in the failed group were significantly higher than in the control group (p < 0.001). Survival analysis showed a failure rate in the patients with Articular Surface Replacement of 9.8% at five years, compared with <1% at five years for the Conserve Plus and 1.5% at ten years for the Birmingham Hip Resurfacing. Two ARMD patients had relatively low wear of the retrieved components. Increased wear from the metal-on-metal bearing surface was associated with an increased rate of failure secondary to ARMD. However, the extent of tissue destruction at revision surgery did not appear to be dose-related to the volumetric wear.

▶ It may seem that I select a disproportionate number of hip topics related to metal-on-metal bearing surfaces. This is, in my mind, the single most important topic in hip replacement surgery today. This important contribution studied a very large sample of patients with long-term surveillance and of 3 different designs. The findings are important. The survival rate is directly related to head size and varies according to implant design and manufacturer (Fig 2 in the original article). The overall concentrations are also markedly different in the 3 groups and directly correlate to implant failure (Fig 3 in the original article). What is of special interest is the lack of correlation of failure with soft-tissue reaction. This implies that the type 5 hypersensitive reaction is very host dependent and probably not too common.

B. F. Morrey, MD

Acetabular UHMWPE Survival and Wear Changes With Different Manufacturing Techniques
Meding JB, Keating EM, Davis KE (St Francis Hosp, Mooresville, IN)
Clin Orthop Relat Res 469:405-411, 2011

Background.—Polyethylene wear may be affected by the type of polyethylene resin, manufacturing technique, degree of thermal stabilization, and sterilization technique.

Questions/Purposes.—We therefore compared femoral head penetration into the PE and cup survival using the same cup system with different PE resins, manufacturing, and sterilization techniques.

Methods.—Our study group consisted of 1912 THAs performed using the same uncemented cup and identical 28-mm cobalt-chrome heads. The polyethylene varied as follows: Group 1 (94 cups), GUR 4150 resin, ram-extruded, sterilized in air, no barrier packaging; Group 2 (74 cups), same as Group 1 but sterilized in argon; Group 3 (75 cups), Himont 1900 resin, compression-molded bar stock, sterilized in argon, no barrier

TABLE 1.—Polyethylene Manufacturing Techniques

Group	Sterilized In	Bar Stock	Barrier Packaging	Resin	Crosslinked
1 (n = 94)	Air	Ram-extruded	No	GUR 4150	No
2 (n = 74)	Argon	Ram-extruded	No	GUR 4150	No
3 (n = 75)	Argon	ICM*	No	Himont 1900	No
4 (n = 620)	Argon	ICM*	Yes	Himont 1900	No
5 (n = 711)	Argon	ICM*	Yes	GUR 1050	No
6 (n = 338)	Argon	ICM*	Yes then No	GUR 1050	Yes

*Isostatic Compression Molding.

packaging; Group 4 (620 cups), same as Group 3 except with barrier packing; Group 5 (711 cups), GUR 1050 resin, compression-molded bar stock, sterilized in argon gas with barrier packaging; and Group 6 (338 cups), GUR 1050 resin, compression-molded bar stock, sterilized in argon with barrier packaging, irradiated with 50 kGy, heated below melting temperature, machined, and finally placed in nonbarrier packaging with gas plasma sterilization. Minimum followup was 2 years (average, 7 years; range, 2–17 years).

Results.—Femoral head penetration averaged 0.05 mm per year for Groups 5 and 6 and was substantially lower than for Groups 1 to 4. Cup survival was higher at seven years in Groups 3, 4, and 5, and at 10 years in group 4 when compared to groups 1, 2, and 3.

Conclusions.—We observed lower FHP rates and higher cup survival with polyethylene machined from direct compression-molded bar stock, sterilized in argon gas, with barrier packaging.

Level of Evidence.—Level III Therapeutic study. See Guidelines for Authors for a complete description of levels of evidence (Table 1).

▶ This is an interesting and important study, as it investigates the influence of manufacturing technique on the wear rate, measured by head penetration. It is timely, as the hard metal/metal bearing is being reassessed because of increasing concerns around the issue of host response. It is noteworthy to observe that the series of manufacturing variables studied here do make a difference (Table 1). This is a very important observation. That the study is primarily of non—cross-linked poly does lessen its direct applicability to the current clinical setting. In addition, other variables such as different head sizes and cup orientation were not considered. Nonetheless, the central message is clear—manufacturing parameters such as substrate resin and sterilization can make a difference in the performance of the implant.

B. F. Morrey, MD

Aseptic Lymphocyte-Dominated Vasculitis-Associated Lesion: A Clinicopathologic Review of an Underrecognized Cause of Prosthetic Failure
Watters TS, Cardona DM, Menon KS, et al (Duke Univ Med Ctr, Durham, NC)
Am J Clin Pathol 134:886-893, 2010

It is estimated that 35% of total hip arthroplasties (THAs) involve a second-generation metal-on-metal (MOM) prosthesis. A novel complication has appeared in a subset of patients with MOM THAs that is described as an aseptic, lymphocyte-dominated vasculitis-associated lesion (ALVAL). The clinical features of ALVAL are nonspecific, but patients complain of pain and may develop "pseudotumors." It is hypothesized that metal ions are released from the prosthesis and form haptens with native proteins that elicit a type IV hypersensitivity response in the local soft tissues. Histopathologic descriptions of ALVAL are similar to those of failed arthroplasty in general, with the addition of a dense perivascular inflammatory infiltrate that is the hallmark of ALVAL. We report 3 cases of ALVAL with clinical, radiographic, and histologic findings. Accurate assessment is crucial because an intraoperative diagnosis of chronic

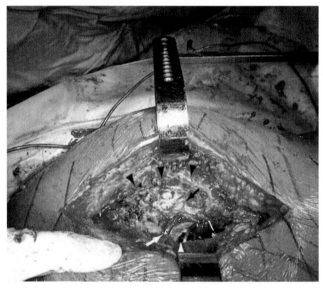

FIGURE 1.—Intraoperative photograph of the large "pseudotumor" adjacent to the prosthesis. The large black arrow denotes the scar tissue and fascia (black arrowheads). Also visible within the incision are the rim of the acetabular (white arrowhead) and the femoral head components (white arrow). (Reprinted from Watters TS, Cardona DM, Menon KS, et al. Aseptic lymphocyte-dominated vasculitis-associated lesion: a clinicopathologic review of an underrecognized cause of prosthetic failure. *Am J Clin Pathol.* 2010;134:886-893. ©(2010) American Society for Clinical Pathology.)

inflammation suggestive of ALVAL will necessitate a replacement of the prosthetic component surfaces (Fig 1).

▶ I was drawn to this report like you can't imagine. I have had the unpleasant experience to take care of several patients with aseptic, lymphocyte-dominated vasculitis-associated lesion. This impact can range from moderate to disastrous. This experience is included primarily to draw the attention of the orthopedic surgeon to the condition. In addition to the pseudotumor reported in the soft tissue (Fig 1), this may also occur in the bone in the form of osteolysis. It appears to be an example of a hypersensitivity reaction, type IV. The frequency is not common—1% or so—but this may be an underestimate. To date, there is no reliable screen to determine the vulnerability of a patient to this process, although patch test for the probable offenders, cobalt and chromium, is a possible screening option. This is a serious concern that surrounds all metal-on-metal implants. Beware!

B. F. Morrey, MD

Catastrophic failure due to aggressive metallosis 4 years after hip resurfacing in a woman in her forties — a case report
von Schewelov T, Sanzén L (Lund Univ, Sweden)
Acta Orthop 81:402-404, 2010

Background.—In the 1970s hip resurfacing techniques were developed to minimize bone resection, wear, and the risk of dislocation. However, these devices were associated with a high failure rate and fell out of favor. In the 1990s hip resurfacing techniques were reintroduced and showed promising short-term results. Serious complications with this implant type are increasingly being reported, however. A case involving a Birmingham metal-on-metal hip resurfacing implant was documented.

Case Report.—Woman, 42, had a hip resurfacing procedure to address osteoarthritis secondary to mild hip dysplasia. She began experiencing mild discomfort and instability in the hip within 4 years and demonstrated radiographically visible aggressive periprosthetic osteolysis and progressive pain 6 months later. The blood levels of cobalt and chromium were grossly elevated, reflecting the influence of the implant.

At surgery there was a massive aggressive metallosis in and around the joint that had eroded half of the cervical neck. Metallosis had fixed the acetabular component in about 55 degrees of abduction and 45 degrees of anteversion. Black-stained granulation tissue was present around the rim of the prosthesis. An area about 2 cm in diameter was the only intact bone remaining; this was detached, showing that the acetabulum was extensively eroded.

A thin unicortical shell was all that remained of the anterior column, and a thin bone bridge was the remnant of the posterior column. Fibrous tissue was found at the site of an elliptical 2.5 × 3 cm defect in the medial wall. Putting the two prosthetic components together revealed obvious macroscopic asymmetry of the articulation, a sign of excessive wear.

Structural allografts and impaction bone grafts were used to reconstruct the acetabulum. The posterior and cranial defects were replaced by a large rim mesh. Surgeons implanted a cemented cross-linked Marathon polyethylene cup and Corail stem to complete the procedure.

Conclusions.—Metal-on-metal articulation hip resurfacing is associated with serious complications and an increased risk of revision. Among the complications are periprosthetic soft tissue destruction, osteolysis, pseudo-tumors, and infiltrates of lymphocytes and plasma cells, perhaps representing an immunologic response to metal debris. The term aseptic lymphocytic vasculitis-associated lesion (ALVAL) has been applied in some cases. Patients may also have high levels of cobalt, chromium, and molybdenum in their blood. The systemic effects of these metals have not been identified. The revision risk is increased in relation to the head size of the surface replacement, especially when the acetabular component is in excessive abduction and/or anteversion, as seen in the case described.

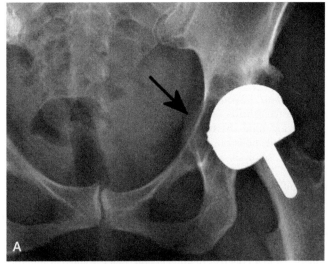

FIGURE 1.—A. View of the lower pelvis before revision. Note the marked abduction angle of the cup and the destruction around both implants with protrusion of metallosis into the pelvis (arrow). (Reprinted from von Schewelov T, Sanzén L. Catastrophic failure due to aggressive metallosis 4 years after hip resurfacing in a woman in her forties — a case report. *Acta Orthop.* 2010;81:402-404. Reprinted by permission of Taylor and Francis Group.)

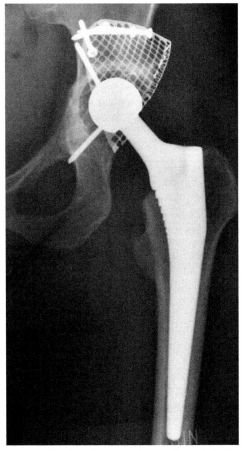

FIGURE 5.—Postoperatively. (Reprinted from von Schewelov T, Sanzén L. Catastrophic failure due to aggressive metallosis 4 years after hip resurfacing in a woman in her forties — a case report. *Acta Orthop.* 2010;81:402-404. Reprinted by permission of Taylor and Francis Group.)

The edge loading of the bearing surface in these cases is increased, leading to greater production of metal wear particles. Older men and women (over age 60 years) are also at increased risk for revision. To be successful with metal-on-metal articulation, patients must be carefully selected and implant positioning should be meticulous. Even so, great caution is advised (Figs 1a and 5).

▶ I rarely select case reports. However, this report is only one of an increasing number that document the potential severe allergic type reactions that have been associated with the metal-on-metal devices. While this report is of an osteolytic expression, Fig 1a, other expressions include the dreaded aseptic lymphocytic vasculitis-associated reaction (ALVAR). If detected early, the osteolytic hyperreaction is often effectively managed, Fig 5. However, in our experience, the management of ALVAR is much more difficult as this attacks and destroys soft tissue, including the abductors. This article closes with a well-stated admonition to use metal-on-metal designs with caution. I agree.

B. F. Morrey, MD

Arthroprosthetic Cobaltism: Neurological and Cardiac Manifestations in Two Patients with Metal-on-Metal Arthroplasty: A Case Report
Tower SS (Anchorage Fracture and Orthopedic Clinic, AK)
J Bone Joint Surg Am 92:2847-2851, 2010

Background.—Early failure of metal-on-metal hip arthroplasties can damage tissues and compromise the ability to perform later revisions. Failure is monitored by measuring serum cobalt levels. Normal cobalt levels are about 0.19 μg/L, with most persons having less than 0.41 μg/L. Excessive cobalt exposure is indicated by levels over 1 μg/L, toxic levels exceed 5 μg/L, and levels over 7 μg/L may indicate periprosthetic metallosis. High cobalt levels associated with beer additives, industrial exposure, or medicinal use damage to multiple organs, causing tinnitus, vertigo, deafness, blindness, optic nerve atrophy, convulsions, headaches, peripheral neuropathy, cardiomyopathy, and hypothyroidism. At least six cases of cobaltism related to arthroplasty implants have been reported. Two cases were detailed.

Case Reports.—Case 1: Man, 49, had a metal-on-metal hip replacement to manage osteoarthritis. Shell diameter was 60 mm, and femoral head diameter was 53 mm. After initial improvement, he developed progressive hip pain with activity. At 3 months, he had axillary rashes, and at 11 months he had dyspnea, progressive hip pain, a large periprosthetic fluid collection, and a serum cobalt level of 50 μg/L. After 18 months the patient complained of anxiety, headaches, irritability, fatigue, tinnitus, and hearing loss; his cobalt level was 35 μg/L. His condition continued to deteriorate, with pain at rest, hip creaking, hand tremor, incoordination, cognitive decline, depression, visual changes, and optic nerve atrophy. The cobalt level at 36 months was 122 μg/L. Revision arthroplasty was performed after 43 months, when his cobalt levels were 83 μg/L in serum, 2.2 μg/L in cerebrospinal fluid (CSF), and 3200 μg/L in joint fluid. The patient demonstrated diastolic dysfunction, with metallosis, necrosis, and lymphocytic infiltrates noted on pathologic testing. The depths of wear in the most worn quadrants of the liner were an estimated 400, 306, and 381 μm, using the three measuring techniques. Sequential roundness scans indicated maximum wear at the rim diminishing to nearly zero 20° into the liner. The femoral head had several burnished areas. The patient's hip pain, affect, cognition, hearing, exercise tolerance, tremor, and professional productivity improved 11 months after the revision and his tinnitus and visual symptoms stabilized. He had five prosthetic dislocations, only two of which required reduction under general anesthesia.

Case 2: Man, 49, required a metal-on-metal hip replacement to treat failed resurfacing of the femoral head. The acetabular shell diameter was 56 mm, and the femoral head diameter was 49 mm. One year later the patient complained of cognitive decline, vertigo, hearing loss, groin pain, rashes, and dyspnea; his serum cobalt level was 23 µg/L. A revision was done 40 months after the initial revision arthroplasty, when the patient's serum cobalt level was 23 µg/L and the joint fluid level was 3300 µg/L. Pathologic evaluation identified gross metallosis, an acellular fibrous pseudocapsule, and no lymphocytic infiltrates. Scratches were seen on the acetabular shell but no visible eccentricity, although the femoral head had an equatorial wear scar. The patient's condition improved over the next 7 months but he needed a hip reduction under sedation.

Conclusions.—Patients with metal-on-metal hip implants at highest risk for cobaltism have shell malposition or persistent hip pain, renal impairment, and Articular Surface Replacement (ASR) implants. Both of the patients reported had hip pain caused by periprosthetic metallosis, neurologic impairment, and cardiac symptoms resulting from high cobalt levels. The wear pattern in the first patient suggests edge loading caused by prosthetic malposition; the pattern in the second patient suggests inadequate bearing clearance. Revision arthroplasties were complicated by instability, which is more common in hips revised because of metallosis. Although metal-on-metal hips are popular, patients are at risk for cobaltism if bearings wear excessively or renal function declines. About 43% of American adults age 40 to 59 years and 74% of adults over age 70 years have acquired impaired renal function.

▶ Although I usually do not select case reports, this is reviewed, as it underscores several important points. Cobalt toxicity is well known but not by orthopedists. The systemic manifestations affect numerous organ systems, including the neurological and cardiac systems. In this instance, the effects came about because of technical errors of insertion resulting in impingement. The last paragraph of the report is most important: recognize the problem and perform early revision. It also serves to point out that some designs and design concepts are less forgiving, especially when dealing with hard bearing surfaces.

B. F. Morrey, MD

Do Ion Levels In Hip Resurfacing Differ From Metal-on-metal THA at Midterm?

Moroni A, Savarino L, Hoque M, et al (Bologna Univ, Italy; Rizzoli Orthopaedic Inst, Bologna, Italy)
Clin Orthop Relat Res 469:180-187, 2011

Background.—Metal-on-metal Birmingham hip resurfacing (MOM-BHR) is an alternative to metal-on-metal total hip arthroplasty (MOM-THA), especially for young and/or active patients. However, wear resulting in increased serum ion levels is a concern.

Questions/Purposes.—We asked whether (1) serum chromium (Cr), cobalt (Co), and molybdenum (Mo) concentrations would differ between patients with either MOM-BHR or MOM-THA at 5 years, (2) confounding factors such as gender would influence ion levels; and (3) ion levels would differ at 2 and 5 years for each implant type.

Patients and Methods.—Ions were measured in two groups with either MOM-BHR (n = 20) or MOM-THA (n = 35) and a mean 5-year followup, and two groups with either MOM-BHR (n = 15) or MOM-THA (n = 25) and a mean 2-year followup. Forty-eight healthy blood donors were recruited for reference values.

Results.—At 5 years, there were no differences in ion levels between patients with MOM-BHR or MOM-THA. Gender was a confounding factor, and in the MOM-BHR group at 5 years, Cr concentrations were greater in females compared with those of males. Mean ion levels were similar in patients with 2 and 5 years of followup for each implant type. Ion levels in patients were sevenfold to 10-fold higher than in controls.

Conclusions.—As the metal ion concentrations in the serum at 5 years were in the range reported in the literature, we do not believe concerns regarding excessive metal ion levels after MOM-BHR are justified.

Level of Evidence.—Level III, therapeutic study. See the Guidelines for Authors for a complete description of level of evidence.

▶ We reviewed and picked this article on the same day we reviewed the information regarding oncogenesis from the Swedish joint replacement registry. While the difference in ion shed between the anatomic-sized resurfacing and the low-friction arthroplasty dimension-sized head is of interest, the gender-specific differences and the absolute elevation of the ion content are of particular value. I have no idea how the 10-fold increase in ion concentration at 5 years can be considered of no consequence, as do these authors!

B. F. Morrey, MD

A Prospective Randomized Trial of Mini-Incision Posterior and Two-Incision Total Hip Arthroplasty

Della Valle CJ, Dittle E, Moric M, et al (Rush Univ Med Ctr, Chicago, IL)
Clin Orthop Relat Res 468:3348-3354, 2010

Background.—The two-incision approach to THA has been controversial, with some authors reporting its use is associated with a rapid recovery whereas others report no differences in outcomes and a higher risk of perioperative complications secondary to increased surgical complexity.

Questions/Purposes.—We therefore compared early postoperative variables including pain, length of stay, functional recovery, complications, and complexity of the mini-posterior and two-incision approaches to THA.

Patients and Methods.—We prospectively enrolled 72 patients scheduled for THA and randomized them into two groups: mini-incision posterior approach and the two-incision approach. Preoperative teaching, anesthetic protocols, implants used, and rehabilitation pathways were identical for both groups. All variables were assessed at a maximum of 1 year postoperatively.

Results.—All key outcomes were similar in the two groups: mean visual analog scale (VAS) scores for pain during the first 3 postoperative days and the first 6 weeks, total narcotic requirements in the hospital and during the first 6 weeks, mean length of stay (51 hours versus 48 hours), and mean Harris hip scores and SF-12 scores. Achievement of functional milestones was similar between the two groups. There was one reoperation in each group. Mean operative time was longer for patients in the two-incision group (98 minutes versus 77 minutes), however the accuracy of component positioning was similar.

Conclusions.—We found no differences in perioperative outcomes between these two approaches for THA. Variables other than the surgical approach including perioperative protocols, patient expectations, and the patient's general health may have a greater effect on outcomes such as pain during the early postoperative period, functional recovery, and length of hospital stay. The use of small incisions for THA was safe as was a shortened hospital stay in selected patients.

▶ This article is included just to reinforce the information that has been conveyed in the past. In spite of additional experience, refinement of technique, and possibly improved patient selection, minimally invasive techniques seem to offer no added value. This may be concluded with certainty with the reported technique, and my interpretation of the literature is that this remains true in general. Given the learning curve, high success rate of conventional techniques, and increased complications, at least in the early stages, minimally invasive techniques are to be reserved by those developing them, by those investigating their value, or by those surgeons with demonstrated superior outcomes from such a procedure.

B. F. Morrey, MD

A comparison of hemiarthroplasty with total hip replacement for displaced intracapsular fracture of the femoral neck: A randomised controlled multicentre trial in patients aged 70 years and over

van den Bekerom MPJ, Hilverdink EF, Sierevelt IN, et al (Academic Med Ctr, Amsterdam, the Netherlands)

J Bone Joint Surg [Br] 92-B:1422-1428, 2010

The aim of this study was to analyse the functional outcome after a displaced intracapsular fracture of the femoral neck in active patients aged over 70 years without osteoarthritis or rheumatoid arthritis of the hip, randomised to receive either a hemiarthroplasty or a total hip replacement (THR). We studied 252 patients of whom 47 (19%) were men, with a mean age of 81.1 years (70.2 to 95.6). They were randomly allocated to be treated with either a cemented hemiarthroplasty (137 patients) or cemented THR (115 patients). At one- and five-year follow-up no differences were observed in the modified Harris hip score, revision rate of the prosthesis, local and general complications, or mortality. The intra-operative blood loss was lower in the hemiarthroplasty group (7% > 500 ml), THR group (26% > 500 ml) and the duration of surgery was longer in the THR group (28% > 1.5 hours *versus* 12% > 1.5 hours). There were no dislocations of any bipolar hemiarthroplasty than in the eight dislocations of a THR during follow-up.

Because of a higher intra-operative blood loss ($p < 0.001$), an increased duration of the operation ($p < 0.001$) and a higher number of early and late dislocations ($p = 0.002$), we do not recommend THR as the treatment of choice in patients aged ≥ 70 years with a fracture of the femoral neck in

TABLE 4.—Outcome Measures at Five Years Follow-Up

	HA[†] (n = 137)	THR[‡] (n = 115)	p-Value
Mean modified HHS (range)*	71.9 (33 to 99)	75.2 (45 to 96)	0.22
Mean HHS pain (range)	38.6 (10 to 44)	40.1 (20 to 44)	
Mean HHS function (range)	18.6 (4 to 35)	20.1 (7 to 33)	
Mortality (%)	61 (44)	71 (54)	0.09
Revision operations (%)	6 (4)	2 (2)	0.29 (Fischer exact)
Dislocation of prosthesis (%)	0	8 (7)	0.002
Radiological findings (%)			
Loosening of femoral component	5 (4)	1 (1)	
Loosening of acetabular component	Not applicable	0	
Polyethylene wear	Not applicable	0	
Osteoarthritis at the acetabulum	14 (10)	Not applicable	
Protrusio acetabuli	4 (3)	1 (1)	
Fracture/fissure at the acetabulum	3 (2)	1 (1)	
Heterotopic ossification	14 (10)	17 (15)	

*The total modified Harris Hip score (HHS) was converted to a maximum of 100 points.
†HA, hemiarthroplasty.
‡THR, total hip replacement.
§Mean modified HHS: students *t*-test; mortality: chi-squared test; revision operations, dislocation of prosthesis: Fisher's exact test.

the absence of advanced radiological osteoarthritis or rheumatoid arthritis of the hip (Table 4).

▶ Although one must always consider differences in culture and patient attitude, this study remains compelling. We continue to discuss the topic of this prospective study, and I feel the findings here will add another nail in the coffin of total hip for all. The methodology is sound; the sample size of 137 hemireplacements and 115 total replacements is ample to draw firm conclusions. The 5-year surveillance offers an opportunity to determine long-term follow-up for this elderly population. The prolonged operative time and increased blood loss is well documented. While I personally feel that 8 dislocations are higher than typically expected, one cannot argue that the hemireplacement group had no dislocations (Table 4). To me, the trump card is that the hemiarthroplasty is less expensive from the perspective of length of stay and acquisition cost. Hence QED.

B. F. Morrey, MD

Comparison of Bipolar Hemiarthroplasty with Total Hip Arthroplasty for Displaced Femoral Neck Fractures: A Concise Four-Year Follow-up of a Randomized Trial
Hedbeck CJ, Enocson A, Lapidus G, et al (Karolinska Institutet, Stockholm, Sweden; Capio St Göran's Hosp, Stockholm, Sweden)
J Bone Joint Surg Am 93:445-450, 2011

We performed a four-year follow-up of a randomized controlled trial involving 120 elderly patients with an acute displaced femoral neck fracture who were randomized to treatment with either a bipolar hemiarthroplasty or a total hip arthroplasty. The difference in hip function (as indicated by the Harris hip score) in favor of the total hip arthroplasty group that was previously reported at one year persisted and seemed to increase with time (mean score, 87 compared with 78 at twenty-four months [p < 0.001] and 89 compared with 75 at forty-eight months [p < 0.001]). The health-related quality of life (as indicated by the EuroQol [EQ-5D$_{index}$] score) was better in the total hip arthroplasty group at the time of each followup, but the difference was significant only at forty-eight months (p < 0.039). These results confirm the better results in terms of hip function and quality of life after total hip arthroplasty as compared with hemiarthroplasty in elderly, lucid patients with a displaced fracture of the femoral neck (Table 2).

▶ We recently reviewed a meta-analysis on the subject of arthroplasty versus fixation for femoral neck fracture. This prospective randomized study addresses the next logical question: Is a total better than a hemi replacement? The answer would appear to be yes, at least regarding the quality-of-life parameters (Fig 2 in the original article, Table 2 [continued portion]). The complication rate is

TABLE 2.—Hip Function*

	4 Months (N=116)			12 Months (N=111)			24 Months (N=101)			48 Months (N=83)		
	Hemiarthroplasty†	Total Hip Arthroplasty	P Value	Hemiarthroplasty	Total Hip Arthroplasty	P Value	Hemiarthroplasty	Total Hip Arthroplasty	P Value	Hemiarthroplasty	Total Hip Arthroplasty	P Value
Total score	77.5 ± 12.4	82.5 ± 11.5	0.011	79.4 ± 12.3	87.2 ± 9.4	<0.001	77.9 ± 12.5	87.2 ± 10.1	<0.001	75.2 ± 15.4	89.0 ± 8.1	<0.001
Pain	40.0 ± 6.6	42.0 ± 4.5	0.121	39.1 ± 5.8	43.1 ± 2.3	<0.001	37.8 ± 6.2	42.7 ± 3.0	<0.001	35.1 ± 7.0	43.0 ± 1.8	<0.001
Function	28.8 ± 8.7	31.9 ± 8.6	0.021	31.6 ± 10.0	35.3 ± 8.8	0.037	31.3 ± 9.2	35.7 ± 8.7	0.024	31.4 ± 10.6	37.2 ± 7.8	0.013
Absence of deformity	4.0 ± 0	4.0 ± 0	1.0	4.0 ± 0	4.0 ± 0	1.0	4.0 ± 0	4.0 ± 0	1.0	4.0 ± 0	4.0 ± 0	1.0
Range of motion	4.7 ± 0.3	4.7 ± 0.3	0.598	4.7 ± 0.3	4.7 ± 0.3	0.435	4.8 ± 0.2	4.8 ± 0.2	0.671	4.7 ± 0.3	4.8 ± 0.1	0.714

Editor's Note: Please refer to original journal article for full references.
*The scores were derived with use of the Harris hip scoring system. The values are given as the mean (and the standard deviation) for all patients who were available at each follow-up interval. The P values pertain to the differences between the groups. The four and twelve-month results were previously published[1].
†The values are missing for two patients.

comparable, including an unbelievable 0% dislocation rate between both groups. The only unanswered question—is the total hip arthroplasty cost-effective?

B. F. Morrey, MD

Cemented Versus Cementless Total Hip Replacements in Patients Fifty-five Years of Age or Older with Rheumatoid Arthritis
Mäkelä KT, Eskelinen A, Pulkkinen P, et al (Turku Univ Central Hosp, Finland; COXA Hosp for Joint Replacement, Tampere, Finland; Univ of Helsinki, Finland; et al)
J Bone Joint Surg Am 93:178-186, 2011

Background.—Results obtained from single-center studies indicate that a cemented total hip replacement is the treatment of choice for the management of patients over fifty-five years of age with rheumatoid arthritis. The aim of this study was to analyze population-based survival rates for cemented and cementless total hip replacements in patients aged fifty-five years or over with rheumatoid arthritis in Finland.

Methods.—Between 1980 and 2006, a total of 6000 primary total hip replacements performed for the management of rheumatoid arthritis in patients who were fifty-five years of age or older were entered in the Finnish Arthroplasty Registry. 4019 of them fulfilled our inclusion criteria and were subjected to analysis. The implants were classified into one of three possible groups: (1) a cementless group (a noncemented proximally porous-coated stem and a noncemented porouscoated press-fit cup), (2) a cemented group 1 (a cemented, loaded-taper stem combined with a cemented, all-polyethylene cup), or (3) a cemented group 2 (a cemented, composite-beam stem with a cemented, all-polyethylene cup).

Results.—Cementless stems and cups, analyzed separately, had a significantly lower risk of revision for aseptic loosening than cemented implants in patients who were fifty-five years of age or older with rheumatoid arthritis. The fifteen-year survival rate of cementless total hip replacements (80%) was comparable with the rates of the cemented groups (86% in cemented group 1 and 79% in cemented group 2) when revisions for any reason were used as the end point.

Conclusions.—Cementless and cemented total hip replacements produced comparable long-term results in patients who were fifty-five years of age or older with rheumatoid arthritis.

Level of Evidence.—Therapeutic Level III. See Instructions to Authors for a complete description of levels of evidence.

▶ As might be imagined, an article about cement fixation will of necessity not originate in the United States. The findings of this Finnish registry study (1) validate the utility of the registry and (2) provide valuable decision-making information. While the results of the cementless and the cemented fixation survival were comparable, overall, the cementless fixation did slightly better in this age group (Fig 2B in the original article). This is in fact similar to findings from the Mayo Clinic demonstrating that the outcome of cemented fixation is equal or even superior to uncemented designs of the 1990s in patients older than 65 years. Nonetheless, the selection will continue to be based on surgeon preference and other less-scientific factors. Too bad.

B. F. Morrey, MD

Hip Dislocation: Are Hip Precautions Necessary in Anterior Approaches?
Restrepo C, Mortazavi SMJ, Brothers J, et al (Thomas Jefferson Univ Hosp, Philadelphia, PA)
Clin Orthop Relat Res 469:417-422, 2011

Background.—In 2005, we reported removal of functional restriction after primary THA performed through the anterolateral approach did not increase the incidence of dislocation.

Questions/Purposes.—To develop a current practice guideline, we evaluated the incidence of early dislocation after primary THA after implementation of a no-restriction protocol.

Methods.—Between January 2005 and December 2007, 2532 patients (2764 hips; 1541 women, 1223 men; mean age, 63.2 years [28−98 years]) underwent primary THA at our institution. Bilateral THA was performed in 232 patients (464 hips). The direct anterior or anterolateral approach was used in all patients. Femoral head size was 28, 32, or 36 mm. Patients were given no traditional functional restrictions postoperatively, such as use of elevated seats, abduction pillows, and restriction from driving. All patients received standard care at the judgment of the attending surgeon. One hundred forty-six patients missed followup appointments despite efforts to be contacted by telephone. The remaining 2386 of 2532 patients (94%) had a minimum followup of 6 months (mean, 14.2 months; range, 6−34 months).

Results.—Four known dislocations occurred in the followed cohort of 2386 patients with 2612 hips (0.15%) at a mean of 5 days (3−12 days) postoperatively, none related to high-impact trauma. One dislocation occurred in a patient with a history of developmental dysplasia of the hip, two dislocations occurred while at the toilet (one with a previous hip fracture treated with a modular system), and one dislocation was idiopathic.

Conclusions.—We confirmed a low incidence of dislocation after primary THA in the absence of early postoperative restrictions. We conclude a no-restriction protocol does not increase the incidence of early dislocation after primary THA.

Level of Evidence.—Level II, therapeutic study. See the Guidelines for Authors for a complete description of levels of evidence.

▶ I have long had a personal interest in this subject. I am attracted to the science of the study in that it asks a specific question, has adequate numbers to address the question asked, and answers the question studied. What isn't emphasized in the title is that all this is possible, in my opinion, because of the inherent stability of the anterior approach. Even more subtle is the lack of value of the larger head. The 28-mm dimension is as stable as the 36-mm dimension. The only issue might be the question of whether longer surveillance would change the findings. In my experience, no.

B. F. Morrey, MD

A Monoblock Porous Tantalum Acetabular Cup Has No Osteolysis on CT at 10 Years
Moen TC, Ghate R, Salaz N, et al (Northwestern Univ Feinberg School of Medicine, Chicago, IL; Northwestern Orthopaedic Inst, Chicago, IL)
Clin Orthop Relat Res 469:382-386, 2011

Background.—Aseptic osteolysis has been the single most important factor limiting the longevity of a THA. A great deal of attention has been focused on the development of implants and materials that minimize the development of osteolysis. The monoblock porous tantalum acetabular cup was designed to minimize osteolysis, but whether it does so is unclear.

Questions/Purposes.—We evaluated the incidence of osteolytic lesions after THA using a monoblock porous tantalum acetabular component.

Methods.—We retrospectively reviewed 51 patients who had a THA using a monoblock porous tantalum acetabular cup. At a minimum of 9.6 years postoperatively (average, 10.3 years; SD, 0.2 years; range, 9.6−10.8 years), a helical CT scan of the pelvis using a metal suppression protocol was obtained. This scan was evaluated for the presence of osteolysis.

Results.—We found no evidence of osteolysis on CT scan at an average of 10.3 years.

Conclusions.—Osteolysis appears not to be a major problem at 10 years with this monoblock porous tantalum acetabular component, but longer term followup will be required to determine whether these findings persist.

Level of Evidence.—Level IV, therapeutic study. See Guidelines for Authors for a complete description of levels of evidence.

▶ The monoblock trabecular metal acetabular component was a popular device used in the late 1990s. This implant has been shown to be a durable device. The disadvantages of the implant include difficulties in searching the implant fully and the lack of modularity. The latter impairs its versatility. The authors have demonstrated good long-term performances in this device largely because of the elimination of backside wear. More modern trabecular metal implants have demonstrated versatility and usefulness in a variety of difficult reconstructive situations. This particular implant is demonstrating good midterm results despite the use of conventional polyethylene.

C. P. Beauchamp, MD

Cementless Femoral Fixation in Total Hip Arthroplasty

Khanuja HS, Vakil JJ, Goddard MS, et al (Sinai Hosp of Baltimore, MD; Orthopaedicare, Willow Grove, PA)
J Bone Joint Surg Am 93:500-509, 2011

A number of cementless femoral stems are associated with excellent long-term survivorship.

Cementless designs differ from one another in terms of geometry and the means of obtaining initial fixation.

Strict classification of stem designs is important in order to compare results among series.

Loosening and thigh pain are less prevalent with modern stem designs.

Stress-shielding is present in most cases, even with newer stem designs (Table 1).

▶ This is an excellent review article and clearly reflects the knowledge and insight of the senior author. The means of classifying the considerable variation among these designs are logical and helpful (Table 1). The illustrations of the

TABLE 1.—Classification System of Cementless Femoral Stem Designs

General Category	Type	Geometry	Description	Location of Fixation
Straight stems				
Tapered proximal fixation	1	Single wedge	Narrows medially-laterally. Proximally coated. Flat stem, thin in anterior-posterior plane	Metaphyseal
Tapered proximal fixation	2	Double wedge, metaphyseal filling	Narrows distally in both medial-lateral and anterior-posterior planes. Wider than Type 1. Fills metaphyseal region	Metaphyseal
Tapered proximal fixation	3A	Tapered, round	Rounded tapered conical stem with porous coating at proximal two-thirds	Metaphyseal-diaphyseal junction
Tapered distal fixation	3B	Tapered, splined	Conical taper with longitudinal raised splines	Metaphyseal-diaphyseal junction and proximal diaphyseal
Tapered distal fixation	3C	Tapered, rectangular	Rectangular cross section with four-point rotational support in metaphyseal-diaphyseal region	Metaphyseal-diaphyseal junction and proximal diaphyseal
Distally fixed	4	Cylindrical, fully coated	Extensive porous coating. Proximal collar to enhance proximal bone oading and axial stability	Primarily diaphyseal
Modular	5		Metaphyseal and diaphyseal components prepared independently	Metaphyseal and diaphyseal
Curved, anatomic stem	6		Proximal portion is wide in both lateral and posterior planes. Posterior bow in metaphysis, anterior bow in diaphysis	Metaphyseal

various types are also extremely helpful (Fig 1 in the original article). One very important point to make about this review is that it accurately points out the reliability of current generation stems and recognizes the ongoing deficiency of proximal stress shielding. The authors do not discuss the newest generation of cementless designs, those without stems, being entirely metaphyseal fit. Our personal experience indicates that this design does decrease stress shielding. Of necessity, any study using the long-term outcome of uncemented devices will often be describing the results of prior designs, not the current generation.

B. F. Morrey, MD

Association of Osteonecrosis and Failure of Hip Resurfacing Arthroplasty
Zustin J, Sauter G, Morlock MM, et al (Univ Med Ctr Hamburg-Eppendorf, Germany; TUHH Hamburg Univ of Technology, Germany)
Clin Orthop Relat Res 468:756-761, 2010

Osteonecrosis (ON) has been reported in femoral remnants removed after failure of hip resurfacing arthroplasty. Experimental and clinical studies have further described thermal effects of the cementation technique, damage of extraosseous blood vessels, and intraoperative hypoxemia as possible causative factors. We analyzed histologically a series of 123 retrieved specimens with a preoperative diagnosis other than ON to investigate the incidence and extent of advanced ON. ON was found in 88% of cases and associated with 60% (51 of a total of 85) of periprosthetic fractures. The fracture incidence correlated with the extent of ON. Collapse of necrotic tissue in three (2%) cases resulted in disconnection of the bone stock-femoral component. We observed smaller regions of superficial ON in the majority of the remaining femoral remnants with periprosthetic fractures and in hips that failed for reasons other than fracture (Fig 2c, d).

▶ The popularity of resurfacing hip replacement continues to grow. Of the concerns expressed by some, the metal ion issue probably predominates. This is an important study because it provides additional insight into the mechanical

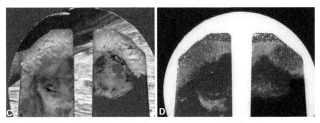

FIGURE 2.—(C) A similar ON lesion with adjacent elastic brownish fibrosis reveals (D) multiple small collapsed bone fragments in the fibrosis in a hip revised for loosening of the femoral component. (With kind permission from Springer Science+Business Media: Zustin J, Sauter G, Morlock MM, et al. Association of osteonecrosis and failure of hip resurfacing arthroplasty. *Clin Orthop Relat Res.* 2010;468: 756-761.)

cause of failure of the resurfacing device. Because osteonecrosis was excluded as a preoperative diagnosis, the changes reported here (Fig 2c, d) have apparently come about from the surgical exposure or from the insult of the implantation. Yet it apparently is an uncommon event, occurring in 1% to 3% of prior reported studies. The surgeon should be aware of this as an inherent potential complication of the resurfacing hip replacement.

B. F. Morrey, MD

Does morbid obesity affect the outcome of total hip replacement?: An analysis of 3290 THRS
McCalden RW, Charron KD, MacDonald SJ, et al (The Univ of Western Ontario, London, Ontario, Canada)
J Bone Joint Surg [Br] 93-B:321-325, 2011

We evaluated the outcome of primary total hip replacement (THR) in 3290 patients with the primary diagnosis of osteoarthritis at a minimum follow-up of two years. They were stratified into categories of body mass index (BMI) based on the World Health Organisation classification of obesity. Statistical analysis was carried out to determine if there was a difference in the post-operative Western Ontario and McMaster Universities osteoarthritis index, the Harris hip score and the Short-Form-12 outcome based on the BMI.

While the pre- and post-operative scores were lower for the group classified as morbidly obese, the overall change in outcome scores suggested an equal if not greater improvement compared with the non-morbidly obese patients. The overall survivorship and rate of complications were similar in the BMI groups although there was a slightly higher rate of revision for sepsis in the morbidly obese group.

Morbid obesity does not affect the post-operative outcome after THR, with the possible exception of a marginally increased rate of infection. Therefore withholding surgery based on the BMI is not justified (Table 3).

▶ This interesting study examines an ongoing and controversial question regarding hip and knee surgery. The data represent a large cohort with reasonably long-term surveillance. While one cannot argue with the data, I do interpret

TABLE 3.—Distribution (Number, %) of Revisions According to the Body Mass Index Groups

	Normal and Underweight (n = 647)	Overweight (n = 1212)	Obese (n = 1225)	Morbidly obese (n = 206)	P-Value*
All revisions	20 (3.1)	42 (3.5)	59 (4.8)	11 (5.3)	0.147
Aseptic revisions	17 (2.6)	40 (3.3)	50 (4.1)	8 (3.9)	0.393
Septic revisions	3 (0.5)	2 (0.2)	9 (0.7)	3 (1.5)	0.061

*statistical significance calculated by Pearson's chi-squared test.

the results somewhat differently than do the authors. First, the patient outcome measurements are not particularly sensitive to the most important questions: survival and complication. In spite of the statement that there is no justification of withholding replacement based on the issue of obesity, the Kaplan-Meier curves are different and worse for the obese patient (Fig 5 in the original article). Further, in spite of the fact that the complication rate of 0.5 for sepsis is not statistically different from the nonobese and the obese rate of 1.5, it is a 3-fold difference (Table 3). This does, or should, represent a meaningful difference for the surgeon and patient. Yet, this article also documents that the improvement in the obese patient is every much as good as in the nonobese patient. This has been documented in prior literature. In my practice, I am aware of the finding of the data conveyed in this article, and of others, and do offer replacement to the morbidly obese, but I clearly discuss the potential increased risks.

B. F. Morrey, MD

Cementless revision for infected total hip replacements
Kim Y-H, Kim J-S, Park J-W, et al (Ewha Womans Univ School of Medicine, Seoul, South Korea)
J Bone Joint Surg [Br] 93-B:19-26, 2011

Our aim was to determine the success rate of repeated debridement and two-stage cementless revision arthroplasty according to the type of infected total hip replacement (THR). We enrolled 294 patients (294 hips) with an infected THR in the study. There were 222 men and 72 women with a mean age of 55.1 years (24.0 to 78.0). The rate of control of infection after the initial treatment and after repeated debridement and two-stage revisions was determined. The clinical (Harris hip score) and radiological results were evaluated. The mean follow-up was 10.4 years (5.0 to 14.0).

The eventual rate of control of infection was 100.0% for early superficial post-operative infection, 98.4% for early deep post-operative infection, 98.5% for late chronic infection and 91.0% for acute haematogenous infection. Overall, 288 patients (98%) maintained a functioning THR at the latest follow-up. All the allografts appeared to be united and there were no failures.

These techniques effectively controlled infection and maintained a functional THR with firm fixation in most patients. Repeated debridement and two-stage or repeated two-stage revisions further improved the rate of control of infection after the initial treatment and increased the likelihood of maintaining a functional THR (Table 7).

▶ This is an impressive study. The authors enrolled a large number of patients and stratified the analysis as a function of the temporal presentation of the infection. The impressive outcomes are certainly encouraging, and would

TABLE 7.—Results in all Types of Infection by Number of Hips (%)

Result	Early Superficial Post-Operative Infection (n = 14)	Early Deep Post-Operative Infection (n = 128)	Late Chronic Post-Operative Infection (n = 130)	Acute Haematogenous Infection (n = 22)	Overall (n = 294)
Successful first treatment	14 (100)	109 (85.1)	112 (86.2)	12 (45.5)	245 (83.0)*
Infection eradicated	14 (100)	126 (98.4)	128 (98.5)	20 (92.0)	288 (98.0)†
Functional hip	14 (100)	126 (98.4)	128 (98.5)	20 (91.0)	288 (98.0)‡

*95% confidence interval, 75.0 to 89.0.
†95% confidence interval, 95.0 to 99.8.
‡95% confidence interval, 89.0 to 99.4.

seem to justify their treatment logic (Fig 1 in the original article). It should be noted, however, that the initial success rate was 83%. That all groups did roughly the same from the perspective of infection control and functional outcome (Table 7) is a bit surprising. I was unable to determine whether the group with negative cultures had any special characteristics, as this is the group that currently causes the greatest concern to most surgeons.

B. F. Morrey, MD

Acetabular Reconstruction with Impaction Bone-Grafting and a Cemented Cup in Patients Younger than Fifty Years Old: A Concise Follow-up, at Twenty to Twenty-Eight Years, of a Previous Report

Busch VJJF, Gardeniers JWM, Verdonschot N, et al (Radboud Univ Nijmegen Med Centre, The Netherlands)
J Bone Joint Surg Am 93:367-371, 2011

In a previous report, we presented our results of forty-two acetabular reconstructions, performed with use of impaction bone-grafting and a cemented polyethylene cup, in thirty-seven patients who were younger than fifty years and had a minimum of fifteen years of follow-up. The present update study shows the results after twenty to twenty-eight years. Eight additional cups had to be revised—four because of aseptic loosening, three because of wear, and one during a revision of the stem. Three additional cups were considered loose on radiographs. Survivorship of the acetabular reconstructions, with an end point of revision for any reason, was 73% after twenty years and 52% after twenty-five years. With revision for aseptic loosening as the end point, survival was 85% after twenty years and 77% after twenty-five years; for signs of loosening on radiographs, survival was 71% at twenty years and 62% at twenty-five years. In conclusion, our previous results have declined but the technique of using impacted morselized bone graft and a cemented cup is useful for the purpose of restoring bone stock in young patients whose acetabular defects require primary or revision total hip arthroplasty.

▶ Of interest, I selected a prior report from this group that revealed the viability of the impacted graft after several years. Although the outcome markedly deteriorated from the 20th year onward (Fig 1 in the original article), the final result is still quite acceptable. The main feature is to recognize that the revision procedure was performed in a young, therefore higher risk, population. What was disappointing to me was the lack of detail of how the failed revision was managed. If the impaction grafting reconstituted viable bone stock, then a second revision with an uncemented shell and highly cross-linked liner would be expected to be highly successful for long term.

B. F. Morrey, MD

5 Total Knee Arthroplasty

Introduction

The section on total knee arthroplasty is similar to the hip in that this is such a successful operation. It is somewhat difficult to know what may be the most relevant additional or new information that might be provided to the general orthopedic surgeon. Questions relating to the patella and the extensor mechanism are some of the most vexing that still confront the knee replacement surgeon, and these have been addressed in this volume. Notably absent is navigation as an adjunct in knee joint replacement. This has not been emphasized this year, not because it is not important, but navigation has not appreciated any substantive new information compared with previous years. Navigation is worthwhile in improving the accuracy, particularly in the frontal plane; however, the cost-effectiveness of the technology is yet to be defined. Thrombophlebitis remains a major issue, both in regard to hip and knee replacement, and it is covered in the YEAR BOOK largely in the general orthopedic section. The efforts at advancing substantive concepts, such as with the mobile bearing knee and the unicompartmental replacement, are also addressed in this year's volume.

Bernard F. Morrey, MD

Hospital Economics of Primary Total Knee Arthroplasty at a Teaching Hospital
Healy WL, Rana AJ, Iorio R (Lahey Clinic Med Ctr, Burlington, MA)
Clin Orthop Relat Res 469:87-94, 2011

Background.—The hospital cost of total knee arthroplasty (TKA) in the United States is a major growing expense for the Centers for Medicare & Medicaid Services (CMS). Many hospitals are unable to deliver TKA with profitable or breakeven economics under the current Diagnosis-Related Group (DRG) hospital reimbursement system.

Questions/Purposes.—The purposes of the current study were to (1) determine revenue, expenses, and profitability (loss) for TKA for all patients and for different payors; (2) define changes in utilization and unit costs associated with this operation; and (3) describe TKA cost control strategies to provide insight for hospitals to improve their economic results for TKA.

Results.—From 1991 to 2009, Lahey Clinic converted a $2172 loss per case on primary TKA in 1991 to a $2986 profit per case in 2008. The improved economics was associated with decreasing revenue in inflation-adjusted dollars and implementation of hospital cost control programs that reduced hospital expenses for TKA. Reduction of hospital length of stay and reduction of knee implant costs were the major drivers of hospital expense reduction.

Conclusions.—During the last 25 years, our economic experience with TKA is concerning. Hospital revenues have lagged behind inflation, hospital expenses have been reduced, and our institution is earning a profit. However, the margin for TKA is decreasing and Managed Medicare patients do not generate a profit. The erosion of hospital revenue for TKA will become a critical issue if it leads to economic losses for hospitals or reduced access to TKA.

Level of Evidence.—Level III, Economic and Decision Analyses. See Guidelines for Authors for a complete description of levels of evidence.

▶ By now, a review of my YEAR BOOK selections and commentary reflects my interest and bias. While I feel it represents enlightened insight, I realize this is open to discussion. Nonetheless, the article allows us to emphasize the prediction of an exponential growth of joint replacements in the next decade, most of the growth being in knee replacement. Unless the orthopedic community understands the threat this poses to the economics of health care delivery, we are in trouble. This nicely done study demonstrates what we also did at Mayo. By instituting standard protocols, competitively bidding the cost of implants, and communicating outcomes data to our colleagues, we were also able to improve the cost basis of our surgery, without compromise of quality. The 2 keys are nicely illustrated here: decrease in the cost of implants and of resources required to do the surgery, and decrease in the length of stay. We must, as a profession, drive toward these goals.

B. F. Morrey, MD

Preoperative Predictors of Returning to Work Following Primary Total Knee Arthroplasty
Styron JF, Barsoum WK, Smyth KA, et al (Case Western Reserve Univ, Cleveland, OH; Cleveland Clinic, OH)
J Bone Joint Surg Am 93:2-10, 2011

Background.—There is little in the literature to guide clinicians in advising patients regarding their return to work following a primary total knee arthroplasty. In this study, we aimed to identify which factors are important in estimating a patient's time to return to work following primary total knee arthroplasty, how long patients can anticipate being off from work, and the types of jobs to which patients are able to return following primary total knee arthroplasty.

Methods.—A prospective cohort study was performed in which patients scheduled for a primary total knee arthroplasty completed a validated questionnaire preoperatively and at four to six weeks, three months, and six months postoperatively. The questionnaire assessed the patient's occupational physical demands, ability to perform job responsibilities, physical status, and motivation to return to work as well as factors that may impact his or her recovery and other workplace characteristics. Two survival analysis models were constructed to evaluate the time to return to work either at least part-time or full-time. Acceleration factors were calculated to indicate the relative percentage of time until the patient returned to work.

Results.—The median time to return to work was 8.9 weeks. Patients who reported a sense of urgency about returning to work were found to return in half the time taken by other employees (acceleration factor = 0.468; p < 0.001). Other preoperative factors associated with a faster return to work included being female (acceleration factor = 0.783), self-employment (acceleration factor = 0.792), higher mental health scores (acceleration factor = 0.891), higher physical function scores (acceleration factor = 0.809), higher Functional Comorbidity Index scores (acceleration factor = 0.914), and a handicap accessible workplace (acceleration factor = 0.736). A slower return to work was associated with having less pain preoperatively (acceleration factor = 1.132), having a more physically demanding job (acceleration factor = 1.116), and receiving Workers' Compensation (acceleration factor = 4.360).

Conclusions.—Although the physical demands of a patient's job have a moderate influence on the patient's ability to return to work following a primary total knee arthroplasty, the patient's characteristics, particularly motivation, play a more important role.

▶ As we increase the rate of performing knee replacement at a break neck rate, more and more procedures are being performed on the working aged patient. The study is therefore worthwhile, but the findings are a bit intuitive. Those who possess a greater motivation return more rapidly. That workers' compensation continues to be the readily identified negative factor is no surprise, but this study quantifies this negative impact factor. It is worthy to note that less pain before the surgery is a negative factor, at least as related to return to work.

B. F. Morrey, MD

Do Residents Perform TKAs Using Computer Navigation as Accurately as Consultants?

Schnurr C, Eysel P, König DP (LVR Clinic of Orthopedic Surgery, Viersen, Germany; Univ of Cologne, Germany)
Orthopedics 34:1-7, 2011

The implantation of a total knee arthroplasty (TKA) is a milestone in a resident's surgical training. Studies demonstrate higher loosening rates after TKA by inexperienced surgeons. Alignment outliers should be avoided to achieve a long implant survival. Therefore, our study questioned whether residents implant knee prostheses using computer navigation as accurately as experienced consultants.

The data for 662 consecutive TKAs were analyzed retrospectively. The operations were performed by 4 consultants (n=555) and 5 residents under supervision by a consultant (n=107). Cutting errors were recorded from the navigation data. The postoperative mechanical axis and operation time were recorded. Operation time was significantly prolonged if residents performed the operation vs consultants (139 vs 122 minutes, respectively). The analysis of cutting errors within each surgeon's first 20 navigated operations resulted in no significant difference between residents and consultants. During the subsequent operations, a trend toward a more accurate placement of the prosthesis was detected for consultants. The rate of outliers with a mechanical axis deviation >2° was low and did not significantly differ between residents and consultants (3.7% vs 2.3%, respectively).

Our study shows that residents implant their first TKA using computer navigation as accurately as experienced consultants. However, the residents' operations take longer and therefore incur additional costs for the teaching clinic.

▶ Being from an academic institution responsible for resident teaching, we constantly struggle with the ethics of allowing an inexperienced surgeon to perform surgery. The introduction of navigation certainly assists in the objective measurement of placement accuracy. We can conclude from this study that allowing supervised resident surgery does not substantively compromise the technical accuracy of the procedure. In addition to the increased cost from prolonged surgery, we do also have concern about an increased complication rate, even though this was not demonstrated in this study.

B. F. Morrey, MD

What is the Evidence for Total Knee Arthroplasty in Young Patients?: A Systematic Review of the Literature
Keeney JA, Eunice S, Pashos G, et al (Washington Univ School of Medicine, St Louis, MO)
Clin Orthop Relat Res 469:574-583, 2011

Background.—TKA is commonly performed to treat advanced inflammatory and degenerative knee arthritis. With increasing use in younger patients, it is important to define the best practices to enhance clinical performance and implant longevity.

Questions/Purposes.—We systematically reviewed the literature to assess: (1) how TKAs perform in young patients; (2) whether the TKA is a durable procedure for young patients, and (3) what guidance the literature outlines for TKA in young patients.

TABLE 3.—Surgical Techniques and Outcomes in Studies of TKAs in Patients 55 Years and Younger

Study	Level of Evidence	Change in Clinical Score	Change in KS Functional Score	Radiographic Lucency	Reported Failure Mechanisms	Revision Surgeries	Component Survival Rate
Stuart and Rand [34]	IV Retrospective case series	32 points*	Not reported	18%	Patellar revision	2	100%—5 years
Ranawat et al. [28]	IV Retrospective case series	41.3 points†	Not reported	30%	Global radiolucency	2	96%—10 years
Stern et al. [32]	IV Retrospective case series	37 points†	Not reported	22%	Patellar revision	4	94%—6.2 years
Dalury et al. [6]	IV Retrospective case series (prospectively collected)	56 points†	41 points	30%	Patellar fracture or loosening	3	Not reported
Diduch et al. [7]	IV Retrospective case series (prospectively collected)	37 points†	Not reported	9%	Patellar revision	7	87%—18 years
Gill et al. [11]	IV Mixed prospective/ retrospective case series	37.4 points†	Not reported	22%	Infection/aseptic loosening	2	96.5%—18 years
Duffy et al. [10]	IV Retrospective case series	48 points†	15 points	None	Instability/patellar fracture	7	99%—10 years
Lonner et al. [22]	IV Retrospective case series	41 points†	35 points	None	Wear/loosening	3	90.6%—8 years
Hofmann et al. [16]	IV Retrospective case series	31 points†	39 points	None	None reported	0	Not reported
Mont et al. [24]	IV Retrospective case series	40 points†	Not reported	20%	Pain	1	Not reported
Crowder et al. [4]	IV Retrospective case series	48 points†	Not reported	None	Wear/osteolysis	6	100%—15 years
Tai and Cross [35]	IV Retrospective case series	47 points†	26 points	None	None reported	2	97.5%—12 years
Duffy et al. [9]	IV Retrospective case series	56 points†	26 points	3.8%	Instability/wear/osteolysis	11	85%—15 years

Editor's Note: Please refer to original journal article for full references.
*Hospital for Special Surgery.
†Knee Society clinical score.

Methods.—We searched the literature between 1950 and 2009 for all studies reporting on TKAs for patients younger than 55 years that documented clinical and radiographic assessments with a minimum 2-year followup. Thirteen studies, reporting on 908 TKAs performed for 671 patients, met these criteria.

Results.—Mean Knee Society clinical and functional scores increased by 47 and 37 points, respectively. Implant survivorship was reported between 90.6% and 99% during the first decade and between 85% and 96.5% during the second decade of followup. The literature does not direct specific techniques for TKA for young patients.

Conclusions.—TKA provides surgeon-measured clinical and functional improvements with a moderate increase in second-decade implant failures. Improvements in study design and reporting will be beneficial to guide decisions regarding implant selection and surgical technique.

Level of Evidence.—Level IV, therapeutic study. See Guidelines for Authors for a complete description of levels of evidence (Table 3).

▶ Because the clinical outcomes of total knee replacement are so reliable, there are less issues to discuss than in the past. One exception to this, however, is that of the long-term outcome in the young patient. Because few practices have sufficient numbers to address this question in a definitive fashion, an analytical review of the literature is appropriate. The methodology is becoming familiar to the orthopedic surgeon (Fig 1 in the original article). This review documents and quantifies what we tell our patients, specifically, the long-term survival is not as good in the young patient (Table 3). The reader is advised to note the survival rates that are reported and, especially, the wide range from the different authors. What remains to be demonstrated is whether the differences are because of the reporting criteria, the design of the implant, or the skill of the surgeon. I suspect it is a combination of all 3 variables.

B. F. Morrey, MD

A Prospective Randomized Study of Minimally Invasive Total Knee Arthroplasty Compared with Conventional Surgery
Wülker N, Lambermont JP, Sacchetti L, et al (Tübingen Univ Hosp, Germany; Univ Hosp CHU André Vesalé, Montigny-le-Tilleul, Belgium; General Hosp, Modena, Italy; et al)
J Bone Joint Surg Am 92:1584-1590, 2010

Background.—Despite intense debate regarding whether minimally invasive techniques for total knee arthroplasty improve clinical outcomes over standard techniques, few prospective randomized trials addressing this debate are available in the literature. We therefore designed this multicenter study to assess the overall safety and effectiveness of a minimally invasive approach without the use of computer navigation in comparison with conventional knee arthroplasty.

Methods.—We prospectively randomized 134 patients (101 women and thirty-three men, with an average age of 70.1 years) to undergo surgery for total knee arthroplasty with use of either minimally invasive knee instruments (sixty-six patients) or a standard approach (sixty-eight patients). The follow-up period was one year.

Results.—On the basis of our sample size, no significant difference was detected between the groups in any of the relevant clinical areas assessed: total range of motion, Knee Society total and function scores, and visual analog scores for pain and activities of daily living. Patients who underwent minimally invasive surgery had a longer mean surgical time (by 5.6 minutes) and had less mean blood loss (by 17 mL). Radiographic measurements demonstrated reliable implant positioning in both groups. Seven patients in each group had an adverse event related to their procedure.

Conclusions.—On the basis of the numbers, no significant advantage to minimally invasive total knee arthroplasty over a conventional technique was observed. Greater sample sizes and a longer follow-up period are required to fully determine the long-term safety and efficacy of this minimally invasive surgical technique.

▶ This article is included just to reinforce the information that has been conveyed in the past. In spite of additional experience, refinement of technique, and possibly improved patient selection, minimally invasive techniques seem to offer no added value. This may be concluded with certainty with the reported technique, and my interpretation of the literature is that this remains true in general. Given the learning curve, high success rate of conventional techniques, and increased complications, at least in the early stages, minimally invasive techniques are to be reserved by those developing them, by those investigating their value, or by those surgeons with demonstrated superior outcomes from such a procedure.

B. F. Morrey, MD

Changes in hip fracture rate before and after total knee replacement due to osteoarthritis: a population-based cohort study

Prieto-Alhambra D, Javaid MK, Maskell J, et al (Univ of Oxford, UK; et al)
Ann Rheum Dis 70:134-138, 2011

Objectives.—Patients with knee osteoarthritis have an increase in bone mass but no corresponding decrease in risk of fracture. This study describes the rates of hip fracture in subjects with knee osteoarthritis before and after having a total knee replacement (TKR), compared with matched controls.

Methods.—A population-based prospective cohort study was conducted. The study population included, from the General Practice Research Database (UK), patients 40 years and older, undergoing TKR between 1986 and end-2006 for knee osteoarthritis as 'cases' (n = 20 033). Five disease-free controls (n = 100 165) were randomly selected, and matched for age, gender and practice. Hip fractures were ascertained using READ codes, and yearly rates of hip fracture and rate differences were calculated for the 5 years before and after surgery, using Poisson regression. Stratified analyses were performed by age and history of fracture.

Results.—Hip fracture rates were non-significantly reduced compared with controls before the operation. In the year after TKR, risk increased significantly (RR 1.58; 95% CI 1.14 to 2.19). Rates then declined to equal those of controls by 3 years, and continued decreasing until the end of follow-up; corresponding RR were not significant. The increased risk is greatest in younger ages and in those without previous fracture.

Conclusions.—The association between knee osteoarthritis and fractures is time-dependent, which may explain the current controversy in the literature. The association is also modified by TKR: subjects have a higher rate of hip fracture than matched controls after TKR, although the rates may eventually decrease.

▶ As more and more joint replacements are preformed, and as the procedures are done in the older patient, studies such as this become relevant. This is especially true from a demographic public health perspective. I suspect few of us have considered the increased risk of a patient undergoing knee replacement for having a hip fracture. Nonetheless, this well-conceived and well-conducted study demonstrates just that. What does it mean? I might advise my patient that the risk is very slightly increased in the first couple of years after surgery in those settings where such information would be of value and would be heeded.

B. F. Morrey, MD

Fast-track surgery for bilateral total knee replacement
Husted H, Troelsen A, Otte KS, et al (Hvidovre Univ Hosp, Copenhagen, Denmark)
J Bone Joint Surg [Br] 93-B:351-356, 2011

Bilateral simultaneous total knee replacement (TKR) has been considered by some to be associated with increased morbidity and mortality. Our study analysed the outcome of 150 consecutive, but selected, bilateral simultaneous TKRs and compared them with that of 271 unilateral TKRs in a standardised fast-track setting. The procedures were performed between 2003 and 2009.

Apart from staying longer in hospital (mean 4.7 days (2 to 16) versus 3.3 days (1 to 25)) and requiring more blood transfusions, the outcome at three months and two years was similar or better in the bilateral simultaneous TKR group in regard to morbidity, mortality, satisfaction, the range of movement, pain, the use of a walking aid and the ability to return to work and to perform activities of daily living. Bilateral simultaneous

TKR can therefore be performed as a fast-track procedure with excellent results.

▶ The question of the safety of bilateral knee replacement under the same anesthetic remains controversial. This article does not definitively answer the question. The sample size may not be large enough to definitively address the safety issue because complications occur at such a low rate. But this is an adequate experience to demonstrate efficacy, and it clearly underscores the advantages from a patient recovery perspective. I have performed bilateral knee replacement for more than 30 years and continue to do so. I should mention that I do use an extramedullary alignment system on these patients.

B. F. Morrey, MD

Comparison Between Standard and High-Flexion Posterior-Stabilized Rotating-Platform Mobile-Bearing Total Knee Arthroplasties: A Randomized Controlled Study
Choi WC, Lee S, Seong SC, et al (Seoul Natl Univ Hosp, South Korea)
J Bone Joint Surg Am 92:2634-2642, 2010

Background.—A high-flexion posterior-stabilized rotating-platform mobile-bearing prosthesis was designed in an attempt to improve the range of motion after total knee arthroplasty without compromising the theoretical advantages of the posterior-stabilized rotating-platform mobile-bearing system. The aim of this study was to compare the outcomes of standard and high-flexion posterior-stabilized rotating-platform mobile-bearing total knee arthroplasties.

Methods.—One hundred and seventy knees were randomly allocated to receive either a standard (n = 85) or a high-flexion (n = 85) posterior-stabilized rotating-platform mobile-bearing prosthesis and were followed prospectively for a minimum of two years. Ranges of motion, functional outcomes determined with use of standard scoring systems, and radiographic measurements were assessed. In addition, patients' abilities to perform activities requiring deep knee flexion and patient satisfaction were evaluated with use of questionnaires.

Results.—The average postoperative maximal flexion was 130° for the knees with the standard design and 128° for those with the high-flexion design, and the difference was not significant. The two prosthetic designs also did not differ significantly with regard to the Knee Society scores; Hospital for Special Surgery (HSS) scores; or the scores on the pain, stiffness, and function subscales of the Western Ontario and McMaster Universities Osteoarthritis Index (WOMAC). In addition, the numbers of knees able to perform deep-flexion-related activities and the rates of patient satisfaction were similar in the two study groups.

Conclusions.—This prospective randomized study revealed no significant differences between standard and high-flexion posterior-stabilized

TABLE 2.—Comparison of Postoperative Ranges of Knee Motion Between the Groups

	Intention-to-Treat Population			Per-Protocol Population		
	Standard (N = 85)	High Flexion (N = 85)	P Value	Standard (N = 74)	High Flexion (N = 76)	P Value
Flexion contracture* *(deg)*	2 ± 3.9 (0-10)	2 ± 3.6 (0-15)	0.705[†]	1 ± 3.9 (0-10)	2 ± 3.8 (0-15)	0.212[†]
Active maximal flexion* *(deg)*	130 ± 10.4 (100-150)	128 ± 11.1 (95-150)	0.281[†]	130 ± 10.7 (100-150)	128 ± 11.5 (95-150)	0.384[†]
Total range of motion* *(deg)*	129 ± 11.6 (95-150)	127 ± 12.6 (90-150)	0.278[†]	129 ± 11.7 (95-150)	126 ± 13.0 (90-150)	0.261[†]

*The values are presented as the mean and the standard deviation with the range in parentheses.
[†]Student t test.

rotating-platform mobile-bearing total knee prostheses in terms of clinical or radiographic outcomes or range of motion at a minimum of two years postoperatively (Table 2).

► Because the total knee arthroplasty is such a successful operation, it is difficult to improve on the results of the generic condylar design. The prospect that the mobile-bearing concept would improve motion and decrease wear has not, to date, proven to be a reality. In addition, the potential to improve motion by design, as opposed to technique, has also been the source of interest in recent years. This study tests the hypothesis: improved function from a high-flex mobile-bearing knee. Unfortunately, as with the majority of other studies, these expectations are not realized when compared with a standard design (Table 2). The sample size is adequate; the follow-up is rather abbreviated, averaging only 28 months. So, the issue of improved wear cannot be addressed with this study. However, it does, once again, confirm that the hoped-for value of this design has not been realized in practice.

B. F. Morrey, MD

A Second Decade Lifetable Survival Analysis of the Oxford Unicompartmental Knee Arthroplasty
Price AJ, Svard U (Nuffield Orthopaedic Centre, Headington, Oxford, UK; Skaraborgs Sjukhus Kärnsjukhuset, Skövde, Sweden)
Clin Orthop Relat Res 469:174-179, 2011

Background.—The role of unicompartmental arthroplasty in managing osteoarthritis of the knee remains controversial. The Oxford medial unicompartmental arthroplasty employs a fully congruent mobile bearing intended to reduce wear and increase the lifespan of the implant. Long-term second decade results are required to establish if the design aim can be met.

Questions/Purposes.—We report the (1) 20-year survivorship for the Oxford mobile bearing medial unicompartmental knee arthroplasty; (2) reasons for the revisions; and (3) time to revision.

Methods.—We reviewed a series of 543 patients who underwent 682 medial Oxford meniscal bearing unicompartmental knee arthroplasties performed between 1983 and January 2005. The mean age at implantation was 69.7 years (range, 48—94 years). The median followup was 5.9 years (range, 0.5 to 22 years). One hundred and forty-one patients (172 knees) died. None were lost to followup. The primary outcome was 20-year survival, a key variable in assessing the longevity of arthroplasty.

Results.—The 16-year all cause revision cumulative survival rate was 91.0% (CI 6.4, 71 at risk) and survival was maintained to 20 years (91.0%, CI 36.2, 14 at risk). There had been 29 revision procedures: 10 for lateral arthrosis, nine for component loosening, five for infection, two bearing dislocations, and three for unexplained pain. In addition, five patients had undergone bearing exchange, four for dislocation and one for bearing fracture. The mean time to revision was 3.3 years (range, 0.3—8.9 years).

Conclusions.—Mobile bearing unicompartmental knee arthroplasty is durable during the second decade after implantation.

Level of Evidence.—Level IV, therapeutic study. See the Guidelines for Authors for a complete description of levels of evidence.

▶ For many, the Oxford unicompartment mobile bearing replacement prosthesis is the classic unireplacement. It represents one of the oldest continuous use unireplacement systems. In addition, it also is an example of one of the oldest mobile bearing joint replacement options (Fig 1 in the original article). The excellent outcomes are truly impressive. This series is of sufficient size and duration to draw meaningful conclusions. In spite of this being a pioneer concept, the > 90% survival at 20 years is truly impressive. The complication rate is also considered modest by any standard. The authors are to be commended for sharing this experience.

B. F. Morrey, MD

Wear Damage in Mobile-bearing TKA is as Severe as That in Fixed-bearing TKA
Kelly NH, Fu RH, Wright TM, et al (Hosp for Special Surgery, NY)
Clin Orthop Relat Res 469:123-130, 2011

Background.—Mobile-bearing TKAs reportedly have no clinical superiority over fixed-bearing TKAs, but a potential benefit is improved polyethylene wear behavior.

Questions/Purposes.—We asked whether extent of damage and wear patterns would be less severe on retrieved mobile-bearing TKAs than on fixed-bearing TKAs and if correlations with patient demographics could explain differences in extent or locations of damage.

Methods.—We performed damage grading and mapping of 48 mobile-bearing TKAs retrieved due to osteolysis/loosening, infection, stiffness, instability or malpositioning. Visual grading used stereomicroscopy to identify damage, and a grade was assigned based on extent and severity. Each damage mode was then mapped onto a photograph of the implant surface, and the area affected was calculated.

Results.—Marked wear damage occurred on both surfaces, with burnishing, scratching, and pitting the dominant modes. Damage occurred over a large portion of both surfaces, exceeding the available articular borders in nearly 30% of implants. Wear of mobile-bearing surfaces included marked third-body debris. Damage on tibiofemoral and mobile-bearing surfaces was not correlated with patient BMI or component alignment. Damage on mobile-bearing surfaces was positively correlated with length of implantation and was greater in implants removed for osteolysis or instability than in those removed for stiffness or infection.

Conclusions.—Each bearing surface in mobile-bearing implants was damaged to an extent similar to that in fixed-bearing implants, making the combined damage score higher than that for fixed-bearing implants. Mobile-bearing TKAs did not improve wear damage, providing another argument against the superiority of these implants over fixed-bearing implants.

▶ And so it goes. I, and others, felt the mobile-bearing knee would represent a true substantive advance over the last great total knee design breakthrough, the generic condylar design. This expectation has not been realized clinically, as patients did not exhibit any improved motion with any of the designs. The improved wear characteristics have also not been realized clinically. This retrieval study offers the sobering but logical explanation. In spite of the polishing and design features, the mobile bearing tends to wear on both surfaces (Fig 2a-d in the original article). Hence, more wear and more debris. Too bad.

B. F. Morrey, MD

The John Insall Award: Control-matched Evaluation of Painful Patellar Crepitus After Total Knee Arthroplasty
Dennis DA, Kim RH, Johnson DR, et al (Colorado Joint Replacement, Denver; Denver-Vail Orthopedics, Parker, CO; et al)
Clin Orthop Relat Res 469:10-17, 2011

Background.—Patellar crepitus (PC) is reported in up to 14% of subjects implanted with cruciate-substituting total knee arthroplasty (TKA). Numerous etiologies of PC have been proposed.

Questions/Purposes.—We determined when painful PC typically occurs postoperatively and compared patients undergoing primary TKA who developed painful PC requiring subsequent surgery with a matched group without this complication to identify clinical, radiographic, and surgical variables associated with this complication.

Methods.—From the databases of two institutions (greater than 4000 TKAs), we identified 60 patients who required surgery for painful PC from 2002 to 2008. This group was then compared with an identified control group of 60 TKA subjects without PC who were matched for the key variables of age, gender, and body mass index to determine clinical, radiographic, and surgical factors associated with the development of PC.

Results.—The mean time to presentation of PC was 10.9 months. The incidence of PC correlated with a greater number of previous knee surgeries, decreased patellar component size, decreased composite patellar thickness, shorter preoperative and postoperative patellar tendon length, increased posterior femoral condylar offset, use of smaller femoral components and thicker tibial polyethylene inserts, and placement of the femoral component in a flexed posture.

Conclusions.—Many of the factors associated with an increased incidence of postoperative PC such as shortened patellar tendon length, use of smaller patellar components, decreased patellar composite thickness, and increased posterior femoral condylar offset may all increase quadriceps tendon contact forces against the superior aspect of the intercondylar box, increasing the risk of fibrosynovial proliferation and entrapment within the intercondylar region of the femoral component. Based on these findings, the authors recommend use of larger patellar components when possible, avoid oversection of the patella or increasing posterior femoral condylar offset, and advising patients preoperatively who have had previous knee surgery or demonstrate a shortened patellar tendon length of an increased risk of development of postoperative patellar crepitus.

Level of Evidence.—Level III, therapeutic study. See Guidelines for Authors for a complete description of levels of evidence.

▶ For the record, I avoid the posterior cruciate—substituting posterior-stabilized (PS) knee design. An article will be published in the *Journal of Bone & Joint Surgery, American Volume* this year that justifies this practice. Regardless, patellar symptoms are well recognized with the PS knee, and this comprehensive study does shed some light as to the reasons. Numerous correlations were made, but at the end of the day, the surgeon can control the patella implant size and the composite thickness to some extent. I find it interesting that the authors do not offer as an additional solution, in the high-risk patient, the characteristics they nicely assess, simply to avoid the PS design.

B. F. Morrey, MD

Management of Intraoperative Medial Collateral Ligament Injury During TKA

Lee G-C, Lotke PA (Univ of Pennsylvania, Philadelphia)
Clin Orthop Relat Res 469:64-68, 2011

Background.—Intraoperative injuries to the medial collateral ligament are often unrecognized and failure to appropriately manage ligament loss may result in knee instability and loosening.

Questions/Purposes.—We compared the functional scores in patients with iatrogenic injury to the medial collateral ligament (MCL) treated with additional constraint to those without.

Methods.—We retrospectively reviewed the records of all 1478 patients (1650 knees) who underwent primary TKA between 1998 and 2004. Thirty-seven patients (2.2%) had recognized intraoperative injury to the MCL; the remaining 1441 patients (1613 knees) served as controls. We attempted to repair the ligament in 14 patients; increased prosthetic constraint over that planned was used in 30 of the 37 patients. We determined Knee Society scores (KSS) in all patients. Three patients were lost to

TABLE 1.—Clinical Results after Intraoperative Medial Collateral Ligament (MCL) Injury

Clinical Outcome	Study Group MCL Injury (n = 37)	Control Group No MCL Injury (n = 1613)	Constraint Only MCL Injury + TCIII (n = 30)
KS pain	81	91	88
	p < 0.01		p = 0.19
KS function	74	87	83
	p < 0.01		p = 0.10

MCL = Medial collateral ligament; KS = Knee Society.

followup. The minimum followup was 36 months (average, 54 months; range, 36−120 months).

Results.—The mean KSS for all MCL injury knees for pain and function averaged 81 and 74 points, respectively, compared with 91 and 87 for the control group. However, in the 30 knees in which the MCL insufficiency was treated with increased constraint, the mean scores for pain and function increased to 88 and 83 points, respectively. Four of the seven patients treated without increased prosthetic constraint were revised for instability; no revisions for instability were performed in the 37 patients treated with additional constraint.

Conclusions.—Recognition of MCL injury during TKA is crucial, since using nonstabilizing inserts was associated with residual instability requiring revision.

Level of Evidence.—Level IV, therapeutic study. See Guidelines for Authors for a complete description of levels of evidence (Table 1).

▶ While uncommon, the release of the medial collateral ligament during total knee replacement is problematic at best. This retrospective study does, however, direct our thought process and implant design selection. The authors clearly show that leaving the deficiency or repairing it tends to be unsuccessful. Fortunately, the ligament-stabilizing design, available in all comprehensive systems, does effectively address the problem. So, if it occurs, alter the plan and use a more constrained design—but not a hinged implant.

B. F. Morrey, MD

Deep Vein Thrombosis After Total Knee Arthroplasty in Asian Patients Without Prophylactic Anticoagulation
Chung L-H, Chen W-M, Chen C-F, et al (Taipei Veterans General Hosp, Taiwan, Republic of China)
Orthopedics 34:1-5, 2011

Deep vein thrombosis (DVT) is an important complication following total knee arthroplasty (TKA). However, the incidence of DVT is generally underestimated due to subclinical or minor symptoms and signs. In

Western countries, prophylactic agents against DVT are administered routinely after TKA. However, in Asia, no regular prophylaxis is generally given to patients undergoing TKA.

This article presents a prospective study evaluating the incidence of DVT in 724 consecutive Taiwanese patients who underwent TKA without prophylactic anticoagulation therapy. Of these, 328 patients (45.3%) showed positive Homan's sign with calf swelling >3 cm. Ultrasonographic examination revealed the overall incidence of DVT to be 8.6% (62/724). The incidence of DVT was significantly higher in women ($P=.035$), in patients who underwent bilateral TKA ($P=.002$), and in patients with a body mass index ≥ 30 kg/m^2 ($P=.026$). The incidence of DVT appeared to be increased in patients with higher tourniquet time; however, the difference was not statistically significant. In all of the suspected cases of DVT, the symptoms subsided after the administration of enoxaparin with uneventful follow-up. No patient developed pulmonary embolism.

Our results showed a relatively high incidence of DVT in an Asian population following TKA. We therefore consider that following TKA, prophylactic anticoagulation therapy should be administered to high-risk patients.

▶ Because the topic of deep vein thrombosis prophylaxis is one of the most controversial in the orthopedic literature, this study caught my attention. The main benefit is to note that routine avoidance by medication is not practiced in Taiwan. Of particular note is that the findings of the ultrasound prompted the authors to begin the practice of prophylaxis; there were zero clots detected without this treatment. There were no pulmonary embolic complications. Hence, I actually think their study justifies not beginning this treatment program. However, in this country, malpractice issues force our hand.

B. F. Morrey, MD

The Mark Coventry Award: Diagnosis of Early Postoperative TKA Infection Using Synovial Fluid Analysis
Bedair H, Ting N, Jacovides C, et al (Harvard Med School, Boston, MA; Rush Univ Med Ctr, Chicago, IL; Thomas Jefferson Univ School of Medicine, Philadelphia, PA)
Clin Orthop Relat Res 469:34-40, 2011

Background.—Synovial fluid white blood cell count is useful for diagnosing periprosthetic infections but the utility of this test in the early postoperative period remains unknown as hemarthrosis and postoperative inflammation may render standard cutoff values inaccurate.

Questions/Purposes.—We evaluated the diagnostic performance of four common laboratory tests, the synovial white blood cell count, differential, C-reactive protein, and erythrocyte sedimentation rate to detect infection in the first 6 weeks after primary TKA.

Methods.—We reviewed 11,964 primary TKAs and identified 146 that had a knee aspiration within 6 weeks of surgery. Infection was diagnosed in 19 of the 146 knees by positive cultures or gross purulence. We compared demographic information, time from surgery, and the laboratory test values between infected and noninfected knees to determine if any could identify infection early postoperatively. Receiver operating characteristic curves were constructed to determine optimal cutoff values for each of the test parameters.

Results.—Synovial white blood cell count (92,600 versus 4200 cells/µL), percentage of polymorphonuclear cells (89.6% versus 76.9%), and C-reactive protein (171 versus 88 mg/L) were higher in the infected group. The optimal synovial white blood cell cutoff was 27,800 cells/µL (sensitivity, 84%; specificity, 99%; positive predictive value, 94%; negative predictive value, 98%) for diagnosing infection. The optimal cutoff for the differential was 89% polymorphonuclear cells and for C-reactive protein 95 mg/L.

Conclusions.—With a cutoff of 27,800 cells/µL, synovial white blood cell count predicted infection within 6 weeks after primary TKA with a positive predicted value of 94% and a negative predictive value of 98%. The use of standard cutoff values for this parameter (~ 3000 cells/µL) would have led to unnecessary reoperations.

Level of Evidence.—Level II, diagnostic study. See Guidelines for Authors for a complete description of levels of evidence.

▶ I personally am very much attracted to this type of study and report. It has direct and apparently valid application to the clinical practice. This article raises the bar regarding the threshold for white blood cells per microliter. The prior standard of 3000 cells/µL appears far too low based on these data. The surgeon should consider that counts below 27 000 or 27 500 are less worrisome for infection. The findings of the other inflammatory markers are also of interest. The real message is that there is no single parameter that we can completely rely on. The surgeon should be familiar with the thresholds for each of the 4 tests discussed herein.

B. F. Morrey, MD

6 Shoulder

Introduction

Topics of the shoulder continue to relate to issues of rotator cuff disease, instability, and a contrast of arthroscopic versus open reconstruction. This year's selections follow the same theme since these are the most relevant issues. We have provided some information regarding shoulder replacement, but we have intentionally limited the more sophisticated contributions relating to the reverse shoulder and complications of shoulder arthroplasty. The indications and role of the reverse shoulder replacement design, however, are included since it is felt that this is an important emerging option and an awareness of which the orthopedic surgeon would find of value.

Bernard F. Morrey, MD

Measuring shoulder injury function: Common scales and checklists
Slobogean GP, Slobogean BL (Univ of British Columbia, Vancouver, Canada; British Columbia Children's Hosp, Vancouver, Canada)
Injury 42:248-252, 2011

The increasing shift towards patient-centred healthcare has lead to an emergence of patient-reported outcome instruments to quantify functional outcomes in orthopaedic patients. Unfortunately, selecting an instrument for use in a shoulder trauma population is often problematic because most shoulder instruments were initially designed for use with chronic shoulder pathology patients. To ensure an instrument is valid, reliable, and sensitive to clinical changes, it is important to obtain psychometric evidence of its use in the target population.

Four commonly used shoulder outcome instruments are reviewed in this paper: American Shoulder and Elbow Surgeons Standardized Shoulder Assessment Form (ASES); Constant–Murley shoulder score (CMS); Disabilities of Arm, Shoulder, and Hand (DASH); Oxford Shoulder Score (OSS). Each instrument was reviewed for floor or ceiling effects, validity, reliability, responsiveness, and interpretability. Additionally, evidence of each instrument's psychometric properties was sought in shoulder fracture populations.

Based on the current literature, each instrument has limited amounts of evidence to support their use in shoulder trauma populations. Overall,

TABLE 1.—Summary of Outcome Instruments

Instrument	Scored Domains	Number of Scored Items	Percentage Contribution to Final Score	Examples of Published Use in Shoulder Fracture Populations
ASES	Pain	1	50%	Clavicle[9,32,34]
	ADLs	10	50%	Proximal humerus[49]
Constant	Pain	1	15%	Clavicle[7,33]
	ADLs	7	20%	Glenoid neck[39]
	ROM	4	40%	Proximal humerus[3,13,47]
	Strength	1	25%	
DASH	ADLs	21	70%	Clavicle[46]
	Social activities	1	3%	Proximal humerus[21]
	Work activities	1	3%	Scapula[23,25]
	Symptoms	5	17%	
	Sleeping	1	3%	
	Confidence	1	3%	
Oxford	Pain	4	33%	Glenoid neck[39]
	ADLs	8	67%	Proximal humerus[3,24]

ADLs − activities of daily living; ASES − American Shoulder and Elbow Surgeons Subjective Shoulder Assessment; Constant − Constant–Murley shoulder score; DASH − Disabilities of Arm, Shoulder, and Hand; Oxford − Oxford Shoulder Score.

Editor's Note: Please refer to original journal article for full references.

psychometric evaluations in isolated shoulder fracture populations remain scarce, and clinicians must remember that an instrument's properties are defined for the population tested and not the instrument. Therefore, caution must always be exercised when using an instrument that has not been fully evaluated in trauma populations (Table 1).

▶ This study addresses an issue of increasing relevance, not just to the shoulder, but also to the musculoskeletal system in general. How do we assess function, true impairment, and relevant improvement with intervention? This was a carefully designed study intending to answer this question using existing shoulder assessment tools. The authors point out that the most commonly used methods to assess status or function were not based on injury but rather on disease and intervention. As such, the existing tools (Table 1) are somewhat inadequate to accurately depict injury status. This issue is well known. Clearly, one tool cannot address all circumstances. The manner of documenting the status of the shoulder function after a brachial plexus injury cannot be the same as that to assess the performance of a professional baseball player with shoulder symptoms. This represents a work in progress.

B. F. Morrey, MD

Frozen shoulder: the effectiveness of conservative and surgical interventions—systematic review
Favejee MM, Huisstede BMA, Koes BW (Erasmus Univ Med Ctr, Rotterdam, The Netherlands)
Br J Sports Med 45:49-56, 2011

Background.—A variety of therapeutic interventions is available for restoring motion and diminishing pain in patients with frozen shoulder. An overview article concerning the evidence for the effectiveness of these interventions is lacking.

Objective.—To provide an evidence-based overview regarding the effectiveness of conservative and surgical interventions to treat the frozen shoulder.

Methods.—The Cochrane Library, PubMed, Embase, Cinahl and Pedro were searched for relevant systematic reviews and randomised clinical trials (RCTs). Two reviewers independently selected relevant studies, assessed the methodological quality and extracted data. A best-evidence synthesis was used to summarise the results.

Results.—Five Cochrane reviews and 18 RCTs were included studying the effectiveness of oral medication, injection therapy, physiotherapy, acupuncture, arthrographic distension and suprascapular nerve block (SSNB).

Conclusions.—We found strong evidence for the effectiveness of steroid injections and laser therapy in short-term and moderate evidence for steroid injections in mid-term follow-up. Moderate evidence was found in favour of mobilisation techniques in the short and long term, for the effectiveness of arthrographic distension alone and as an addition to active physiotherapy in the short term, for the effectiveness of oral steroids compared with no treatment or placebo in the short term, and for the effectiveness of SSNB compared with acupuncture, placebo or steroid injections. For other commonly used interventions no or only limited evidence of effectiveness was found. Most of the included studies reported short-term results, whereas symptoms of frozen shoulder may last up to 4 years. High quality RCTs studying long-term results are clearly needed in this field.

▶ Although decreasing in frequency, the frozen shoulder remains a frequently encountered problem. It continues to be a source of pain and frustration for the patient and an enigma for the surgeon. It is one of those interesting problems for which we have little explanation. This carefully constructed article reviews a vast amount of literature and confirms the modalities we have come to rely on: steroid injection, manipulation, and arthroscopic-assisted releases. One point of emphasis not usually considered is the potential for substantive chronicity, up to 4 years. This condition is begging for an explaination, but it does not appear to be near at hand.

B. F. Morrey, MD

Cigarette Smoking Increases the Risk for Rotator Cuff Tears

Baumgarten KM, Gerlach D, Galatz LM, et al (Orthopedic Inst, Sioux Falls, SD; Washington Univ School of Medicine, St Louis, MO)
Clin Orthop Relat Res 468:1534-1541, 2010

There is little available evidence regarding risk factors for rotator cuff tears. Cigarette smoking may be an important risk factor for rotator cuff disease. The purpose of this study was to determine if cigarette smoking correlates with an increased risk for rotator cuff tears in patients who present with shoulder pain. A questionnaire was administered to 586 consecutive patients 18 years of age or older who had a diagnostic shoulder ultrasound for unilateral, atraumatic shoulder pain with no history of shoulder surgery. Three hundred seventy-five patients had a rotator cuff tear and 211 patients did not. Data regarding cigarette smoking were obtained for 584 of 586 patients. A history of smoking (61.9% versus 48.3%), smoking within the last 10 years (35.2% versus 30.1%), mean duration of smoking (23.4 versus 20.2 years), mean packs per day of smoking (1.25 versus 1.10 packs per day), and mean pack-years of smoking (30.1 versus 22.0) correlated with an increased risk for rotator cuff tear. We observed a dose-dependent and time-dependent relationship between smoking and rotator cuff tears. We observed a strong association between smoking and rotator cuff disease. This may indicate smoking is an important risk factor for the development of rotator cuff tears.

Level of Evidence.—Level III, prognostic study. See Guidelines for Authors for a complete description of levels of evidence.

▶ I seem to gravitate to certain topics, one of which is the evil of smoking. This study would seem to provide sufficient evidence to support the correlation of smoking to the development of rotator cuff disease. Who would have guessed it? What's next?

B. F. Morrey, MD

Platelet-Rich Plasma Augmentation for Arthroscopic Rotator Cuff Repair: A Randomized Controlled Trial

Castricini R, Longo UG, De Benedetto M, et al (Ospedale Civile, Jesi, Italy; Campus Bio-Medico Univ, Via Alvaro del Portillo, Rome, Italy; Villa Maria Cecilia Hosp—GVM Care & Res, Cotignola-Ravenna, Italy; et al)
Am J Sports Med 39:258-265, 2011

Background.—After reinsertion on the humerus, the rotator cuff has limited ability to heal. Growth factor augmentation has been proposed to enhance healing in such procedure.

Purpose.—This study was conducted to assess the efficacy and safety of growth factor augmentation during rotator cuff repair.

TABLE 3.—Details of Constant Score for Each Group[a]

Constant Score	Group 1 (Without Augmentation With Platelet-Rich Fibrin Matrix [PRFM]) Preoperative	Postoperative	Group 2 (With PRFM Augmentation) Preoperative	Postoperative
Shoulder pain	3.1 (0-5)	14.3 (10-15)	3.6 (0-5)	14.3 (10-15)
Activities of daily living	10.1 (8-12)	18.8 (14-20)	9.8 (6-12)	19.3 (16-20)
Range of movement	26.5 (12-39)	38.8 (26-40)	26 (16-32)	39.1 (36-40)
Strength	3.2 (1-9)	16.5 (4-25)	2.6 (0-6)	15.7 (4-24)
Total score	42.9 (22-55)	88.4 (54-100)	42 (30-53)	88.4 (72-99)

[a]Average values are given, with the numbers in parentheses indicating the range of values.

Study Design.—Randomized controlled trial; Level of evidence, 1.

Methods.—Eighty-eight patients with a rotator cuff tear were randomly assigned by a computer-generated sequence to receive arthroscopic rotator cuff repair without (n = 45) or with (n = 43) augmentation with autologous platelet-rich fibrin matrix (PRFM). The primary end point was the postoperative difference in the Constant score between the 2 groups. The secondary end point was the integrity of the repaired rotator cuff, as evaluated by magnetic resonance imaging. Analysis was on an intention-to-treat basis.

Results.—All the patients completed follow-up at 16 months. There was no statistically significant difference in total Constant score when comparing the results of arthroscopic repair of the 2 groups (95% confidence interval, -3.43 to 3.9) ($P = .44$). There was no statistically significant difference in magnetic resonance imaging tendon score when comparing arthroscopic repair with or without PRFM ($P = .07$).

Conclusion.—Our study does not support the use of autologous PRFM for augmentation of a double-row repair of a small or medium rotator cuff tear to improve the healing of the rotator cuff. Our results are applicable to small and medium rotator cuff tears; it is possible that PRFM may be beneficial for large and massive rotator cuff tears. Also, given the heterogeneity of PRFM preparation products available on the market, it is possible that other preparations may be more effective (Table 3).

▶ We have discussed the hot issue of platelet-rich plasma (PRP) in previous selections. We chose to include this randomized study to highlight the central issue. In spite of the enthusiasm demonstrated by patients, surgeons, and especially the orthopedic industry, PRP is not a panacea. In this specific study, the addition of PRP offers no added value to the traditional repair of the rotator cuff. The real take-home message is that the use of PRP, like bone growth supplements, is a costly adjunct. Its use should be predicated on demonstrated value and that alone.

B. F. Morrey, MD

The Arthroscopic Management of Partial-Thickness Rotator Cuff Tears: A Systematic Review of the Literature

Strauss EJ, Salata MJ, Kercher J, et al (Rush Univ Med Ctr, Chicago, IL)

Arthroscopy 27:568-580, 2011

Purpose.—There is currently limited information available in the orthopaedic surgery literature regarding the appropriate management of symptomatic partial-thickness rotator cuff tears.

Methods.—A systematic search was performed in PubMed, EMBASE, CINAHL (Cumulative Index to Nursing and Allied Health Literature), and the Cochrane Central Register of Controlled Trials of all published literature pertaining to the arthroscopic management of partial-thickness rotator cuff tears. Inclusion criteria were all studies that reported clinical outcomes after arthroscopic treatment of both articular-sided and bursal-sided lesions using a validated outcome scoring system and a minimum of 12 months of follow-up. Data abstracted from the selected studies included tear type and location (articular *v* bursal sided), treatment approach, postoperative rehabilitation protocol, outcome scores, patient satisfaction, and postoperative imaging results.

Results.—Sixteen studies met the inclusion criteria and were included for the final analysis. Seven of the studies treated partial-thickness rotator cuff tears with debridement with or without an associated subacromial decompression, 3 performed a takedown and repair, 5 used a transtendon repair technique, and 1 used a transosseous repair method. Among the 16 studies reviewed, excellent postoperative outcomes were reported in 28.7% to 93% of patients treated. In all 12 studies with available preoperative baseline data, treatment resulted in significant improvement in shoulder symptoms and function. For high-grade lesions, the data support arthroscopic takedown and repair, transtendon repairs, and transosseous repairs, with all 3 techniques providing a high percentage of excellent results. Debridement of partial-thickness tears of less than 50% of the tendon's thickness with or without a concomitant acromioplasty also results in good to excellent surgical outcomes; however, a 6.5% to 34.6% incidence of progression to full-thickness tears is present.

Conclusions.—This systematic review of 16 clinical studies showed that significant variation is present in the results obtained after the arthroscopic management of partial-thickness rotator cuff tears. What can be supported by the available data is that tears that involve less than 50% of the tendon can be treated with good results by debridement of the tendon with or without a formal acromioplasty, although subsequent tear progression may occur. When the tear is greater than 50%, surgical intervention focusing on repair has been successful. There is no evidence to suggest a differential in outcome for tear completion and repair versus transtendon repair of these lesions because both methods have been shown to result in favorable outcomes.

TABLE 3.—Study Demographics of Articles Included in Current Systematic Review of Arthroscopic Management of Partial-Thickness Rotator Cuff Tears

Author	Year	No. of Shoulders	Mean Age (yrs)	Tear Type	Treatment	Mean Follow-Up (mo)	% Follow-Up
Spencer[32]	2010	20	41	Articular sided	TT repair	29	100%
Castricini et al.[21]	2009	33	53.3	Articular sided	TT repair	33	94%
Castagna et al.[20]	2009	70	56.7	Articular sided	TT repair	32.4	77%
Kamath et al.[25]	2009	47	53	A3 tears	TD and repair	39	89.4%
Porat et al.[29]	2008	51	59.7	Articular sided	TD and repair	42.4	70.6%
Liem et al.[27]	2008	46	59.2	A1 and A2 tears	Debridement with SAD	50.3	100%
Tauber et al.[33]	2008	16	NR	A2 and A3 tears	TO repair	18	100%
Reynolds et al.[30]	2008	82	25.6	Articular sided	Debridement without SAD	39.2	41.5%
Deutsch[23]	2007	46	49	A3 tears (33) and bursal sided (8)	TD and repair	38	89.1%
Kartus et al.[26]	2006	33	51.5	A2 tears (13), bursal sided (10), both (3)	Debridement with SAD	101	79%
Waibl and Buess[34]	2005	22	45	Articular sided	TT repair	16	100%
Ide et al.[24]	2005	17	42	A3 tears	TT repair	39	100%
Budoff et al.[19]	2005	98	45	Articular sided (51), bursal sided (1), both (27)	Debridement with and without SAD	114	80.6%
Park et al.[28]	2003	49	52	Articular sided (24), bursal sided (13)	Debridement with SAD	42	75.5%
Cordasco et al.[22]	2002	107	55	Articular sided (63), bursal sided (14)	Debridement with SAD	52.7	72%
Snyder et al.[31]	1991	38	42	Articular sided (27), bursal sided (7)	Debridement with and without SAD	23	81.6%

Abbreviations: TT, transtendon; TD, takedown; NR, not reported; SAD, subacromial decompression; TO, transosseous.
Editor's Note: Please refer to original journal article for full references.

Level of Evidence.—Level IV, systematic review of Level IV studies (Table 3).

▶ The authors conducted a detailed review of the literature on a controversial issue—management of the partial rotator cuff tear. This is not a meta-analysis. Yet the topic is relevant and controversial. Subject to their interpretation, it would seem that the literature does support simple debridement for tears involving < 50% of the tendon thickness. What is more uncertain is the value of subacromial decompression (probably not much added value). What is more certain is, regardless of the treatment used, the poorer outcomes are associated with longer surveillance (Table 3).

B. F. Morrey, MD

Pathomechanisms and Complications Related to Patient Positioning and Anesthesia During Shoulder Arthroscopy
Rains DD, Rooke GA, Wahl CJ (Univ of Washington, Seattle)
Arthroscopy 27:532-541, 2011

The lateral decubitus and beach-chair positions each offer unique benefits to the shoulder surgeon with respect to visualization, efficiency, and ease during arthroscopic shoulder procedures. The purpose of this article was to comprehensively review the reports and studies documenting independent and dependent complications related to patient positioning and anesthesia during arthroscopic shoulder surgery. The lateral decubitus position has been associated with the potential for peripheral neurapraxia, brachial plexopathy, direct nerve injury, and airway compromise. The beach-chair position has been associated with cervical neurapraxia, pneumothorax, and the potential for end-organ hypoperfusion injuries (when deliberate hypotension is used). Potentially concerning are hypotensive bradycardic events, which may be relatively common in association with the use of epinephrine-containing interscalene anesthetics in beach chair—positioned patients. Irrigant complications (fluid spread, ventricular tachycardia) are avoidable risks not unique to either specific position. Although minor transient anesthetic- and position-related complications (neurapraxia, hypotension) may occur in as many 10% to 30% of patients, major complications such as end-organ damage or permanent impairments are exceedingly rare. Regardless of position, complications are almost uniformly avoidable if surgeon and anesthetist exercise care and prudent attention to position and anesthetic choices. The purpose of this article is to review the potential for position- and anesthesia-related complications and acquaint the shoulder surgeon with the proposed pathophysiologic mechanisms that can lead to them (Tables 1 and 2).

▶ This review article is included this year as it highlights an important issue for the surgeon performing arthroscopic shoulder surgery. Although nerve injury

TABLE 1.—Position-Related Complications During Shoulder Arthroscopy

Beach Chair	Lateral Decubitus
HBE (interscalene block) (4%-29%)	Temporary paresthesia (10%)
Cervical neurapraxia (rare)	Permanent neurapraxia (2.5%)
Air embolism/pneumothorax (reported)	Risk of musculotendinous nerve injury (5-o'clock portal) (rare)
Cerebral hypoperfusion event (reported)	Fluid-related obstructive airway compromise (reported)

TABLE 2.—Interscalene Block Anesthesia

Risks/Complications	Benefits
Brachial plexus neurapraxia/transient neuropathy	Decreased concentrations of anesthetics
Inadvertent spinal/epidural anesthesia	Less postoperative nausea
Seizure	Decreased postoperative analgesic requirements
Cardiac arrest	Decreased hospital admission rates
HBE	Shortened postanesthesia stays
Adjacent nerve blockade	
Phrenic nerve	
Laryngeal nerve	
Sympathetic chain	

associated with positioning is uncommon, when it occurs it is devastating. This article does a nice job of pointing out the differences between the beach chair and lateral decubitus positions (Table 1). It would seem that the beach chair is probably inherently the safest position, but not dramatically better than the carefully positioned and protected lateral decubitus position. The choice of anesthetic is also discussed along with the advantages and disadvantages (Table 2). This serves as a nice reminder and a nice review.

B. F. Morrey, MD

Position and Duration of Immobilization After Primary Anterior Shoulder Dislocation: A Systematic Review and Meta-Analysis of the Literature
Paterson WH, Throckmorton TW, Koester M, et al (Campbell Clinic-Univ of Tennessee Dept of Orthopaedics, Memphis; Slocum Ctr for Orthopedics and Sports Medicine,Eugene; et al)
J Bone Joint Surg Am 92:2924-2933, 2010

Background.—Immobilization after closed reduction has long been the standard treatment for primary anterior dislocation of the shoulder. To determine the optimum duration and position of immobilization to prevent recurrent dislocation, a systematic review of the relevant literature was conducted.

Methods.—Of 2083 published studies that were identified by means of a literature review, nine Level-I and Level-II studies were systematically reviewed. The outcome of interest was recurrent dislocation. Additional calculations were performed by pooling data to identify the ideal length and position (external or internal rotation) of immobilization.

Results.—Six studies (including five Level-I studies and one Level-II study) evaluated the use of immobilization in internal rotation for varying lengths of time. Pooled data analysis of patients younger than thirty years old demonstrated that the rate of recurrent instability was 41% (forty of ninety-seven) in patients who had been immobilized for one week or less and 37% (thirty-four of ninety-three) in patients who had been immobilized for three weeks or longer (p = 0.52). An age of less than thirty years at the time of the index dislocation was significantly predictive of recurrence in most studies. Three studies (including one Level-I and two Level-II studies) compared recurrence rates with immobilization in external and internal rotation. Analysis of the pooled data demonstrated that the rate of recurrence was 40% (twenty-five of sixty-three) for patients managed with conventional sling immobilization in internal rotation and 25% (twenty-two of eighty-eight) for those managed with bracing in external rotation (p = 0.07).

Conclusions.—Analysis of the best available evidence indicates there is no benefit of conventional sling immobilization for longer than one week for the treatment of primary anterior shoulder dislocation in younger patients. An age of less than thirty years at the time of injury is significantly predictive of recurrence. Bracing in external rotation may provide a clinically important benefit over traditional sling immobilization, but the difference in recurrence rates did not achieve significance with the numbers available.

▶ Once again I include a meta-analysis on a common and controversial subject. The methodology is explained (Fig 1 in the original article). Our understanding is that the younger patient is at risk for recurrence. This analysis confirms this, and places the age at risk not at 20 years, but those younger than 30 years! Less well recognized is the finding that there is no documented benefit of protection for more than 1 week. A third observation of value is that in recent years, there has been interest and suggestions that immobilization in external rotation provides superior outcomes, especially regarding recurrence and motion. This analysis could not confirm this specific recommendation, but there was a tendency in that direction.

B. F. Morrey, MD

Pain Relief for Reduction of Acute Anterior Shoulder Dislocations: A Prospective Randomized Study Comparing Intravenous Sedation With Intra-articular Lidocaine

Cheok CY, Mohamad JA, Ahmad TS (Penang Adventist Hosp, Malaysia; Selangor Specialist Hosp, Malaysia; Univ of Malaya, Kuala Lumpur)
J Orthop Trauma 25:5-10, 2011

Objectives.—The aim was to compare the effectiveness of intra-articular lidocaine (IAL) versus intravenous Demerol and Diazepam (IVS) in reduction of acute anterior shoulder dislocation.

Design.—This is a prospective randomized study.

Setting.—Emergency room setting.

Patients.—Thirty-one dislocations reduced with IVS, whereas 32 patients were reduced using IAL.

Main Outcome Measurements.—The visual analog pain scale was used before analgesic administration and during the closed manipulative reduction. Length of time since dislocation, frequency of dislocation, ease of reduction, patient satisfaction, adverse effects, and duration of hospitalization were recorded.

Results.—The IVS group had a 100% success rate, whereas the IAL group had a 19% (six of 32) failure rate ($P = 0.024$). However, there was no significant difference in terms of pain relief ($P = 0.23$) or patient satisfaction ($P = 0.085$) between both groups. In addition, patients in the IAL group had a shorter duration of hospitalization and no reported complications, whereas the intravenous group had a longer hospital stay and a 29% complication rate. The cost of IAL was 32% less than the cost for IVS.

Conclusion.—IAL was more cost effective than the IVS method. IAL provided adequate pain relief and fewer complications and is a viable

TABLE 2.—Successful Reduction, Complication, Patients' Satisfaction, and Duration of Hospitalization Between the IVS and IAL Groups

Feature	IVS (N = 31)	IAL (N = 32)	P Value
Reduction*			
Successful	31 (100)	26 (81)	0.024[‡]
Failed	0 (0)	6 (19)	
Complication*			
Yes	9 (29)	0 (0)	0.001[‡]
No	22 (71)	32 (100)	
Satisfaction*			
Yes	28 (90)	22 (69)	0.09[‡]
No	3 (10)	10 (31)	
Duration of hospitalization (hours)[†]	8.1 (3.6)	2.2 (2.8)	0.00[§]

IVS, Demerol and Diazepam; IAL, intra-articular lidocaine.
Numbers in bold indicate statistical significance.
*Number of patients (%).
[†]Values are mean (standard deviation).
[‡]Fisher exact test.
[§]Student *t* test.

option for analgesia during reduction of acute shoulder dislocation (Table 2).

▶ The question and conclusions are not uniquely asked or answered. However, this is a nice clinical study that is prospective and randomized. In addition, it provides a power analysis to justify the sample size. Hence, the findings and conclusions are scientifically sound. And they are readily summarized, remembered, and can be acted upon (Table 2). Intra-articular lidocaine is effective and probably the treatment of choice as an analgesic in reduction of the dislocated shoulder.

B. F. Morrey, MD

Arthroscopic Capsulolabral Revision Repair for Recurrent Anterior Shoulder Instability
Bartl C, Schumann K, Paul J, et al (Ulm Univ, Germany; Spital Davos, Switzerland; Technical Univ Munich, Germany)
Am J Sports Med 39:511-518, 2011

Background.—Open capsulolabral repair is still considered the standard revision procedure for a failed anterior shoulder instability repair. To date, only a few studies have evaluated the outcome of arthroscopic revision instability repair.

Purpose.—This study was undertaken to assess the clinical outcome and postoperative sports activity level of arthroscopic revision stabilization using defined inclusion criteria and a standardized operative revision technique.

Study Design.—Case series; Level of evidence, 4.

Methods.—Fifty-six patients with recurrent anterior shoulder instability after an anatomic index procedure (open or arthroscopic) were included in the study. Arthroscopic revision repair was performed by a single surgeon using standardized suture anchor repair technique via an anteroinferior 5:30-o'clock approach. Patients were evaluated after a mean follow-up of 37 months (range, 25-72 months) with the Rowe, the Constant score, and the Simple Shoulder Test (SST). Return to sports, including sports level and discipline, were evaluated with a sports activity assessment tool.

Results.—For the revision repair, a minimum of 3 anchors were placed in the lower glenoid half. Recurrent instability after the revision procedure was found in 6 cases (11%). There were 4 recurrent instability cases caused by trauma and 2 atraumatic cases. Arthroscopic revision repair did not result in an additional loss of external rotation or additional subscapularis muscle insufficiency. The Rowe and Constant scores and the SST were significantly improved by the procedure. Eighty-six percent of the patients rated their result as good or excellent. Sports activity level was significantly improved by the procedure and the majority of patients returned to their previous sports level.

TABLE 3.—Anchor Position at the Primary and Revision Procedure

Anchor Position	No. of Patients
Primary procedure	
1 anchor below equator	30
2 anchors below equator	10
Not used	16
Revision procedure	
3 anchors below equator	54
Additional anchors above equator	27

Conclusion.—Arthroscopic capsulolabral revision repair via the antero-inferior 5:30-o'clock approach achieves results comparable with open revision repairs with a low recurrent instability rate. Arthroscopic revision repair reached a high patient satisfaction, good clinical outcomes, and a high rate of return to sports. The results suggest that arthroscopic revision repair is a viable treatment option for selected patients with a failed index repair (Table 3).

▶ This European experience represents another expression of continued growth and development of arthroscopic technique and expertise. In the past, failed stabilization procedures were thought to require an open revision. The impressive success rate reported herein now demonstrates that arthrotomy is no longer necessary to address the failed stabilization procedure, whether a failed arthroscopic or open procedure. It is of interest to note the relatively large number of patients requiring sutures in the lower capsule in the revision compared with the primary group (Table 3).

B. F. Morrey, MD

Contact Pressure and Glenohumeral Translation Following Subacromial Decompression: How Much Is Enough?
Denard PJ, Bahney TJ, Kirby SB, et al (Oregon Health and Science Univ, Portland)
Orthopedics 33:805, 2010

Subacromial decompression is a common surgical procedure that has historically included coracoacromial ligament resection. However, recent reports have advocated preserving the coracoacromial ligament to avoid the potential complication of anterosuperior escape. The optimal subacromial decompression would achieve a smooth coracoacromial arch and decreased rotator cuff contact pressures while preserving the function of the arch in glenohumeral stability. We hypothesized that a subacromial decompression with a limited acromioplasty with preservation of the coracoacromial ligament can decrease extrinsic pressure on the rotator cuff similar to a coracoacromial ligament resection, without altering gleno-humeral translation.

Three different subacromial decompressions, including a "smooth and move," a limited acromioplasty with coracoacromial ligament preservation, and a coracoacromial ligament resection, were performed on 6 cadaveric specimens with intact rotator cuffs. Glenohumeral translation and peak rotator cuff pressure during abduction were recorded. No change in translation was observed after a smooth and move or a limited acromioplasty. Compared to baseline specimens, anterosuperior translation was increased at 30° of abduction following coracoacromial ligament resection ($P<.05$). Baseline rotator cuff pressure was greatest during abduction with the arm in 30° of internal rotation. Peak rotator cuff pressure decreased up to 32% following a smooth and move, up to 64% following a limited acromioplasty, and up to 72% following a coracoacromial ligament resection. Based on the present study, a limited acromioplasty with coracoacromial ligament preservation may best provide decompression of the rotator cuff while avoiding potential anterosuperior glenohumeral translation.

▶ In spite of rather limited evidence of its true effectiveness, subacromial decompression is one of the most common procedures performed at the shoulder. Hence, some effort to better understand the biomechanic impact as a function of the extent of the procedure is a worthwhile endeavor. This study investigates the hypothesis that a more limited resection, one that preserves the acromioclavicular (a/c) ligament, may be the most desirable to stabilize the humeral head and lessen the glenohumeral contact pressure. The evidence would seem to support the hypothesis (Fig 3 in the original article). Those cadavers with maintenance of the a/c ligament did demonstrate a more stable glenohumeral joint. Preservation of the ligament should be considered when performing the decompression procedure.

B. F. Morrey, MD

7 Elbow

Introduction

The elbow is an interesting section for me since it is one of the areas of my special focus. I have intentionally reviewed and included articles that I think have a more general relevance. Hence, topics relating to trauma and epicondylitis are featured. Hopefully this will provide a useful insight to those who see these common problems. The emergence of joint replacement arthroplasty as a reliable technique is becoming more universally accepted, and the documentation of this reality is included in this year's selections.

Bernard F. Morrey, MD

Revision Arthroscopic Contracture Release in the Elbow Resulting in an Ulnar Nerve Transection: Surgical Technique

Raphael BS, Weiland AJ, Altchek DW, et al (Kerlan Jobe Orthopaedic Clinic, Los Angeles, CA; Hosp for Special Surgery, NY; et al)
J Bone Joint Surg Am 93:100-108, 2011

Background.—Elbow arthroscopy can help remove loose bodies, treat lateral epicondylitis, achieve synovectomy, debride osteophytes, assess instability contracture release, and treat osteochondritis dissecans. Neurovascular complications occur in 0% to 14% of cases, with a few reports of complete nerve transection. Understanding elbow anatomy and how abnormalities affect it can reduce complications related to elbow arthroscopy. Complications can also be minimized by using a systematic approach to the procedure, adequately preparing preoperatively, having all needed equipment readily available, and using proper surgical technique.

Surgical Technique.—An auxiliary block with intravenous sedation is done to achieve regional anesthesia. The patient is in a modified supine-suspended position with the shoulder in 90° of flexion. The forearm and wrist are supported over the chest using a hydraulic arm positioner attached to the bed's contralateral side. Gravity assists in displacing anterior neurovascular structures away from the anterior capsule and keeping the radial nerve anterior. If arthrotomy is needed, the forearm is placed on an armboard.

Portal choice depends on the abnormality. The most commonly used are the anterolateral, midlateral (soft spot), anteromedial, proximal medial, proximal lateral, transtricipital, and accessory posterior lateral. Each portal has risks. The elbow joint is then insufflated with 20 to 30 mL of saline solution injected into the soft spot of the midlateral portal. Distending the articular capsule and flexing the elbow increases the distance between portals and where neurovascular structures are usually found. With joint capsule contracture, displacement is minimal, with insufflation volumes as little as 5 mL.

Anterior Arthroscopy.—After insufflation, a proximal medial or proximal lateral portal will permit diagnostic arthroscopy. The proximal medial portal is 2 cm proximal to the medial epicondyle and 5 mm anterior to the intermuscular septum. Before incision the intermuscular septum is palpated to ensure an anterior portal site, keeping the ulnar nerve posteriorly. A No. 15 scalpel blade is used to incise the skin only, then a blunt hemostat is placed on the anterior humeral surface and passed distally, toward the coronoid tip. This protects the ulnar nerve and avoids the median nerve. The capsule is pierced using a sheath and conical trocar. Via the arthroscope, one can see the radiocapitellar articular and annular ligament. The coronoid tip and medial aspect of the elbow are assessed as the arthroscope is withdrawn. Lateral portals are established under direct visualization with the arthroscope in the joint. Anteromedial portals are 2 cm distal and 2 cm anterior to the medial epicondyle and within 5 mm of the medial antebrachial nerve.

The anterior compartment is seen through the proximal lateral portal initially in patients who have had ulnar nerve transposition, in those being assessed for valgus extension overload, and before medial collateral ligament reconstruction is performed. This permits one to rule out intra-articular abnormalities. The proximal lateral portal is 2 cm proximal to the lateral epicondyle and directly on the anterior humeral surface. The posterior branch of the antebrachial cutaneous nerve is about 6.2 mm from the proximal lateral portal if the skin incision is 1 to 2 mm proximal to the lateral epicondyle. This portal is obtained with the elbow flexed to protect the radial nerve. Elbow arthroscopy can be used in patients who have had ulnar nerve transposition when only laterally based portals can be used. Posteromedial portals are not used to avoid neurovascular injury. Once the anterior arthroscopy is completed, the arthroscope is placed in a midlateral portal. However, use of the midlateral portal is limited to approaching an osteochondral defect of the capitellum. The arthroscope is extended down the elbow gutter with the elbow extended using a posterolateral portal to view the posterior radiocapitellar joint. This allows viewing of the posterior radiocapitellar joint, radioulnar articulation, lateral gutter, trochlea, and trochlear groove. Sometimes a 2.7-mm arthroscope is needed.

Posterior Arthroscopy.—To assess the posterior compartment, the arm is placed in a more extended position and a posterolateral portal is used. The extension reduces tension on the triceps and facilitates placing the trocar toward the olecranon fossa. Multiple options are available for this portal and more than one may be needed. It is located 15 to 20 mm from the mixed and major cutaneous nerves. The first portal is 2 to 3 cm proximal to the olecranon tip and lateral to the triceps tendon. Work is done via a transtricipital portal located in the midline and 2 to 3 cm proximal to the olecranon tip. A motorized shaver can achieve soft tissue debridement of the olecranon fossa, which improves the view of the posterior compartment. Osteophytes are sought throughout the medial, lateral, and central aspects of the olecranon, then abnormalities are assessed in the olecranon fossa, the posteromedial aspect of the humeral condyle, and the medial and lateral gutters.

Capsular Release.—Capsular releases via the arthroscope can be more technically demanding than dealing with conditions not affected by diminished capsular compliance, which reduces intracapsular working space and minimizes displacement of neurovascular structures with insufflation. The arthroscope is placed in the anterior compartment and the joint capsule. Adhesions are released from the anterior humeral aspect, with the arthroscope in the proximal medial portal and using a blunt trocar to define and elevate the capsular attachment from the proximal lateral portal. The oscillating full-radius shaver removes adhesions and achieves debridement of the anterior compartment. Gravity assists suction and reduces the risk of overly aggressive debridement of the lateral aspect of the elbow. When sufficient working space is achieved, the coronoid process is assessed for osteophytes that limit flexion. A motorized burr is used to resect osteophytes from the coronoid tip and clear the coronoid fossa from tissue. The anterior capsulectomy is performed using the full-radius shaver and an up-cutting resector until one can identify the muscular fibers of the brachialis. A lateral capsulotomy is done as an open procedure once the arthroscopic procedure is completed. The arm is placed on an armboard and the proximal lateral portal incorporated into an incision exposing the elbow's lateral aspect.

Similar steps are taken in the posterior compartment, with soft tissue removal from the olecranon fossa and posterior compartment using the full-radius shaver through the transtricipital portal. Care is exercised when the medial gutter is addressed to protect the subcapsular position of the ulnar nerve. Any impinging osteophytes are removed from the olecranon using a motorized burr. Osteophytes may also be removed from the olecranon fossa. Before the procedure is completed, the arm is gently moved through its range of motion to release residual adhesions.

▶ I typically do not include technique topics such as this. This particular article is included for several reasons. It provides an opportunity to stress that not only is the ulnar nerve at risk because of its intimacy with the posterior medial collateral bundle, but with increased use of arthroscopy to address primary osteoarthritis of the elbow, the ulnar nerve is even more at risk. Further, there is an increased recognition of the need to address ulnar nerve compression when dealing with elbow stiffness. When this involves formal translation of the nerve, the ability to safely use the anterior medial portal is compromised (Fig 10 in the original article).

B. F. Morrey, MD

Combination of Arthrolysis by Lateral and Medial Approaches and Hinged External Fixation in the Treatment of Stiff Elbow

Liu S, Fan C-Y, Ruan H-J, et al (Shanghai Jiaotong Univ School of Medicine, People's Republic of China)
J Trauma 70:373-376, 2011

Background.—Various methods are available to treat the stiff elbow. However, there is no consensus on which one is most useful. This study involves the effects of combination of arthrolysis by lateral and medial approaches and hinged external fixation in the treatment of stiff elbow.

Patients.—We treated 12 patients with stiff elbows using a combination of arthrolysis by lateral and medial approaches and hinged external fixation. The arthrolysis was applied to the elbow for complete soft-tissue release, and the hinged external fixation mainly for rehabilitation and stability of the elbow after arthrolysis. With the help of the hinged external fixation, nonsurgical treatment including exercises was effectively performed to maintain the stability and the results of arthrolysis. Before surgery, the mean extension was −35 degrees and the mean flexion 70 degrees. One patient had a loss of 70 degrees in pronation.

Results.—Satisfactory follow-up was given to 11 patients with the mean length of 15 months. The mean postoperative extension was −8 degrees whereas flexion was 122 degrees. Two of 11 patients had a transient ulnar paresthesia and returned to normal after 8-month follow-up. The loss of pronation in one patient reduced to 30 degrees afterward. There were no complicating infections. All patients reported satisfactory effect.

Conclusion.—The combination of arthrolysis by lateral and medial approaches and hinged external fixation in the treatment of stiff elbow is safe and effective.

▶ Because elbow stiffness is the most common complication of elbow fracture, it is helpful to understand its treatment. Today, both arthroscopic and open procedures are advocated and both are effective. Selection is largely based on the experience of the surgeon and the nature of the contracture. This study demonstrates effective improvement in 11 of 12 patients treated by the technique described. I personally also prefer the use of an external fixator in many of these patients for the reasons discussed herein. It protects the joint while allowing early motion. Bottom line, many of these patients can be helped by secondary surgical arthrolysis.

B. F. Morrey, MD

Arthroscopic Restoration of Terminal Elbow Extension in High-Level Athletes

Blonna D, Lee G-C, O'Driscoll SW (Mayo Clinic, Rochester, MN)
Am J Sports Med 38:2509-2515, 2010

Background.—Although most people can lead near-normal lives with a limited but functional arc of elbow motion, athletes may find loss of terminal extension severely impairing.

Hypothesis.—Arthroscopic contracture release is effective in restoring full elbow extension in athletes whose loss of terminal extension impairs their intensities and/or levels of performance in sport.

Study Design.—Case series; Level of evidence, 4.

Methods.—Between 1997 and 2007, 24 athletes (26 elbows; mean age, 38 years [range, 12-58]) whose chief complaint was limited elbow extension (≤35°) underwent arthroscopic release of contractures (average follow-up, 33 months [range, 12-88]). All the patients were classified according to a sport-specific scoring system using the subjective patient outcome for return to sports score and the summary outcome determination score.

Results.—All 26 elbows improved subjectively and objectively with surgery. Of the 26 elbows, 25 were rated by the patients as normal (n = 15) or near-normal (n = 10) at final follow-up. Pain during intense sporting activities was absent in 17, mild and occasional without affecting performance in 6, and severe enough to affect performance in 1. Of the 24 patients (26 elbows), 22 patients (23 elbows) returned to the same sport at the same level of intensity and performance as before injury. Two patients (3 elbows) returned to the same sport but failed to reach their preinjury levels of performance. Extension improved in all patients, with the average flexion contracture decreasing from 27° ± 7° (range, 10°-35°) to 6° ± 9° (range, 10° of hyperextension to 25°; P < .001). Lack of extension was not a residual impairment factor in any patients. Three patients developed delayed-onset ulnar neuropathy after surgery, 2 of which were treated by subcutaneous transposition. All 3 resolved completely, 2 within the first 6 weeks; the other took longer than a year.

Conclusion.—The arthroscopic release of contractures is a predictable technique to achieve a highly functional elbow in athletes.

▶ The value of the arthroscope in treating elbow conditions continues to evolve. That the management can be affected with limited comorbidity is of particular value in the athlete and when dealing with the elbow.

The points of emphasis here are that these are relatively mild contractures. Furthermore, in the athlete, the majority will have some component of impingement pain, which is because of osteophytic changes at the tip of the olecranon. This article also identifies the single most important additional factor in a successful intervention: the presence of ulnar nerve symptoms. This possibility must be specifically investigated. If ulnar nerve symptoms are present, or even if there is a positive Tinel sign, the nerve should be decompressed in site at the time of the scope.

B. F. Morrey, MD

Clinical Assessment of the Ulnar Nerve at the Elbow: Reliability of Instability Testing and the Association of Hypermobility with Clinical Symptoms
Calfee RP, Manske PR, Gelberman RH, et al (Washington Univ School of Medicine at Barnes-Jewish Hosp, St Louis, MO)
J Bone Joint Surg Am 92:2801-2808, 2010

Background.—Ulnar nerve hypermobility has been reported to be present in 2% to 47% of asymptomatic individuals. To our knowledge, the physical examination technique for diagnosing ulnar nerve hypermobility has not been standardized. This study was designed to quantify the interobserver reliability of the physical examination for ulnar nerve hypermobility and to determine whether ulnar nerve hypermobility is associated with clinical symptoms.

Methods.—Four hundred elbows in 200 volunteer participants were examined. Each participant was queried regarding symptoms attributable to the ulnar nerve. Three examiners, unaware of reported symptoms, independently performed a standardized examination of both elbows to assess ulnar nerve hypermobility. Ulnar nerves were categorized as stable or as hypermobile, which was further subclassified as perchable, perching, or dislocating. Provocative maneuvers, consisting of the Tinel test and flexion compression testing, were performed, and structural measurements were recorded. Kappa values quantified the examination's interobserver reliability. Unpaired t tests, chi-square tests, Wilcoxon tests, and Fisher exact tests were utilized to compare data between those with hypermobile nerves and those with stable nerves.

Results.—Ulnar nerve hypermobility was identified in 37% (148) of the 400 elbows. Hypermobility was bilateral in 30% (fifty-nine) of the 200 subjects. For the three examiners, weighted kappa values on the right and left sides were 0.70 and 0.74, respectively. Elbows with nerve hypermobility did not experience a higher prevalence of subjective symptoms (snapping, pain, and tingling) than did elbows with stable nerves. Provocative physical examination testing for ulnar nerve irritability, however, showed consistent trends toward heightened irritability in hypermobile nerves (p = 0.04 to 0.16). Demographic data and anatomic measurements were similar between the subjects with stable nerves and those with hypermobile nerves.

Conclusions.—Ulnar nerve hypermobility occurs in over one-third of the adult population. Utilizing a standardized physical examination, a diagnosis of ulnar nerve hypermobility can be established with substantial interobserver reliability. In the general population, ulnar nerve hypermobility does not appear to be associated with an increased symptomatology attributable to the ulnar nerve.

▶ Ulnar nerve symptomatology is second only to epicondylitis in frequency of elbow pathology. In addition to my interest in this joint, I was also interested in the specific topic, as I personally have bilateral subluxing nerves. That the diagnosis can be made reliable is comforting but not surprising. The clinical relevance is what is important. I completely agree that, given the 33% frequency of occurrence, one might consider this a variation of normal. The interpretation of symptom correlation is less clear. The nerve is clearly more vulnerable to direct blows, and the hypermobility clearly causes irritation in some individuals and with certain occupations. The important message is the same as always. Surgical treatment is on an individual basis. The simple presence of a hypermobile nerve is not a reason to transpose it.

B. F. Morrey, MD

The effect of haematoma aspiration on intra-articular pressure and pain relief following Mason I radial head fractures
Ditsios KT, Stavridis SI, Christodoulou AG (1st Orthopaedic Dept of Aristotle Univ, Thessaloniki, Greece)
Injury 42:362-365, 2011

Background.—The aspiration of the accompanying haematoma by Mason type I radial head fractures is advocated by several authors to achieve an analgesic effect. The purpose of this study was to investigate the effect of haematoma aspiration on intra-articular pressure and on pain relief after Mason I radial head fractures.

Materials and Methods.—A total of 16 patients (10 men and six women, age 23–47 years) with an isolated Mason I radial head fracture were subjected to haematoma paracentesis. Initially, intra-articular pressure was measured by using the Stryker Intra-Compartmental Pressure Monitor System. After haematoma aspiration, a new pressure measurement without moving the needle was performed. Pain before and after haematoma aspiration was evaluated by using an analogue 10-point pain scale.

Results.—Intra-articular elbow pressure prior to haematoma aspiration varied from 49 to 120 mmHg (median, 76.5 mmHg), while following aspiration, it ranged from 9 to 25 mmHg (median, 17 mmHg). The median quantity of the aspired blood was 2.75 ml (range, 0.5–8.5 ml). Patients reported a decrease in the visual analogue score (VAS) for pain from 5.5 (4–8) before to 2.5 (1–4) after aspiration. Decrease for both pressure and pain was statistically significant ($p = 0.005$).

Conclusion.—The formation of an intra-articular haematoma in the elbow joint following an undisplaced Mason I radial head fracture leads to a pronounced increase of the intra-articular pressure accompanied by

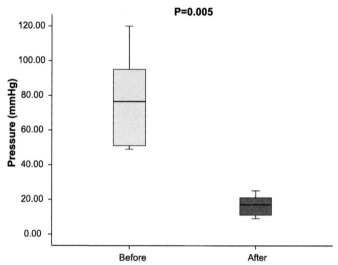

FIGURE 1.—Box-plot of elbow intraarticular pressure before and after aspiration (Wilcoxon signed ranks test $p = 0.005$). Elbow intraarticular pressure decreased significantly after aspiration ($p = 0.005$). (Reprinted from Ditsios KT, Stavridis SI, Christodoulou AG. The effect of haematoma aspiration on intra-articular pressure and pain relief following Mason I radial head fractures. *Injury.* 2011;42:362-365, Copyright 2011, with permission from Elsevier.)

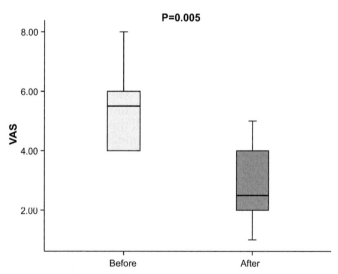

FIGURE 2.—Boxplot of VAS score for pain before and after aspiration (Wilcoxon signed ranks test $p = 0.005$). VAS score for pain decreased significantly after aspiration ($p = 0.005$). (Reprinted from Ditsios KT, Stavridis SI, Christodoulou AG. The effect of haematoma aspiration on intra-articular pressure and pain relief following Mason I radial head fractures. *Injury.* 2011;42:362-365, Copyright 2011, with permission from Elsevier.)

intense pain for the patient. The aspiration of the haematoma results in an acute pressure decrease and an immediate patient relief (Figs 1 and 2).

▶ This is an attractive albeit simple study that offers a scientific basis for clinical practice, that is, evidence-based patient management. I have long practiced and have been an advocate for this type of treatment, not only of the Mason type I, but also for some type II fractures. My experience had suggested a dramatic improvement in a patient's perception of pain, as borne out in this study (Fig 2). The demonstration of a marked reduction in joint pressure is the objective explanation of the finding (Fig 1). If the ultimate treatment plan is to begin early motion, controlling pain would seem to be an essential feature. The one question that remains is the frequency of recurrence of the pain and swelling over the next several days.

B. F. Morrey, MD

8 Sports Medicine

Introduction

As had been mentioned in previous reviews, to many the chapter on sports medicine is synonymous with issues relating to the anterior cruciate ligament (ACL). This is no less true this year. However, as in previous years, I have assiduously attempted to limit the issues referable to the ACL to those that are truly unique or of value. Hence, those numerous articles documenting the success of one technique or another or slight variations in technique are not to be found in this edition. On the other hand, I have attempted to identify sports-related topics of other anatomic parts, particularly the shoulder and the ankle, to be included in this chapter. The reason for this is that it is felt that these are most germane to the practice of the general orthopedic surgeon, and information regarding the ACL and its various expressions is readily available through numerous sources, including those that are commercially based.

Bernard F. Morrey, MD

Orthopaedic In-Training Examination: An Analysis of the Sports Medicine Section
Osbahr DC, Cross MB, Bedi A, et al (Hosp for Special Surgery, NY; Univ of Michigan, Ann Arbor)
Am J Sports Med 39:532-537, 2011

Background.—Since 1963, the Orthopaedic In-Training Examination (OITE) has been administered to orthopaedic residents to assess resident knowledge and measure the quality of teaching within individual programs. The OITE has evolved dramatically over the years and now maintains a standardized format consisting of 275 questions divided among 12 sections.

Purpose.—To provide a detailed analysis of the OITE sports medicine section to identify patterns in question content, recommended references, and resident performance.

Study Design.—Cross-sectional study.

Methods.—All OITE sports medicine questions from 2005 to 2009 were analyzed, and the following data were recorded: resident performance scores, tested topics, type of imaging modalities, tested treatment modalities, taxonomy classification, and recommended references.

Results.—From 2005 to 2009, the sports medicine section composed 7.8% of the OITE. Mean resident performance on the entire OITE as well as on the sports medicine section improved during each year of training. Imaging modalities typically involved questions on radiographs and magnetic resonance imaging and constituted 27.4% of the OITE sports medicine section. Treatment modalities involved 36.8% of the OITE sports medicine section questions, including most treatment questions relating to ligament reconstruction or rehabilitation. The authors' assessment of taxonomy classification showed that recall-type questions were most common; however, mean resident performance was minimally affected by type of taxonomy question. Finally, there were trends noted in recommended references; namely, the *American Journal of Sports Medicine* and *Orthopaedic Knowledge Update: Sports Medicine* were the most commonly and consistently cited journal and review book, respectively.

Conclusion.—The current study provides some unique information relating to content, recommended references, and resident performance on the OITE sports medicine section. It is hoped this information will provide orthopaedic trainees, orthopaedic residency programs, and the American Academy of Orthopaedic Surgeons Evaluation Committee valuable information relating to improving resident knowledge and performance and optimizing sports medicine educational curricula.

▶ I found this study interesting and useful. I have through the years avoided fueling the sports section with articles about the anterior cruciate ligament (ACL). We have always included articles related usually to comparative long-term outcomes, but at the end of the day, how much new can be said about this small structure? Yet this analysis indicates almost 40% of the Orthopedic In-Training Examination relates to ligament issues, that is, the ACL. I also find it interesting that almost 30% of the questions relate to imaging, another area I tend not to emphasize. So in the future, I will consider these 2 areas more carefully in my selection process but will continue to try to offer broad-based subject matter in the sports section.

B. F. Morrey, MD

Osteochondral Lesions of the Knee: A New One-Step Repair Technique with Bone-Marrow-Derived Cells
Buda R, Vannini F, Cavallo M, et al (Rizzoli Orthopaedic Inst, Bologna, Italy)
J Bone Joint Surg Am 92:2-11, 2010

Background.—Usually traumatic in origin, osteochondral lesions of the knee are defects of the cartilaginous surface and underlying subchondral bone. Most involve the medial femoral condyle, and about 40% also have ligamentous or meniscal pathology. Increased stress concentrations at the rims of the osteochondral defect may adversely affect cartilage lifespan. Larger osteochondral lesions cause immediate significant impairment and show symptoms about a decade before degenerative cartilage changes related to idiopathic osteoarthritis. Treatment of osteochondral lesions is usually surgical and aimed at restoring the cartilage's articular surface, reducing the risk of osteoarthritis. Traditional methods include cartilage replacement and cartilage regeneration through autologous chondrocyte implantation, but both methods have drawbacks. A new method using bone marrow—derived mesenchymal stem cell transplantation in a one-step technique overcomes these drawbacks. The validity of the one-step technique was assessed, and the results obtained in 20 patients were reported.

Methods.—The 12 men and 8 women had grade III or IV osteochrondral lesions of the femoral condyle with symptoms of pain, swelling, locking, or giving way. Seven patients also had meniscal injury, six of whom had partial meniscectomy and one meniscal repair. Two had anterior cruciate ligament injury that was reconstructed using semitendinosus and gracilis tendon grafts. Three had femorotibial malalignment that required high tibial osteotomy. Three had osteophytes that were tangentially resected.

The surgical technique used 6 mL of platelet-rich fibrin gel generated from 120 mL of the patient's venous blood collected and processed the day before surgery. A total of 60 mL of bone marrow aspirate was collected and processed in the operating room, removing most erythrocytes and plasma. Patients had a standard knee arthroscopy, identifying the cartilage lesion. A flipped cannula was inserted into the portal ipsilateral to the lesion to allow ingress of surgical instruments and fat pad retraction. Lesion debridement yielded a circular area with regular healthy cartilage margins for biomaterial implantation. A hyaluronic acid membrane provided cell support. The scaffold was filled with 2 mL of bone-marrow concentrate, then loaded onto a device for positioning. The area was covered using overlapping stamp-sized membrane pieces, which were covered with a layer of platelet-rich fibrin to provide growth factors. Implants' stability was assessed from flexion to extension via the arthroscope. Gradual passive and active mobilization activities were begun the day after surgery, progressing at 4 weeks to muscle reinforcement exercises, closed kinetic-chain proprioceptive rehabilitation, static and walking exercises with partial and gradual weight-bearing, and swimming. After 10 weeks, exercises focused on rehabilitating muscular function. After 6 months, patients could perform light running, with a return to high-impact sports after 12 months.

Assessments were done before surgery and 6, 12, 18, and 24 months afterward and included the International Knee Documentation Committee (IKDC) subjective questionnaire and the Knee Injury and Osteoarthritis Outcome Score (KOOS) questionnaire. Patients also had magnetic resonance imaging (MRI) scans postoperatively at 6 and 12 months and at the final evaluation. A second-look arthroscopy and biopsy samples were

TABLE 1.—Different Parameters of the MOCART Score Were Evaluated at the Final Follow-up

Degree of Defect Repair	Integration to the Surrounding Cartilage	Surface of the Repaired Tissue	Structure of the Repaired Tissue	Signal Intensity DPFSE*	Subchondral Lamina	Subchondral Bone	Adhesions	Effusion
Complete (14)	Complete (16)	Intact (14)	Homogeneous (6)	Isointense (13)	Intact (6)	Intact (6)	No (20)	No (17)
Hypertrophy (4)	Incomplete (2)	Damaged (6)	Inhomogeneous (14)	Hyperintense (7)	Not intact (14)	Not intact (14)	Yes (0)	Yes (3)
Incomplete (2)	Defect visible (2)			Hypointense (0)				

*DPFSE = proton-density fast-spin-echo magnetic resonance imaging.

done on the first two patients 12 months after surgery, including staining and immunohistochemical analysis.

Results.—Patients' mean IKDC scores were 32.9 preoperatively and 90.4 postoperatively. KOOS score averages were 47.1 preoperatively and 93.3 postoperatively. Clinical improvement was significant and was not influenced by age at the time of surgery, gender, or size of the cartilage defect. Associated procedures significantly reduced IKDC score after 12 months but did not affect the final outcome. MRI results indicated regeneration of subchondral bone and cartilaginous tissue. KOOS score at 24 months and signal intensity were significantly related. Patients with a hyperintense signal had a mean KOOS score of 89 after 24 months; patients with an iso-intense signal had a mean KOOS score of 96. Safranin-O staining of regenerated tissue demonstrated a proteoglycan-rich matrix, especially in the middle and deep zones. Hematoxylin-eosin staining showed cells homogeneously distributed throughout the tissue. Immunohistochemical analysis was positive for type II collagen but negative for type I collagen. No intra-operative or postoperative complications were seen.

Conclusions.—The one-step technique permits cells to be processed directly in the operating room, avoiding the need for a laboratory, and allows bone marrow—derived mesenchymal stem cell transplantation in a single operation. This technique for repairing osteochondral lesions of the knee produced results comparable to those obtained with autologous chondrocyte implantation. Both IKDC and KOOS scores significantly improved with this approach. Bone and cartilage growth was satisfactory, the defect was almost completely covered, and the graft was well integrated in 80% of patients. The one-step technique was shown to be a satisfactory and reliable approach to treating osteochondral lesions of the knee without the limitations of other methods (Table 1).

▶ I was attracted to this report for several reasons. It represents an improved and simplified technique of a promising technology. The concept is based on the emerging use of growth factors and progenitor cells. It appeared in the *Journal of Bone and Joint Surgery, American Volume*. This is a real accomplishment for an article such as this. It does imply rigorous review and validity, at least in my mind. Also, all these perceptions are realized by this excellent study from the Rizzoli Institute, Italy. The technique is clearly described and nicely illustrated. More importantly, the outcomes are rigorously assessed and presented (Fig 12A,C in the original article; Table 1). The results are impressive, including evidence for cartilage regrowth with similar mechanical properties as that of the surrounding cartilage. Finally, the durability at 2 years is documented, even in those with more complex associated injuries (Fig 11A,B in the original article).

B. F. Morrey, MD

6-year follow-up of 84 patients with cartilage defects in the knee: Knee scores improved but recovery was incomplete

Løken S, Heir S, Holme I, et al (Oslo Univ Hosp, Norway; Martina Hansens Hosp, Norway; Oslo Sports Trauma Res Ctr, Norway)
Acta Orthop 81:611-618, 2010

Background and Purpose.—The natural history of focal cartilage injury is largely unknown. In this study we investigated 6-year outcomes in patients with arthroscopically verified, focal, full-thickness cartilage injuries of the knee.

Methods.—In a previous report (baseline study) of 993 knee arthroscopies, 98 patients were less than 50 years old at baseline and showed grade 3–4 focal cartilage injury, as assessed with the International Cartilage Repair Society (ICRS) scale. In the present study, 84 of the 98 patients completed follow-ups at median 6.1 (5.3–7.8) years after baseline assessments. At baseline, the patients had undergone different types of cartilage repair (n = 34) or had no treatment or only debridement (n = 64) for their cartilage injury. The follow-up included evaluations with the ICRS knee evaluation form, the Lysholm score, and other knee evaluation tests. 68 patients underwent radiographic assessments with weight bearing.

Results.—Improvements compared to baseline were noted in the average ICRS functional score, visual analog scale (VAS) pain score, and the patients' rating of the function in the affected knee compared to the contra-lateral knee. However, the average ICRS activity level had decreased from baseline. The average Lysholm score was 76 (SD 21). 19 patients had Kellgren-Lawrence grades 2–3 in the affected knee and 6 patients had grades 2–3 in the contralateral knee. There was a statistically significant difference between affected and contralateral knees.

Interpretation.—Patients with arthroscopically diagnosed ICRS grade 3–4 cartilage injuries in the knee may show improvement in knee function over the following 5–8 years, with or without cartilage repair. However, knee function remains substantially affected. Further studies are needed to determine whether cartilage surgery can yield better functional outcomes than non-surgical or less invasive surgical treatments.

▶ This is a very worthwhile study, as it contains a large sample of patients with a relatively homogenous knee cartilage lesion. The management was primarily cartilage repair or debridement only with the contralateral knee serving as the control. Hence, there are adequate numbers in all 3 groups to offer some legitimate observations. That the follow-up methods are detailed and the authors achieved 85% capture of long-term results are also strengths of this study. The minimal 5-year surveillance and mean of over 6-year surveillance lend credibility to their findings and conclusion. In spite of the treatment, the injured knee tends to become stable with time, but the function is not normal. Finally, there is no definite value of the repair to the nonrepair group.

B. F. Morrey, MD

Cartilage from the edge of a debrided articular defect is inferior to that from a standard donor site when used for autologous chondrocyte cultivation
Maličev E, Barlič A, Kregar-Velikonja N, et al (Univ Med Centre, Ljubljana, Slovenia)
J Bone Joint Surg [Br] 93-B:421-426, 2011

The aim of this study was to evaluate the cultivation potential of cartilage taken from the debrided edge of a chronic lesion of the articular surface. A total of 14 patients underwent arthroscopy of the knee for a chronic lesion on the femoral condyles or trochlea. In addition to the routine cartilage biopsy, a second biopsy of cartilage was taken from the edge of the lesion. The cells isolated from both sources underwent parallel cultivation as monolayer and three-dimensional (3D) alginate culture. The cell yield, viability, capacity for proliferation, morphology and the expressions of typical cartilage genes (collagen I, COL1; collagen II, COL2; aggrecan, AGR; and versican, VER) were assessed. The cartilage differentiation indices (COL2/COL1, AGR/VER) were calculated. The control biopsies revealed a higher mean cell yield (1346 cells/mg *vs* 341 cells/mg), but similar cell proliferation, viability and morphology compared with the cells from the edge of the lesion. The cartilage differentiation indices were superior in control cells: COL2/COL1 (threefold in biopsies (non-significant)); sixfold in monolayer cultures (p = 0.012), and 7.5-fold in hydrogels (non-significant), AGR/VER (sevenfold in biopsies (p = 0.04), threefold (p = 0.003) in primary cultures and 3.5-fold in hydrogels (non-significant)).

Our results suggest that the cultivation of chondrocytes solely from the edges of the lesion cannot be recommended for use in autologous chondrocyte implantation.

▶ This simple study offers very clinically relevant information. It is convenient to use normal-appearing cartilage donor cells from the proximity of a cartilage lesion. One might theorize that these cells may be diseased. This study proves that they are, or at least they are not as healthy as those from more remote, more normal sites. Little more need be said. QED.

B. F. Morrey, MD

Outcome of Ulnar Collateral Ligament Reconstruction of the Elbow in 1281 Athletes: Results in 743 Athletes With Minimum 2-Year Follow-Up
Cain EL Jr, Andrews JR, Dugas JR, et al (American Sports Medicine Inst, Birmingham, AL; et al)
Am J Sports Med 38:2426-2434, 2010

Background.—The anterior bundle of the ulnar collateral ligament (UCL) is the primary anatomical structure providing elbow stability in overhead sports, particularly baseball. Injury to the UCL in overhead athletes often leads to symptomatic valgus instability that requires surgical treatment.

Hypothesis.—Ulnar collateral ligament reconstruction with a free tendon graft, known as Tommy John surgery, will allow return to the same competitive level of sports participation in the majority of athletes. *Study Design.*—Case series; Level of evidence, 4. *Methods.*—Ulnar collateral reconstruction (1266) or repair (15) was performed in 1281 patients over a 19-year period (1988-2006) using a modification of the Jobe technique. Data were collected prospectively and patients were surveyed retrospectively with a telephone questionnaire to determine outcomes and return to performance at a minimum of 2 years after surgery. *Results.*—Nine hundred forty-two patients were available for a minimum 2-year follow-up (average, 38.4 months; range, 24-130 months). Seven hundred forty-three patients (79%) were contacted for follow-up evaluation and/or completed a questionnaire at an average of 37 months postoperatively. Six hundred seventeen patients (83%) returned to the previous level of competition or higher, including 610 (83%) after reconstruction. The average time from surgery to the initiation of throwing was 4.4 months (range, 2.8-12 months) and the average time to full competition was 11.6 months (range, 3-72 months) after reconstruction. Complications occurred in 148 patients (20%), including 16% considered minor and 4% considered major. *Conclusion.*—Ulnar collateral ligament reconstruction with subcutaneous ulnar nerve transposition was found to be effective in correcting valgus elbow instability in the overhead athlete and allowed most athletes (83%) to return to previous or higher level of competition in less than 1 year.

▶ Quite frankly, this is the article and study for which I have been waiting. This clearly is the most extensive experience in the world for this operation. It is noteworthy that the technique did not change much through the years and always includes translocation of the nerve. The interested reader must read this monumental work in its entirety. The salient features include an 83% success rate of return to normal function. That 34% needed attention to some additional pathology may not be well appreciated. Furthermore, about 7% required additional surgery, usually (5%) to remove the posterior medial impingement osteophyte. There is far too much information to summarize. Thank you, Dr Andrews and fellows, for this contribution.

B. F. Morrey, MD

A Systematic Review on the Treatment of Acute Ankle Sprain: Brace versus Other Functional Treatment Types
Kemler E, van de Port I, Backx F, et al (Univ Med Centre Utrecht, the Netherlands; et al)
Sports Med 41:185-197, 2011

Ankle injuries, especially ankle sprains, are a common problem in sports and medical care. Ankle sprains result in pain and absenteeism from work and/or sports participation, and can lead to physical restrictions such as ankle instability. Nowadays, treatment of ankle injury basically consists of taping the ankle. The purpose of this review is to evaluate the effectiveness of ankle braces as a treatment for acute ankle sprains compared with other types of functional treatments such as ankle tape and elastic bandages.

A computerized literature search was conducted using PubMed, EMBASE, CINAHL and the Cochrane Clinical Trial Register. This review includes randomized controlled trials in English, German and Dutch, published between 1990 and April 2009 that compared ankle braces as a treatment for lateral ankle sprains with other functional treatments. The inclusion criteria for this systematic review were (i) individuals (sports participants as well as non-sports participants) with an acute injury of the ankle (acute ankle sprains); (ii) use of an ankle brace as primary treatment for acute ankle sprains; (iii) control interventions including any other type of functional treatment (e.g. Tubigrip™, elastic wrap or ankle tape); and (iv) one of the following reported outcome measures: re-injuries, symptoms (pain, swelling, instability), functional outcomes and/or time to resumption of sports, daily activities and/or work. Eight studies met all inclusion criteria. Differences in outcome measures, intervention types and patient characteristics precluded pooling of the results, so best evidence syntheses were conducted. A few individual studies reported positive outcomes after treatment with an ankle brace compared with other functional methods, but our best evidence syntheses only demonstrated a better treatment result in terms of functional outcome. Other studies have suggested that ankle brace treatment is a more cost-effective method, so the use of braces after acute ankle sprains should be considered. Further

TABLE 1.—The PEDro Scale[32]a

Criteria	Yes	No
1. Eligibility criteria were specified	1	0
2. Subjects were randomly allocated to groups (in a crossover study, subjects were randomly allocated in order in which treatments were received)	1	0
3. Allocation was concealed	1	0
4. The groups were similar at baseline regarding the most important prognostic indicators	1	0
5. There was blinding of all subjects	1	0
6. There was blinding of all therapists who administered the therapy	1	0
7. There was blinding of all assessors who measured at least one key outcome	1	0
8. Measures of at least one key outcome were obtained from >85% of the subjects initially allocated to groups	1	0
9. All subjects for whom outcome measures were available received the treatment or control condition as allocated or, where this was not the case, data for at least one key outcome were analysed by 'intent to treat'	1	0
10. The results of between-group statistical comparisons are reported for at least one key outcome	1	0
11. The study provides both point measures and measures of variability for at least one key outcome	1	0

Editor's Note: Please refer to original journal article for full references.
aTotal score is calculated using items 2–11 (range 0–10).

research should focus on economic evaluation and on different types of ankle brace, to examine the strengths and weaknesses of ankle braces for the treatment of acute ankle sprains (Table 1).

▶ There were multiple reasons this article was selected. The first was to expose those less familiar with systemic literature reviews to some of the methodology that this entails (Table 1). The second was to highlight that in spite of the frequency and body of literature, fewer than 10 articles satisfied the study inclusion criteria. Third, I was genuinely interested in the conclusions. However, I was disappointed because the conclusions were typical of analytical reviews of the orthopedic literature and no definite conclusions can be drawn. Yet there is a suggestion of the superiority of the more formal Aircast-type support. Finally, the observation of the cost-effectiveness of the management that will ultimately be required is on target—but I fear a long way off.

B. F. Morrey, MD

Accuracy of the Anterior Apprehension Test as a Predictor of Risk for Redislocation After a First Traumatic Shoulder Dislocation

Safran O, Milgrom C, Radeva-Petrova DR, et al (Hadassah Univ Hosp, Jerusalem, Israel; et al)
Am J Sports Med 38:972-975, 2010

Background.—The treatment options for a first traumatic shoulder dislocation in a young patient are either nonoperative care or primary surgery. It would be valuable to find patient-specific assessments that could predict the risk for redislocation in these patients and thereby identify those who would benefit from primary surgery.

Hypothesis.—The supine apprehension test, performed after completion of physical therapy in first traumatic shoulder dislocators, can predict risk for redislocation. Patients with a positive test would be at very high risk for redislocation and therefore would be candidates for primary surgery.

Study Design.—Cohort study (prognosis); Level of evidence, 2.

Methods.—Men aged 17 to 27 years who sustained first traumatic shoulder dislocations were treated in a shoulder immobilizer for 4 weeks and then treated according to a physical therapy protocol. At the 6-week follow-up, an anterior apprehension test was performed to assess risk of redislocation. Follow-up of patients was done at 3 months, 6 months, 1 year, and 2 years. Follow-up continued yearly for up to another 2 years.

Results.—Fifty-two men with a mean age of 20.3 years (standard deviation, 2.5) participated. Seventy-nine percent were combat soldiers. Twenty-four participants (46.2%) sustained redislocation. The minimum follow-up period was 24 months (range, 24-48 months; mean, 39.6 months). Redislocations were sustained in 36.8% of participants with negative apprehension tests and 71.4% with positive tests $(P=.03)$. The odds ratio was 4.285 (95% confidence interval, 1.129-16.266). The sensitivity of the apprehension test was 41.7% and the specificity was 85.7%.

Conclusion.—The anterior apprehension test performed 6 to 9 weeks after a first traumatic dislocation is not a definitive tool to predict risk for recurrent dislocation. It can, however, categorize patients into groups at higher and lower risk for recurrence. The redislocation rate found in this study is less than that of previous reports.

▶ I am drawn to studies that seem to be well constructed and offer a practical useful conclusion. Hence this contribution is useful, as it helps the clinician and patients have some general idea of what might be expected based on the early-term examination that reveals apprehension for recurrent shoulder dislocation.

While the numbers are not conclusive, it does offer some insight regarding the relevance of apprehension in the early healing stages.

This is possibly more valuable and considerably less expensive than an MRI study.

B. F. Morrey, MD

Does Arthroscopic Partial Meniscectomy Result in Knee Osteoarthritis? A Systematic Review With a Minimum of 8 Years' Follow-up
Petty CA, Lubowitz JH (Ochsner Med Ctr, LA; Taos Orthopaedic Inst, NM)
Arthroscopy 27:419-424, 2011

Purpose.—Our purpose is to test the hypothesis that arthroscopic partial meniscectomy results in knee osteoarthritis at long-term follow-up.

Methods.—We systematically reviewed PubMed search terms "meniscus AND arthritis AND knee" and "meniscectomy AND arthritis AND knee" and included English-language, Levels I to IV evidence studies reporting either radiographic or clinical osteoarthritis outcome measures with a minimum of 8 years' follow-up after partial arthroscopic meniscectomy.

Results.—Five studies met the inclusion criteria. All reported both radiographic and clinical measures. All studies compared the normal, contralateral knee as a radiographic control, but none included a clinical control group. Follow-up ranged from 8 to 16 years. In all studies operative knees showed a statistically significant incidence of radiographic signs of osteoarthritis compared with control knees. However, clinical symptoms of osteoarthritis were not observed. Furthermore, clinical outcomes did not correlate with radiographic findings.

Discussion.—Our results show that radiographic signs of osteoarthritis are significant at 8 to 16 years' follow-up after knee arthroscopic partial meniscectomy, but clinical symptoms of knee arthritis were not observed. Limitations include absence of clinical control groups and heterogeneity of reported outcome measures. Future research of higher levels of evidence and with longer-term follow-up is required to determine whether the radiographic signs ultimately foreshadow clinical symptoms in patients after arthroscopic partial meniscectomy.

Conclusions.—Radiographic signs of osteoarthritis are significant at 8 to 16 years' follow-up after knee arthroscopic partial meniscectomy, but clinical symptoms of knee arthritis are not significant.
Level of Evidence.—Systematic review of Level IV clinical evidence and Levels II and III radiographic evidence.

▶ What I learned early on as a resident was the association between meniscectomy and arthritis of the knee. It should be noted that there is a recognized difference between the radiographic evidence of arthritis (arthrosis?) and symptomatic osteoarthritis. This analysis of the literature again demonstrates that even partial meniscectomy is associated with image changes of the involved knee. Lacking a clinical control, the interpretation is difficult. What it means for me is that even partial meniscus removal will not prevent radiographic changes, but it may alter the clinical phenomenon of symptomatic arthritis.

B. F. Morrey, MD

Meniscal Repair for Radial Tears of the Midbody of the Lateral Meniscus
Choi N-H, Kim T-H, Son K-M, et al (Eulji Med Ctr, Seoul, Korea; St Mary's Hosp, Cheong-ju, Korea; United Hosp, Seoul, Korea; et al)
Am J Sports Med 38:2472-2476, 2010

Background.—Radial meniscal tears historically have been treated by partial meniscectomy, although they are more biomechanically detrimental than longitudinal tears. Clinical results after meniscal repair for radial tears of the midbody of the lateral meniscus have been reported rarely.
Study Design.—Case series: Level of evidence, 4.
Methods.—Fourteen consecutive patients who had radial tears of the midbody of the lateral meniscus underwent arthroscopic repair. Inclusion criteria were radial tears involving the red-red or red-white zone. All patients underwent all-inside meniscal repair using absorbable sutures. Postoperative evaluation was performed using joint-line tenderness, McMurray test, range of motion, and follow-up magnetic resonance imaging (MRI) scan at 6 months postoperatively. Lysholm knee score and Tegner activity level were evaluated at last follow-up. In 4 patients, second-look arthroscopies were performed.
Results.—The average follow-up was 36.3 months. No patient had joint-line tenderness. Three patients complained of pain or a click on McMurray test. The mean follow-up range of motion was 138.6°. Follow-up MRI scans demonstrated that 5 (35.7%) menisci were healed, 8 (57.1%) were partially healed, and 1 (7.1%) was not healed. The follow-up Lysholm score was 94.7 (range, 81-100; standard deviation [SD] = 6.4) and Tegner score was 5.7 (range, 3-7; SD = 1.4). Second-look arthroscopies in 4 patients showed partial healing of meniscal tears.

Conclusion.—Meniscal repair for radial tears of the midbody of the lateral meniscus may be an effective, alternative treatment to partial meniscectomy.

▶ This study suffers from a small sample size and short follow-up. However, it does address an important and relatively uncommon issue of managing the radial midbody lateral meniscus tear. The increasing awareness of the adverse impact of partial meniscectomy justifies investigation of alternate strategies. While it would have been much more desirable to have second-look arthroscopies in more than 4 patients, the overall outcomes are encouraging. This report does justify a more aggressive approach to repair for this lesion.

B. F. Morrey, MD

Can the Reparability of Meniscal Tears Be Predicted With Magnetic Resonance Imaging?

Bernthal NM, Seeger LL, Motamedi K, et al (David Geffen School of Medicine at UCLA; et al)
Am J Sports Med 39:506-510, 2011

Background.—Historically, magnetic resonance imaging (MRI) has been very useful in diagnosing meniscal tears but not as valuable in predicting whether a meniscal tear is reparable. Given that several recent studies suggested that MRI can be used to predict tear reparability, the topic has resurfaced as a controversy in the orthopaedic and radiology literatures.

Hypothesis.—Experienced musculoskeletal radiologists can use MRI to predict the reparability of meniscal tears with good to excellent accuracy using the same arthroscopic criteria used by surgeons intraoperatively.

Study Design.—Cohort study (diagnosis); Level of evidence, 3.

Methods.—Fifty-eight patients with meniscal tears treated with repair were matched by age and sex with 61 patients with tears treated with meniscectomy. Two senior musculoskeletal radiologists independently and blindly reviewed preoperative MRI of these 119 meniscal tears. Using established arthroscopic criteria, the radiologists were asked to grade each tear 0 to 4, with 1 point for each of the following: a tear larger than 10 mm, within 3 mm of the meniscosynovial junction, greater than 50% thickness, and with an intact inner meniscal fragment. Only a tear with a score of 4 would be predicted to be reparable.

Results.—The 2 radiologists' ability to correctly estimate reparability was poor, with 58.0% and 62.7% correct predictions ($\kappa = 0.155$ and 0.250, respectively). Interrater reliability assessment showed that the raters agreed on a score of 4 (reparable) versus <4 (not reparable) 73.7% of the time ($\kappa = 0.434$) but came to identical scores only 38.1% of the time ($\kappa = 0.156$). Determining the status of the inner fragment was the most predictive individual criterion and the only one to reach statistical significance ($\chi^2 = 14.9$, $P < .001$).

TABLE 3.—Predictors for Meniscal Repair, %

	Accuracy	Sensitivity	Specificity	Predictive Value Positive	Predictive Value Negative
Examiner 1	58	48	67	58	58
Examiner 2	63	45	80	68	60
Mean	60	47	74	63	59

Conclusion.—Magnetic resonance imaging is not an effective or efficient predictor of reparability of meniscal tears with the current arthroscopic criteria (Table 3).

▶ This is a simple, timely, and relevant study. With the increasing use and therefore dependency on diagnostic imaging, especially MRI, there is a corresponding tendency to look for this modality to help predict treatment optimization. The injured knee is probably the most common indication for extremity MRI. It is logical to ask whether this technique can be of sufficient accuracy and specificity as to predict the success of meniscus repair. The answer is no. Unfortunately, it looks as if the surgeon will be burdened with having to exercise judgment for this decision (Table 3).

B. F. Morrey, MD

Biological Knee Reconstruction: A Systematic Review of Combined Meniscal Allograft Transplantation and Cartilage Repair or Restoration
Harris JD, Cavo M, Brophy R, et al (The Ohio State Univ Med Ctr, Columbus; Washington Univ School of Medicine, St Louis, MO)
Arthroscopy 27:409-418, 2011

Purpose.—Combined meniscal allograft transplantation (MAT) and cartilage repair or restoration is a recognized treatment for patients with painful, meniscus-deficient knees and full-thickness cartilage damage. The purpose of this systematic review was to compare outcomes after combined MAT and cartilage repair/restoration with the outcomes of isolated MAT or cartilage repair/restoration.

Methods.—Multiple databases were searched with specific inclusion and exclusion criteria for clinical outcome studies after combined MAT and cartilage repair or restoration.

Results.—Six studies were identified for inclusion. In total 110 patients underwent combined MAT/cartilage repair or restoration (medial compartment in 66 and lateral compartment in 44). Patients underwent MAT and either autologous chondrocyte implantation (n = 73), osteochondral allograft (n = 20), osteochondral autograft transfer (n = 17), or microfracture (n = 3). Thirty-six patients underwent additional concurrent surgeries (high tibial or distal femoral osteotomy, cruciate or collateral

TABLE 1.—Inclusion and Exclusion Criteria

Inclusion Criteria	Exclusion Criteria
Studies reporting clinical outcomes after combined MAT and cartilage repair/restoration	Studies not reporting clinical outcomes after combined MAT and cartilage repair/restoration
Studies that address symptomatic meniscus-deficient compartment(s) and full-thickness or nearly full-thickness ipsi-compartmental cartilage damage	Studies reporting MAT and combined cartilage repair/restoration in meniscus-deficient knees for superficial cartilage damage
Minimum 2 years' clinical follow-up	Studies reporting prophylactic MAT in meniscus-deficient knees
Level I, II, III, or IV evidence	Studies reporting MAT and cartilage defect debridement only
English language	Studies reporting meniscus replacement with collagen meniscus implant
Human subjects	Studies with <2 years' clinical follow-up
Study publication date of January 1, 1950, to February 18, 2010	Level V evidence Non—English language

NOTE. The PubMed search was performed on February 18, 2010. On the basis of application of these criteria, 6 studies were identified for inclusion.

ligament reconstruction, and hardware removal). All clinical outcomes were improved at final follow-up (mean, 36 months). In 4 of 6 studies, overall outcomes of combined surgery were equivalent to those of either procedure performed in isolation. In 2 studies outcomes of combined surgery were not as good as those of either procedure performed in isolation. Failure occurred in 12% of patients who underwent combined MAT and cartilage restoration, and they required revision surgery. Most failures (85%) of combined surgery were due to failure of the MAT (as opposed to the cartilage technique). One-half of all patients required at least 1 surgery after the index procedure before final follow-up.

Conclusions.—Clinical outcomes after combined MAT and cartilage repair/restoration are similar to those after either procedure in isolation. Despite low rates of complications and failures, there is a high rate of subsequent surgery after combined MAT and cartilage repair or restoration.

Level of Evidence.—Level IV, systematic review of Level IV studies (Table 1).

▶ This contribution is important because it addresses an issue that is both important and for which the answer is not known. How should one manage the patient with a meniscus-deficient knee in the face of early arthritis? The question is addressed by a systematic review of the literature, a review technique I strongly favor. Even with this, only 6 studies could be included that satisfied their inclusion and exclusion criteria (Table 2). And these 6 studies yielded only a little over 100 patients. By the time one stratifies the outcomes by variations of the 2 procedures, the sample sizes are quite small. Nonetheless, as of today, in spite of the logic to address all the pathologic components, the outcomes are no better than addressing one or the other. This can and hopefully will change with time.

B. F. Morrey, MD

Anatomic Reconstruction of the Posterolateral Corner of the Knee: A Case Series With Isolated Reconstructions in 27 Patients

Jakobsen BW, Lund B, Christiansen SE, et al (Univ Hosp of Aarhus, Denmark)
Arthroscopy 26:918-925, 2010

Purpose.—This study presents clinical results of a case series of isolated reconstruction of the posterolateral corner (PLC) with a new technique that aims to reconstruct the lateral collateral ligament (LCL), popliteus tendon, and popliteofibular ligament.

Methods.—From 1997 to 2005, 27 patients available for follow-up with isolated posterolateral instability were treated with primary reconstruction of the LCL and PLC. The median age was 28 years, and there were 16 male patients. Of the patients, 26% had remaining instability after anterior or posterior cruciate ligament reconstruction. All underwent reconstruction with a novel technique addressing both the LCL and the PLC by use of hamstring autografts. Follow-up was more than 24 months, and patients were examined by an independent observer using the International Knee Documentation Committee objective measures and subjective Knee Injury and Osteoarthritis Outcome Scores.

Results.—In our series 95% of patients with isolated lateral rotatory instability had rotatory stability after PLC reconstruction. On the basis of International Knee Documentation Committee scoring, 71% were normal or nearly normal. Subjective Knee Injury and Osteoarthritis Outcome Scores were comparable to scores in patients after meniscectomy. One patient had a deep infection, but none had any peroneal nerve injury.

Conclusions.—This case series presents a new method for combined reconstruction of the LCL and the PLC. Despite the extensiveness of procedure, complications were low. The technique restores lateral stability clinically at 2 years' follow-up.

Level of Evidence.—Level IV, therapeutic case series (Fig 2).

▶ Although the sample size is small, the rarity of reports and information regarding deficiencies of the posterolateral corner justifies this review. The authors correctly point out that precisely because this is an uncommon problem, there is little information regarding the preferred technique, but what is reported produces quite unpredictable results. I was impressed that the authors used pure clinical indicators for recommending surgery and found MRI imaging of no predictive value in patient selection. Several outcome tools were used to provide some confidence that the proposed technique was as successful as clinically assumed to be the case. Although the reconstruction is somewhat complex (Fig 2), the favorable results do justify its consideration. Use of allograft tissue is also a positive consideration.

B. F. Morrey, MD

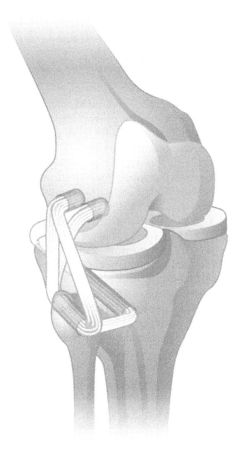

FIGURE 2.—The posterolateral reconstruction is shown at the lateral aspect of the knee. The reconstruction consist of 2 parts. First, a gracilis autograft sling is placed through the proximal fibula to the LCL insertion point at the lateral femoral condyle to reconstruct the LCL. Second, a semitendinosus autograft is used to reconstruct both the popliteus tendon and popliteofibular ligament. The popliteus tendon is reconstructed by a graft strand going from the drill hole opening at the posterolateral tibial condyle to the popliteus tendon insertion point at the femoral condyle. The popliteofibular ligament is reconstructed by a graft strand starting from the posterior aspect of the proximal fibula to the popliteus tendon insertion point at the femoral condyle. Resorbable interference screws are used for fixation of the graft in the femoral drill holes. (Reprinted from Arthroscopy: The Journal of Arthroscopic and Related Surgery, Jakobsen BW, Lund B, Christiansen SE, et al. Anatomic reconstruction of the posterolateral corner of the knee: a case series with isolated reconstructions in 27 patients. *Arthroscopy*. 2010;26:918-925, with permission from the Arthroscopy Association of North America.)

Posterolateral corner injuries of the knee: A serious injury commonly missed

Pacheco RJ, Ayre CA, Bollen SR (Bradford Teaching Hosps NHS Foundation Trust, UK)
J Bone Joint Surg [Br] 93-B:194-197, 2011

We retrospectively reviewed the hospital records of 68 patients who had been referred with an injury to the posterolateral corner of the knee to a specialist knee surgeon between 2005 and 2009. These injuries were diagnosed based on a combination of clinical testing and imaging and arthroscopy when available. In all, 51 patients (75%) presented within 24 hours of their injury with a mean presentation at eight days (0 to 20) after the injury. A total of 63 patients (93%) had instability of the knee at presentation. There was a mean delay to the diagnosis of injury to the posterolateral corner of 30 months (0 to 420) from the time of injury. In all, the injuries in 49 patients (72%) were not identified at the time of the initial presentation, with the injury to the posterolateral corner only recognised in those patients who had severe multiple ligamentous injuries. The correct diagnosis, including injury to the posterolateral corner, had only been made in 34 patients (50%) at time of referral to a specialist knee clinic. MRI correctly identified 14 of 15 injuries when performed acutely (within 12 weeks of injury), but this was the case in only four of 15 patients in whom it was performed more than 12 weeks after the injury.

Our study highlights a need for greater diligence in the examination and investigation of acute ligamentous injuries at the knee with symptoms of instability, in order to avoid failure to identify the true extent of the injury at the time when anatomical repair is most straightforward.

▶ We recently had a grand rounds discussion on injury to the posterolateral corner of the knee. This article nicely documents 2 main issues. Of all the cases, 75% are initially missed with the first evaluation. And even by the time of referral, 50% are still without a proper diagnosis. We include this article to highlight these findings. However, the limitations should also be noted. The actual diagnosis of lateral corner injury is not standardized in this study. Further, and in my mind most importantly, the implications for treatment are not completely explained, thereby documenting that a missed diagnosis does result in persistent instability.

B. F. Morrey, MD

A Comparison of the Effect of Central Anatomical Single-Bundle Anterior Cruciate Ligament Reconstruction and Double-Bundle Anterior Cruciate Ligament Reconstruction on Pivot-Shift Kinematics

Bedi A, Musahl V, O'Loughlin P, et al (Hosp for Special Surgery, NY)
Am J Sports Med 38:1788-1794, 2010

Background.—Biomechanical differences between anatomical double-bundle and central single-bundle anterior cruciate ligament reconstruction using the same graft tissue have not been defined.

Purpose.—The purpose of this study was to compare these reconstructions in their ability to restore native knee kinematics during a reproducible Lachman and pivot-shift examination.

Study Design.—Controlled laboratory study.

Methods.—Using a computer-assisted navigation system, 10 paired knees were subjected to biomechanical testing with a standardized Lachman and mechanized pivot-shift examination. The navigation system recorded the 3D motion path of a tracked point at the center of the tibia, center of the medial tibial plateau, and center of the lateral tibial plateau with each maneuver. The testing protocol consisted of evaluation in the intact state, after complete anterior cruciate ligament transection, after medial and lateral meniscectomy, and after anterior cruciate ligament reconstruction with (1) a single-bundle center-center or (2) anatomical double-bundle technique. Repeated-measures analysis of variance with a post hoc Tukey test was used to compare the measured translations with each test condition.

Results.—A significant difference in anterior translation was seen with Lachman examination between the anterior cruciate ligament- and medial and lateral meniscus-deficient condition compared with both the double-bundle and single-bundle center-center anterior cruciate ligament reconstruction ($P < .001$); no significant difference was observed between reconstructions. The double-bundle construct was significantly better in limiting anterior translation of the lateral compartment compared with the single-bundle reconstruction during a pivot-shift maneuver (2.0 ± 5.7 mm vs 7.8 ± 1.8 mm, $P < .001$) and was not significantly different than the intact anterior cruciate ligament condition (2.7 mm ± 4.7 mm, $P > .05$).

Discussion.—Although double-bundle and single-bundle, center-center anterior cruciate ligament reconstructions appear equally effective in controlling anterior translation during a Lachman examination, analysis of pivot-shift kinematics reveals significant differences between these surgical reconstructions. An altered rotational axis resulted in significantly greater translation of the lateral compartment in the single-bundle compared with double-bundle reconstruction.

Clinical Relevance.—A double-bundle anterior cruciate ligament reconstruction may be a favorable construct for restoration of knee kinematics in the at-risk knee with associated meniscal injuries and/or significant pivot shift on preoperative examination.

▶ I was prepared to reject this article as another of the numerous that deal with single-bundle versus double-bundle reconstructions. I have my personal views about this subject, but must confine myself to the science. This basic investigation suffers from the inability to know what actually happens with the healing process. However, I selected it because of the interesting conclusion. Their data suggest the double-bundle reconstructive design may be protective to the meniscus. To me, this is the key, as this dictates subsequent arthritis. The real issue is whether the graft will perform as advertised after rehabilitation and with use.

B. F. Morrey, MD

A Long-Term, Prospective, Randomized Study Comparing Biodegradable and Metal Interference Screws in Anterior Cruciate Ligament Reconstruction Surgery: Radiographic Results and Clinical Outcome

Stener S, Ejerhed L, Sernert N, et al (NU Hosp Organisation, Trollhättan/ Uddevalla, Sweden; et al)
Am J Sports Med 38:1598-1605, 2010

Background.—During the past decade, the use of biodegradable implants in anterior cruciate ligament surgery has increased.

Hypothesis.—Poly-L-lactide acid (PLLA) interference screws would render the same clinical results but greater tunnel enlargement than metal screws 8 years after anterior cruciate ligament reconstruction using hamstring tendon (semitendinosus/gracilis) autografts.

Study Design.—Randomized controlled trial; Level of evidence, 1.

Methods.—A randomized series of 77 patients, all with a unilateral anterior cruciate ligament rupture, were divided into 2 groups (PLLA and metal). In both groups, hamstring tendon autografts were used with interference screw fixation at both ends and the patients were examined with standard radiographs, Tegner activity level, Lysholm knee score, single-legged hop test, early C-reactive protein response, and KT-1000 arthrometer knee laxity measurements.

Results.—The preoperative assessments in both groups were similar in terms of gender, clinical tests, and the time from injury to surgery. The patients returned for a radiographic and clinical examination a mean of 96 months (range, 78-120 months) after the index operation. The PLLA group displayed significantly larger bone tunnels on the radiographs than the metal group on the femoral side (mean, 11.4 mm [range, 0-17.8 mm] vs 8.0 mm [range, 0-16.3 mm]; $P < .005$) but not on the tibial side (mean, 10.7 mm [range, 7.8-14.1 mm] vs 10.5 mm [range, 0-20.3 mm]; difference not significant). At follow-up, no significant differences were found between the PLLA and metal groups in terms of knee laxity measurements (median, 1.0 mm [range, −2.0-4.0 mm] vs 1.0 mm [range, −3.0-6.5 mm]), Tegner activity level (median, 7 [range, 3-9] vs 6 [range, 2-9]), or the Lysholm knee score (median, 90 points [range, 51-100] vs 89 points [range, 53-100]). The C-reactive protein values did not differ significantly between the 2 groups except for an increase in the PLLA group compared with the metal group at day 1 postoperatively— 23 mg/L (range, <6-55) vs 9 mg/L (range, <6-55) ($P < .001$).

Conclusion.—There were significantly larger radiographically visible bone tunnels on the femoral side but not on the tibial side in the PLLA group compared with the metal group 8 years after anterior cruciate ligament reconstruction using hamstring tendon autografts. This finding did not correlate with inferior clinical results. Because of the results in the present study, the authors have discontinued the use of PLLA interference screws.

▶ This is a worthwhile contribution because it constitutes a valid prospective study or a clinically relevant topic. In spite of the lack of clinical difference, the enlarged resorption halo at the tibia is sufficiently worrisome as to prompt the authors to abandon this type of screw. A similar study and conclusion were recently reported when fixation of a distal biceps tendon used a similar biodegradable fixation. In this instance, the clinical result was also comparable but was of sufficient concern to prompt the surgeon to discontinue that product as well.

B. F. Morrey, MD

Allograft Anterior Cruciate Ligament Reconstruction in the Young, Active Patient: Tegner Activity Level and Failure Rate
Barrett GR, Luber K, Replogle WH, et al (Mississippi Sports Medicine and Orthopaedic Ctr, Jackson; Oxford Orthopaedics & Sports Medicine, MS; Univ of Mississippi Med Ctr, Jackson)
Arthroscopy 26:1593-1601, 2010

Purpose.—The purpose was to analyze outcomes of nonirradiated, fresh-frozen bone–patellar tendon–bone (BPTB) allograft anterior cruciate ligament (ACL) reconstruction in patients aged under 40 years with regard to activity level (Tegner score).

Methods.—Between 1993 and 2005, 111 patients, aged under 40 years, underwent primary, nonirradiated, fresh-frozen BPTB allograft ACL reconstruction and were retrospectively reviewed. Follow-up was limited to a minimum of 24 months. Patients with concomitant ligament injuries and previous surgeries were excluded. Seventy-eight patients met the inclusion criterion and were available for follow-up. Four hundred eleven patients had BPTB autograft ACL reconstructions and comprised the control group. Failure of the graft was defined as repeat ACL reconstruction because of reinjury or graft failure, 2+ Lachman (no endpoint), any pivot shift, and/or 5-mm side-to-side KT-1000 difference (MEDmetric, San Diego, CA) or greater. Initial examinations, surgical findings, and follow-up examinations were prospectively entered into a computerized relational database. The results were assessed by both objective and subjective measures.

Results.—High-activity allograft patients had a 2.6- to 4.2-fold increase in the probability of graft failure compared with low-activity BPTB allograft patients and low- and high-activity BPTB autograft patients. Patients undergoing BPTB autograft reconstruction reported significantly fewer problems on a visual analog scale and scored significantly higher on the postoperative Tegner activity scale than patients undergoing allograft reconstruction.

Conclusions.—The active allograft group is 2.6 to 4.2 times more likely to fail compared with low-activity allografts and low- and high-activity autografts. We conclude that fresh-frozen BPTB allografts should not be used in young patients who have a high Tegner activity score because of their higher risk of failure.

Level of Evidence.—Level III, retrospective comparative study.

▶ The sports-related literature is replete with articles regarding the anterior cruciate ligament (ACL). I find myself avoiding most such studies as, in the final analysis, being irrelevant. This study caught my attention, as it represents an interesting question that is relevant to the sports practice of ACL surgery. Concern regarding the durability of allograft tissue has long been voiced, but there have been little data to direct one's thinking. I personally have used allografts at the elbow for medial collateral ligament and lateral ulnar collateral ligament reconstruction for years. Hence, this experience with a reasonable sample of more than 100 patients with long-term surveillance is worth consideration. I think it wise to note the high incidence of failure in the young active patient. And, of course, it is the patient younger than 40 years who is active, that is, the exact type of patient most often operated on. Consequently, I think we can rely on the conclusion: don't use a bone-patellar tendon-bone allograft for this type of patient.

B. F. Morrey, MD

Factors Explaining Chronic Knee Extensor Strength Deficits after ACL Reconstruction
Krishnan C, Williams GN (Rehabilitation Inst of Chicago, IL; Univ of Iowa)
J Orthop Res 29:633-640, 2011

Persistent quadriceps muscle weakness is common after anterior cruciate ligament (ACL) reconstruction. The mechanisms underlying these chronic strength deficits are not clear. This study examined quadriceps strength in people 2–15 years post-ACL reconstruction and tested the hypothesis that chronic quadriceps weakness is related to levels of voluntary quadriceps muscle activation, antagonistic hamstrings moment, and peripheral changes in muscle. Knee extensor strength and activation were evaluated in 15 ACL reconstructed and 15 matched uninjured control subjects using an interpolated triplet technique. Electrically evoked contractile properties were used to evaluate peripheral adaptations in the quadriceps muscle. Antagonistic hamstrings moments were predicted using a practical mathematical model. Knee extensor strength and evoked torque at rest were significantly lower in the reconstructed legs ($p < 0.05$). Voluntary activation and antagonistic hamstrings activity were similar across legs and between groups ($p > 0.05$). Regression analyses indicated that side-to-side differences in evoked torque at rest explained 71% of the knee extensor strength differences by side ($p < 0.001$). Voluntary activation and antagonistic hamstrings moment did not contribute significantly ($p > 0.05$). Chronic quadriceps weakness in this sample was primarily related to peripheral changes in the quadriceps muscle, not to levels of voluntary activation or antagonistic hamstrings activity.

▶ The overall excellent success rate of anterior cruciate ligament reconstruction represents a real advancement in the development of sports medicine over the last several decades. Yet chronic quadriceps muscle weakness is known to persist indefinitely. Although the weakness is usually mild, even subclinical, the etiology is not well understood. This nice study does document that the source of the problem is at the muscle tendon unit, and not neurologically or centrally controlled. It seems this finding might aid in the development of more focused rehabilitative programs.

B. F. Morrey, MD

Prompt Operative Intervention Reduces Long-Term Osteoarthritis After Knee Anterior Cruciate Ligament Tear
Richmond JC, Lubowitz JH, Poehling GG
Arthroscopy 27:149-152, 2011

Background.—When preparing scientific articles, authors have many opportunities to introduce "spin," which is specific reporting that can distort the interpretation of results and mislead readers. Spin can occur because of ignorance of the scientific issues, unconscious bias, or a willful intent to deceive. An example was seen in the *New England Journal* article, "A Randomized Trial of Treatment for Acute Anterior Cruciate Ligament Tears." Although a carefully planned randomized controlled trial of early or delayed reconstructive surgery for acute anterior cruciate ligament (ACL) tears in active patients was conducted, the conclusion that the two approaches yield the same results should be rejected because it fails to consider important secondary outcome measures.

Methods and Results.—The participants were active Swedish adults age 18 to 35 years. The primary outcome measure was the Knee Injury and Osteoarthritis Outcome Score (KOOS). The KOOS results were similar after 2 years, but in fact, 39% of the patients in the delayed-surgery group had to have ACL reconstruction because of instability. When the authors stated that there was no difference in outcome at 2 years between operative and nonoperative approaches, they ignored the surgery that was needed by a third of the nonoperative group. Seeing that a nonoperative approach would yield the same result might persuade physicians to "avoid surgery" initially for young active athletes, only to have them develop instability that requires repair and limits their ultimate ability to participate in active sports. The Tegner Activity Scale (TAS), a measure of one's ability to participate in increasingly demanding athletics, was not considered in this conclusion, yet TAS scores showed dramatic differences between the two study groups, with the average surgical patient able to return to recreational cutting sports but the average nonoperative patient limited to jogging on uneven ground.

Analysis.—Return to function is an extremely important outcome measure for patients with a torn ACL, but preventing osteoarthritis is a more important measure. Meniscectomy is one of the most important factors determining long-term function and osteoarthritis risk in knees. Meniscal status is a strong, primary determinant of function and risk of osteoarthritis within 10 years of ACL surgery. The literature clearly shows that the way to decrease the risk of knee osteoarthritis is to lower the rate of meniscectomy. Many patients who "avoid surgery" initially eventually develop symptomatic meniscal tears that require meniscectomy and increase their risk for osteoarthritis. A more accurate conclusion would be that prompt operative intervention reduces the long-term risk for osteoarthritis after ACL tear.

Conclusions.—Quality of life is a critical issue in managing ACL injuries. The best possible outcome is returning the patient to preinjury activity levels. Delaying surgery tends to significantly increase the rate of damage to the meniscus, the articular cartilage, or both and limits eventual functional levels. Operative treatment is a standard of care for patients with ACL tears who want to avoid degenerative joint disease and optimize functional status.

▶ This is the first editorial I have selected for review in the YEAR BOOK since I have been an editor, that is, over 10 years. I included this one because I liked the way it was written, and I liked the message because it got it right. Because we are so busy, we may get lulled into a state that lets others do our thinking for us. Hence, when a prestigious journal such as the *New England Journal of Medicine* reports on the lack of evidence for the value of an anterior cruciate ligament (ACL) reconstruction, we take notice. And we should. But we must be aware that, whether we like it or not, some have agendas. Actually, I suppose we all have an agenda of some sort. This editorial does a nice job of systematically critiquing this article and points out that there is an established role for an ACL reconstruction. It certainly lessens the likelihood of subsequent meniscal injury and that of secondary osteoarthritis. That said, not all ACL-deficient knees need reconstruction. And we are learning which do and which do not. Hopefully, we will follow this information in our practice.

B. F. Morrey, MD

Anterior Cruciate Ligament Reconstruction Improves Activity-Induced Pain in Comparison With Pain at Rest in Middle-Aged Patients With Significant Cartilage Degeneration

Kim S-J, Park K-H, Kim S-H, et al (Yonsei Univ Health System, Seoul, Korea)
Am J Sports Med 38:1343-1348, 2010

Background.—Recent reports revealed that outcomes of anterior cruciate ligament (ACL) reconstruction in middle- or old-age patients are comparable with those of young patients. However, in case of concomitant arthrosis in the affected knee, there has been a paucity of literature regarding the outcomes of ACL reconstruction. We studied the level of improvement in pain originating from significant cartilage degeneration in middle-aged ACL-deficient patients after ACL reconstruction. We divided the pain into pain at rest and activity-induced pain.

Hypothesis.—The activity-induced pain would be more improved by ACL reconstruction than the pain at rest.

Study Design.—Case series; Level of evidence, 4.

Methods.—We studied 36 patients who had undergone arthroscopic isolated ACL reconstruction for functional instability with significant cartilage degeneration grade III or IV without mensical injury. All patients had activity-induced pain; 20 of these patients also had pain at rest. To assess the pain level, the visual analog scale (VAS) was employed, in addition to radiologic and clinical evaluations such as the Lachman test, KT-2000 arthrometer, and pivot shift test. The mean age of the patients was 48.6 years (range, 41-61 years); mean follow-up was 46.7 months (range, 27-74 months).

Results.—The preoperative mean VAS of the activity-induced pain (4.1 ± 1.0; range, 2-6) showed significant improvement at the most recent follow-up (2.0 ± 1.0; range, 0-4; $P < .0001$). However, the preoperative mean VAS of the pain at rest (2.9 ± 0.9; range, 2-5) did not improve significantly at the most recent follow-up (2.5 ± 0.8; range, 1-4; $P = .149$). The Lachman test, KT-2000 arthrometer, and pivot shift test showed significant improvement compared with preoperative outcomes ($P < .0001$). There was no significant difference in radiologic assessment between preoperative and postoperative outcomes ($P = .082$).

Conclusion.—Anterior cruciate ligament reconstruction in middle-aged patients with significant cartilage degeneration is effective in reducing activity-induced pain and instability. Even though all patients had less than severe arthritic changes on preoperative radiographs, the pain at rest did not improve after ACL reconstruction.

▶ In addition to the findings that pain with activity was improved more than pain at rest, the most interesting issues for me with this article are the inclusion criteria. These are exclusively those of arthritis and status of the meniscus, not degree of instability. For me the central question is, "What is bothering the patient more—instability or arthritis symptoms?" If both are contributing to the patient's pain, most physicians today would stabilize the knee but do an upper tibial osteotomy to unload the arthritic compartment. The results from this study would suggest more is necessary in this type of knee pain than just anterior cruciate ligament reconstruction.

B. F. Morrey, MD

Cost-Effectiveness of Anterior Cruciate Ligament Reconstruction: A Preliminary Comparison of Single-Bundle and Double-Bundle Techniques
Paxton ES, Kymes SM, Brophy RH (Washington Univ School of Medicine, St Louis, MO)
Am J Sports Med 38:2417-2425, 2010

Background.—There has been growing interest in anatomical reconstruction of the anterior cruciate ligament (ACL), including the use of double-bundle (DB) reconstruction techniques.

Hypothesis.—The DB technique will not be cost-effective when compared with single-bundle (SB) reconstruction.

Study Design.—Economic and decision analysis; Level of evidence, 1.

Methods.—A decision-analysis model with input values derived from the literature was used to estimate the cost-effectiveness of DB ACL reconstruction compared with SB ACL reconstruction. Effectiveness was based on the revision rate and the postoperative International Knee Documentation Committee (IKDC) score.

Results.—Sixty-four percent of DB knees result in an IKDC score of A, compared with 54% of SB knees. The incremental cost-effectiveness ratio of a DB reconstruction compared with an SB reconstruction was $6416 per quality adjusted life year in the baseline scenario and $64 371 per quality adjusted life year in the alternate scenario. The model is very sensitive to the proportions of IKDC A outcomes. The model is also sensitive to the utility values assigned to IKDC A and B outcomes and is less sensitive to the marginal cost of a DB reconstruction.

Conclusion.—This preliminary analysis based on published clinical results to date shows DB ACL reconstruction may be cost-effective, despite increased upfront cost. More research is needed to confirm whether there is any difference in the distribution of IKDC outcomes between the 2 techniques. Perhaps more importantly, the lack of any other demonstrated clinical benefit from the DB technique questions the clinical relevance of this difference in IKDC scores.

Clinical Relevance.—Revision data and longer term outcomes after DB reconstruction and more reliable clinical utility data are needed to definitively compare the cost-effectiveness of DB and SB ACL reconstruction. Studies of ACL reconstruction and other sports medicine procedures should report the distribution of outcomes data to facilitate future analyses of clinical effectiveness.

▶ This important contribution is of value as much for the topic being addressed as the conclusions. The orthopedic community must begin to question the cost-effectiveness of our interventions. I would encourage the reader to review the entire article, as it introduces the cost-effective methodology, one that is not intuitive to the orthopedic surgeon. Note that the conclusion is a function of the end point metric; if this is wrong, the conclusion is wrong. Notice the emphasis of the value of the procedure and the somewhat arbitrary definition of what constitutes this important variable. I commend the authors for addressing the issue and bringing this type of analysis to our attention.

B. F. Morrey, MD

Adductor Tenotomy in the Management of Groin Pain in Athletes
Robertson IJ, Curran C, McCaffrey N, et al (Mater Misericordiae Hosp, Dublin, Ireland; Dublin City Univ, Ireland)
Int J Sports Med 32:45-48, 2011

This study evaluates the efficacy of adductor longus tenotomy in athletes with chronic tendinopathy refractory to conservative management. In a retrospective case series we report our experience with 109 male athletes who underwent unilateral adductor tenotomy during the period 2000–2005, all of whom responded to a detailed questionnaire. The criterion for tenotomy was chronic adductor origin pain which prevented training or playing (Level 4), limited training or playing (Level 3), or affected performance (Level 2) and which had failed to respond to conservative management including rest, rehabilitation and/or local steroid injection. Level 1 performance is classified as optimal performance with no pain. 99 of the 109 patients (91%) reported improvement. Best results were achieved in patients with maximum discomfort preoperatively (Level 4) with 32 of 38 (84%) patients returning to Level 1 performance. In conclusion, adductor tenotomy in athletes with severely incapacitating pain (Level 3/4) which fails to respond to conservative management offers the best opportunity of returning to competitive sport (Table 2).

▶ Although this study originates from Ireland and may not be completely applicable to practice in the United States, it was included for several reasons. Not all may be familiar with this treatment option. In addition, the problem may be somewhat specific to soccer, but it is a common generic problem with all athletics. Further, it is well recognized to often be refractory to treatment.

TABLE 2.—Pre- and Post-op Pain Severity Levels

Pre-op		Post-op			
		Level 1	Level 2	Level 3	Level 4
Level 4	38	32	6	0	0
Level 3	60	42	15	2	1
Level 2	11	4	1	5	1

Thus, that this simple procedure seems to be quite safe and effective is worth noting (Table 2). One might also speculate as to whether the success rate would hold true for other sport-specific injuries.

B. F. Morrey, MD

9 Foot and Ankle

Introduction

The chapter on the foot and ankle is an interesting section for me since it probably represents the broadest spectrum of anatomy and pathology. It includes topics relating to the toes, midfoot, hindfoot, and ankle. The problems with the diabetic foot, of course, are major concerns for the general orthopedic surgeon. However, in this year's volume, I have attempted to define those techniques that seem to be effective in the various anatomic regions of the foot and ankle. A passing recognition of the status of ankle joint replacement is also included in this year's foot and ankle section. This is an area that is rapidly expanding, and we have made an effort to document those surgical techniques that seem to be of value and have stood the test of time, particularly as they relate to ankle joint replacement and its alternative—ankle fusion.

Bernard F. Morrey, MD

Are the feet of obese children fat or flat? Revisiting the debate
Riddiford-Harland DL, Steele JR, Baur LA (Univ of Wollongong, New South Wales, Australia; Univ of Sydney Discipline of Paediatrics and Child Health, New South Wales, Australia)
Int J Obes 35:115-120, 2011

Objective.—There is debate as to the effects of obesity on the developing feet of children. We aimed to determine whether the flatter foot structure characteristic of obese primary school-aged children was due to increased medial midfoot plantar fat pad thickness (fat feet) or due to structural lowering of the longitudinal arch (flat feet).

Methods and Procedures.—Participants were 75 obese children (8.3 ± 1.1 years, 26 boys, BMI 25.2 ± 3.6 kg m^{-2}) and 75 age- and sex-matched non-obese children (8.3 ± 0.9 years, BMI 15.9 ± 1.4 kg m^{-2}). Height, weight and foot dimensions were measured with standard instrumentation. Medial midfoot plantar fat pad thickness and internal arch height were quantified using ultrasonography.

Results.—Obese children had significantly greater medial midfoot fat pad thickness relative to the leaner children during both non-weight bearing (5.4 and 4.6 mm, respectively; $P < 0.001$) and weight bearing (4.7 and 4.3 mm, respectively; $P < 0.001$). The obese children also displayed a lowered medial longitudinal arch height when compared to their leaner counterparts (23.5 and 24.5 mm, respectively; $P = 0.006$).

Conclusion.—Obese children had significantly fatter and flatter feet compared to normal weight children. The functional and clinical relevance of the increased fatness and flatness values for the obese children remains unknown.

▶ Because obesity has become endemic in America, this is a very timely and relevant study. The question of the presence and relevance of a flat foot in a child is an age-old one. With the problem of obesity, it has assumed new proportions (no pun intended). This study was well conceived and conducted; hence, I think we can trust the findings and conclusion. So the answer to the question of whether this is a fat or flat foot is yes! This assessment found both to be present in the obese patient. The next concern is the management. Ideally, this would be to lose weight. Not in America!

So I fear we will be faced with an increasing incidence of obese children with foot pain. No surprise.

B. F. Morrey, MD

Autologous Platelets Have No Effect on the Healing of Human Achilles Tendon Ruptures: A Randomized Single-Blind Study
Schepull T, Kvist J, Norrman H, et al (Linköping Univ, Sweden)
Am J Sports Med 39:38-47, 2011

Background.—Animal studies have shown that local application of platelet-rich plasma (PRP) stimulates tendon repair. Preliminary results from a retrospective case series have shown faster return to sports.

Hypothesis.—Autologous PRP stimulates healing of acute Achilles tendon ruptures.

Study Design.—Randomized controlled trial; Level of evidence, 2.

Methods.—Thirty patients were recruited consecutively. During surgery, tantalum beads were implanted in the Achilles tendon proximal and distal to the rupture. Before skin suture, randomization was performed, and 16 patients were injected with 10 mL PRP (10 times higher platelet concentration than peripheral blood) whereas 14 were not. With 3-dimensional radiographs (roentgen stereophotogrammetric analysis; RSA), the distance between the beads was measured at 7, 19, and 52 weeks while the patient resisted different dorsal flexion moments over the ankle joint, thereby estimating tendon strain per load. An estimate of elasticity modulus was calculated using callus dimensions from computed tomography. At 1 year, functional outcome was evaluated, including the heel raise index and Achilles Tendon Total Rupture Score. The primary effect variables were elasticity modulus at 7 weeks and heel raise index at 1 year.

Results.—The mechanical variables showed a large degree of variation between patients that could not be explained by measuring error. No significant group differences in elasticity modulus could be shown. There was no significant difference in heel raise index. The Achilles Tendon Total Rupture Score was lower in the PRP group, suggesting a detrimental effect. There was a correlation between the elasticity modulus at 7 and 19 weeks and the heel raise index at 52 weeks.

Conclusion.—The results suggest that PRP is not useful for treatment of Achilles tendon ruptures. The variation in elasticity modulus provides biologically relevant information, although it is unclear how early biomechanics is connected to late clinical results.

▶ This useful prospective randomized study offers important insights. The use of platelet-rich plasma (PRP) is one of the hot topics in orthopedics today. It is safe, so it is being extensively used and studied. As demonstrated here, the use of PRP is not always favorable. For tennis elbow, maybe. Not for sure, just maybe. This is a simple clear study that included an adequate sample, with valid measurement tools and adequate follow-up period to offer valid conclusions. Specifically, PRP is not an effective healing adjunct for the repaired Achilles tendon at 1 year. Regardless, this will remain a hot topic. It will be market and hype driven. The best we can do is pay attention to the good studies and their conclusions. This is one of them.

B. F. Morrey, MD

The Majority of Patients With Achilles Tendinopathy Recover Fully When Treated With Exercise Alone: A 5-Year Follow-Up
Silbernagel KG, Brorsson A, Lundberg M (Univ of Delaware, Newark; Univ of Gothenburg, Sweden)
Am J Sports Med 39:607-613, 2011

Background.—Systematic reviews indicate that exercise has the most evidence of effectiveness in treatment of midportion Achilles tendinopathy. However, there is a lack of long-term follow-ups (>4 years).

Purpose.—To evaluate the 5-year outcome of patients treated with exercise alone and to examine if certain characteristics, such as level of kinesiophobia, age, and sex, were related to the effectiveness of the treatment.

Study Design.—Case series; Level of evidence, 4.

Methods.—Thirty-four patients (47% women), 51 ± 8.2 years old, were evaluated 5 years after initiation of treatment. The evaluation consisted of a questionnaire regarding recovery of symptoms and other treatments, the Victorian Institute of Sports Assessment—Achilles questionnaire (VISA-A) for symptoms, the Tampa Scale for Kinesiophobia, and tests of lower leg function.

Results.—Twenty-seven patients (80%) fully recovered from the initial injury; of these, 22 (65%) had no symptoms, and 5 (15%) had a new occurrence of symptoms. Seven patients (20%) had continued symptoms. Only 2 patients received another treatment (acupuncture and further exercise instruction). When compared with the other groups, the continued-symptoms group had lower VISA-A scores ($P = .008$ to.021) at the 5-year follow-up and the previous 1-year follow-up but not at any earlier evaluations. There were no significant differences among the groups in regard to sex, age, or physical activity level before injury. There was a significant ($P = .005$) negative correlation (-0.590) between the level of kinesiophobia and heel-rise work recovery.

Conclusion.—The majority of patients with Achilles tendinopathy in this study fully recovered in regard to both symptoms and function when treated with exercise alone. Increased fear of movement might have a negative effect on the effectiveness of exercise treatment; therefore, a pain-monitoring model should be used when patients are treated with exercise.

▶ When I read the title of this work, I didn't think this was an article from the United States. So we turn, once again, to other societies to understand the natural history of nonoperative treatment. With the advent of ultrasound, platelet-rich plasma, and the like, our tendency is to increase the tendency to treat more rather than less aggressively. The interesting twist of this study was to analyze the fear of pain or reinjury, kinesiophobia, on outcome. The question does remain whether some form of intervention that is simple, noninvasive, and inexpensive might not ultimately be the treatment of choice for this and other similar tendinopathies.

B. F. Morrey, MD

Operative versus Nonoperative Treatment of Acute Achilles Tendon Ruptures: A Multicenter Randomized Trial Using Accelerated Functional Rehabilitation
Willits K, Amendola A, Bryant D, et al (The Univ of Western Ontario, London, Canada; The Univ of Lowa Hosp and Clinics; The Univ of Western Ontario, London, Canada; et al)
J Bone Joint Surg Am 92:2767-2775, 2010

Background.—To date, studies directly comparing the rerupture rate in patients with an Achilles tendon rupture who are treated with surgical repair with the rate in patients treated nonoperatively have been inconclusive but the pooled relative risk of rerupture favored surgical repair. In all but one study, the limb was immobilized for six to eight weeks. Published studies of animals and humans have shown a benefit of early functional stimulus to healing tendons. The purpose of the present study was to compare the outcomes of patients with an acute Achilles tendon rupture treated with operative repair and accelerated functional rehabilitation with the outcomes of similar patients treated with accelerated functional rehabilitation alone.

Methods.—Patients were randomized to operative or nonoperative treatment for acute Achilles tendon rupture. All patients underwent an accelerated rehabilitation protocol that featured early weight-bearing and early range of motion. The primary outcome was the rerupture rate as demonstrated by a positive Thompson squeeze test, the presence of a palpable gap, and loss of plantar flexion strength. Secondary outcomes included isokinetic strength, the Leppilahti score, range of motion, and calf circumference measured at three, six, twelve, and twenty-four months after injury.

Results.—A total of 144 patients (seventy-two treated operatively and seventy-two treated nonoperatively) were randomized. There were 118 males and twenty-six females, and the mean age (and standard deviation) was 40.4 ± 8.8 years. Rerupture occurred in two patients in the operative group and in three patients in the nonoperative group. There was no clinically important difference between groups with regard to strength, range of motion, calf circumference, or Leppilahti score. There were thirteen complications in the operative group and six in the nonoperative group, with the main difference being the greater number of soft-tissue-related complications in the operative group.

Conclusions.—This study supports accelerated functional rehabilitation and nonoperative treatment for acute Achilles tendon ruptures. All measured outcomes of nonoperative treatment were acceptable and were clinically similar to those for operative treatment. In addition, this study suggests that the application of an accelerated-rehabilitation nonoperative protocol avoids serious complications related to surgical management (Table 3).

▶ The optimum management of the Achilles tendon rupture is a favorite topic of debate. In spite of the data presented, most surgeons seem to prefer operative treatment. As might be expected, this carefully designed, well-controlled prospective study was performed in Canada and possesses an adequate number of subjects to arrive at a definitive conclusion (Fig 1 in the original article). But

TABLE 3.—Complications

Complication	Operative Group	Nonoperative Group
Rerupture	2	3
Deep venous thrombosis	1	1
Pain (substantial)		1
Failure to heal (palpable gap)		1
Achilles tendon tethered to skin	1	
Hypertrophic scar	1	
Superficial infection	4	
Deep infection	1	
Pulmonary embolus	1	
Wound complication (small opening in skin)	2	

the nonoperative group contains a twist—early aggressive functional rehabilitation. With this earlier motion, and more aggressive rehabilitative program, the outcomes favor nonoperative management from the perspective of both rerupture and function (Table 3). So, if the rehabilitative program can be followed, the nonoperative program would seem to be our treatment of choice.

B. F. Morrey, MD

Peroneal tendon subluxation: the other lateral ankle injury
Roth JA, Taylor WC, Whalen J (Mayo Clinic Florida, Jacksonville)
Br J Sports Med 44:1047-1053, 2010

Ankle injuries are a frequent cause of patient visits to the emergency department and orthopaedic and primary care offices. Although lateral ligament sprains are the most common pathologic conditions, peroneal tendon subluxations occur with a similar inversion mechanism. Multiple grades of subluxation have been described with a recent addition of intrasheath subluxation. Magnetic resonance imaging is the best imaging modality to view the peroneal tendons at the retrofibular groove. Currently, point-of-care ultrasound is gaining clinical ground, especially for the dynamic viewing capability to capture an episodic subluxation. Although conservative treatment may be attempted for an acute injury, it has a low rate of success for the prevention of recurrent subluxation. Surgical procedures of various techniques have resulted in excellent recovery rates and faster return to play. The aim of this paper was to give a complete review of the current literature on peroneal tendon subluxation and to propose a clinical algorithm to help guide diagnosis and treatment. The goal of this study was to heighten clinical awareness to improve earlier detection and treatment of this sometimes elusive diagnosis (Fig 7).

▶ As this article indicates in the introductory remarks, subluxation of the peroneal tendons, while not the most common injury, is nonetheless a relatively common source of morbidity. The main issue for the orthopedic surgeon is not so much the diagnosis, which quite frankly is rather easy, but what to do? This review does offer a thoughtful algorithm that helps direct the thought process (Fig 7). Of note, once the subluxation occurs, nonoperative treatment is usually not effective and surgery is indicated.

B. F. Morrey, MD

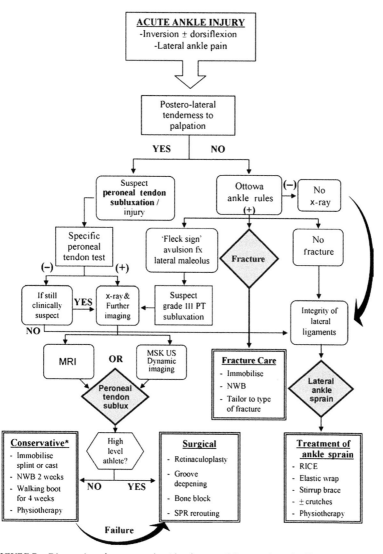

FIGURE 7.—Diagnostic and treatment algorithm for care of the acute lateral ankle injury. The asterisk indicates conservative treatment should be reserved only for acute injuries in the less-active population. fx, fracture; NWB, non–weight bearing; PT, peroneal tendon; RICE, rest, ice, compression, elevation. (Reprinted from Roth JA, Taylor WC, Whalen J. Peroneal tendon subluxation: the other lateral ankle injury. Br J Sports Med. 44:2010;1047-1053, and reproduced with permission from the BMJ Publishing Group.)

Tibiotalocalcaneal Arthrodesis With a Curved, Interlocking, Intramedullary Nail

Budnar VM, Hepple S, Harries WG, et al (Southmead Hosp, Bristol, Avon, UK)
Foot Ankle Int 31:1085-1092, 2010

Background.—Tibiotalocalcaneal fusion with a straight rod has a risk of damaging the lateral plantar neurovascular structures and may interfere with maintaining normal heel valgus position. We report the results of a prospective study of tibiotalocalcaneal (TTC) arthrodesis with a short, anatomically curved interlocking, intramedullary nail.

Material and Methods.—Forty-five arthrodeses in 42 patients, performed between Jan 2003 and Oct 2008, were prospectively followed. The mean followup was 48 (range, 10 to 74) months. The main indications for the procedure were failed ankle arthrodesis with progressive subtalar arthritis, failed ankle arthroplasty and complex hindfoot deformity. The outcome was measured by a combination of pre and postoperative clinical examination, AOFAS hindfoot scores, SF−12 scores and radiological assessment.

Results.—Union rate was 89% (40/45). Eighty-two percent (37/45) reported improvement in pain and 73% (33/45) had improved foot function. Satisfactory hindfoot alignment was achieved in 84% (38/45). Postoperatively there was a mean improvement in the AOFAS score of 37. Complications included a below knee amputation for persistent deep infection, five nonunions, and three delayed unions. Four nails, six proximal and six distal locking screws were removed for various causes. Other complications included two perioperative fractures, four superficial wound infections and one case of lateral plantar nerve irritation.

Conclusion.—With a short, anatomically curved intramedullary nail, we had a high rate of tibiotalocalcaneal fusion with minimal plantar neurovascular complications. We believe a short, curved intramedullary nail,

TABLE 4.—Peri- / Postoperative Complications

Complication		Number
Below-knee amputation		1
Non-union (5)	Ankle Joint	2
	Subtalar Joint	1
	Ankle and subtalar	2
Delayed union		3
Removal of hardware	Removal of nail	4
	Removal of proximal screws	6
	Removal of distal screws	6
Peri-op fracture	Talus	1
	Medial malleolus	1
Infection	Superficial	4
	Deep	1
Deep vein thrombosis		4

with its more lateral entry point, helped maintain hindfoot alignment (Table 4).

▶ There remain few options to reconstruct the ankle. While ankle arthrodesis remains a viable consideration, with rejuvenation in ankle replacement, the technique is largely being performed as a salvage for the failed ankle replacement. This technique-oriented article is used as an example of the trend to use a transcalcaneal approach to access the tibial canal (Figs 8 and 9 in the original article). The rather high complication rate (Table 4) is a reflection of the patient sample being largely that of a salvage for a failed ankle device and is also somewhat reflective of the inherent vulnerability of this anatomic site. For the nondeformed ankle, compression screws remain our preferred treatment.

B. F. Morrey, MD

Limb Salvage In Severe Diabetic Foot Infection

Kim BS, Choi WJ, Baek MK, et al (Yonsei Univ College of Medicine, Seoul, Korea)
Foot Ankle Int 32:31-37, 2011

Background.—The purpose of our study was to determine the efficacy of a management algorithm that includes negative pressure wound therapy (NPWT) in diabetic feet with limb-threatening infection.

Materials and Methods.—Forty-five septic diabetic feet were treated with NPWT between 2006 and 2008. After emergent abscess evacuation, early vascular intervention was performed if necessary. Debridement, with or without partial foot amputation, was followed by NPWT. Wound progress was measured using a digital scanner. A limb was considered salvaged if complete healing was achieved without any or with minor amputation through or below the ankle. The mean followup after complete wound healing was 17 (range, 6 to 35) months.

Results.—Thirty-two cases (71%) were infected with two or more organisms. Negative pressure wound therapy was applied for 26.2 ± 14.3 days. The median time to achieve more than 75% wound area granulation was 23 (range, 4 to 55) days and 104 (range, 38 to 255) days to complete wound healing. Successful limb salvage was achieved in 44 cases (98%); 14 (31%) without any amputation and 30 (67%) with partial foot amputations. Total number of operations per limb was 2.4 ± 1.3. One case of repeated infection and necrosis was managed with a transtibial amputation. There were no complications associated with NPWT.

Conclusion.—This study provides the outcome of a management algorithm which includes NPWT in salvaging severely infected diabetic feet. With emergent evacuation of abscess, early vascular intervention and appropriate debridement, NPWT can be a useful adjunct to the management of limb-threatening diabetic foot infections.

▶ This impressive study reveals successful management in more than 90% of those with ischemic infected diabetic foot ulcers. This is one of the most difficult of all patient populations to manage effectively. The use of negative pressure wound dressings was performed in conjunction with other treatment modalities as indicated (Fig 1 in the original article). Although an impressive success rate is documented, the treatment was conducted for a prolonged period. I was also unable to discern the long-term success rate of this treatment program. It is clearly effective; however, the disease is relentless.

B. F. Morrey, MD

Long-Term Results After Modified Brostrom Procedure Without Calcaneofibular Ligament Reconstruction
Lee KT, Park YU, Kim JS, et al (Eulji Univ School of Medicine, Seoul, Korea; et al)
Foot Ankle Int 32:153-157, 2011

Background.—The short-term results of modified Brostrom procedures (MBP) have been satisfactory. However, the long-term results of anatomical reconstruction have been less frequently reported. We report on our long-term results in our patient group.

Materials and Methods.—Thirty patients with chronic ankle instability who were treated using the MBP without CFL reconstruction from March 1997 to June 1999 were evaluated retrospectively. This consecutive series of patients was comprised of 26 males and four females. The mean age of the patients at the time of operation was 23 years. The mean followup period was 10.6 years. Twenty-four of the 30 were high-level amateur or professional athletes. The operation procedure involved only ATFL imbrication with inferior extensor retinaculum (IER) reinforcement. Clinical outcomes were evaluated by reviewing clinical charts, retrospectively. Functional outcome scores were obtained using the Hamilton scale, a VAS, and AOFAS score at final followup visit, when each patient underwent a physical examination and stress radiography.

Results.—Mean AOFAS score was 91 and the mean VAS at final followup was 87. According to the Hamilton classification, 12 achieved an excellent result, 16 a good result, and two a fair result. Mean anterior translation values at final followup were 6.9 and 6.1 mm on ipsilateral and contralateral sides. Furthermore, mean talar tilt angles were 3.0 and 2.5 degrees for ipsilateral and contralateral sides. Twenty-eight of the 30 patients were restored to pre-injury activity levels.

Conclusion.—The long-term surgical results of the MBP without CFL reconstruction for chronic lateral ankle instability were good to excellent in terms of functional, clinical, and radiographic assessments.

▶ This study was of interest to me primarily because of the long-term surveillance. There is still considerable debate as to the optimum technique for chronic ankle instability. Unlike the original description, the proposed modified Brostrom technique does not address the calcaneofibular ligament (Fig 1 in the original article). Nonetheless, the mean of 10-year follow-up is impressive, as are the results of greater than 90% acceptance and return to a high level of function. Of particular note is the lack of secondary arthrosis and the excellent stability achieved. Both would explain the favorable clinical and objective outcomes.

B. F. Morrey, MD

Total Ankle Replacement Outcome in Low Volume Centers: Short-Term Followup
Reuver JM, Dayerizadeh N, Burger B, et al (Deventer Hosp, Nico Bolkesteinlaan, The Netherlands)
Foot Ankle Int 31:1064-1068, 2010

Background.—The indication for total ankle replacement (TAR) as an alternative to ankle fusion continues to be a much-debated topic. The reported survival of TAR at midterm followup is approximately 90%. The aim of this study was to compare functional outcome and survival of TAR in low volume centers versus high volume centers.

Materials and Methods.—A retrospective cohort study was carried out in four low volume centers. Sixty-four Salto TARs were performed between 2003 and 2007 in 60 patients. Fifty-five (59 TAR) patients were eligible for followup with 28 men. Standardized American Orthopaedic Foot and Ankle Society (AOFAS) scores, patient satisfaction, and range of motion (ROM) were measured. Standardized and dynamic radiographs were used for evaluation of radiolucencies, ROM and component alignment.

Results.—Seven of the 59 ankle prostheses had to be revised: five for loosening and two for deep infection. Three of the five revised for loosening went on to fusion, and in two a revision of one of the components was performed. Both infected ankles were fused. Five patients declined to participate in this study, among these two were TAR failures. Survival with revision as the endpoint was 86% at final followup. The average AOFAS score was 75 (SD ± 15). On dynamic radiographs the ROM was 22 degrees (SD ± 8) in the tibiotalar joint.

Conclusion.—This study demonstrated that functional results of total ankle replacement in low volume centers were comparable to most high

TABLE 1.—Data

Year	Author	Prosthesis	Followup (Years)	Survival	Functional Score
2003	Anderson	STAR	4.3	70%	AOFAS 74 (21–100)
2004	Kofoed*	STAR	9.5	95%	KOFOED 92 ± 7
2004	Buechel*	Buechel-Pappas	12	92%	
2004	Knecht*	Agility	9	89%	
2004	Bonnin*	Salto	3	95–98%	AOFAS 82 ± 16
2004	Valderrabano	STAR	3.7	86.8%	AOFAS 84 (28–100)
2006	San Giovanni**	Buechel-Pappas	8.3	93%	AOFAS 81 (40–92)
2006	Wood	STAR	7.3	80.3%	AOFAS 70 (20–94)
2010	Reuver	Salto	3	86%	AOFAS 75 ± 15

*Authors all well connected to the prosthesis used.
**All rheumatoid arthritis patients.

volume centers but survival was lower especially when we consider our shorter followup than most comparable series (Table 1).

▶ We have intentionally not included much on total ankle replacement in recent volumes, as we felt the designs and data were too much in flux. I believe this is still the case. Yet, this article is included in large measure to provide an opportunity to discuss the current state of this joint replacement. The sample size of 80 is reasonable, but the follow-up averages only a short 36 months. The design is of interest in the manner that it attempts to distribute forces in the tibia in over the talus (Fig 1 in the original article). Of value is the review of the literature with an effort to distinguish reports from those with vested interest in the design and those with no such potential conflict (Table 1). My interpretation is that the newer designs may be a marked step forward, but the techniques are difficult, and long-term surveillance is needed to offer any cogent opinion of the effectiveness of the current designs.

B. F. Morrey, MD

High Rate of Osteolytic Lesions in Medium-Term Followup After the AES Total Ankle Replacement

Kokkonen A, Ikävalko M, Tiihonen R, et al (Rheumatism Foundation Hosp, Heinola, Finland)
Foot Ankle Int 32:168-175, 2011

Background.—Some previous studies have shown a high percentage of early-onset and rapidly progressing osteolysis associated with total ankle arthroplasty (TAA) by the Ankle Evolutive System (AES). The purpose of our study was to analyze medium-term results at our institution.
Materials and Methods.—Altogether 38 TAAs using AES prostheses were carried out between 2003 and 2007. Diagnoses were rheumatoid arthritis (71%), post-traumatic and idiopathic osteoarthritis (29%). The mean age was 54 years, followup 28 months. Tibial and talar components

had hydroxyapatite coating on metal (Co-Cr) components (HA-coated). Since 2005 the design was changed and components were porous coated with titanium and hydroxyapatite (dual-coated).

Results.—Two-year survival was 79% (95% CI: 56 to 98). At followup 34 (89%) primary tibial and talar components were preserved. In 19 (50%) TAAs osteolysis (more than or equal to 2 mm) occurred in the periprosthetic bone area and in nine (24%) comprised large "cyst-like osteolysis". In HA-coated prostheses radiolucent lines (less than or equal to 2 mm) or osteolysis (more than or equal to 2 mm) were detected in 11 (100%) cases and in dual-coated prostheses in 19 (74%) ($p = 0.08$). On the other hand there was more large "cyst-like osteolysis" around the dual-coated prosthesis and lesions were larger ($p = 0.017$). In rheumatoid arthritis osteolysis was detected in 14 (52%) and large "cyst-like osteolysis" in seven (26%) prostheses and in the group of traumatic and idiopathic osteoarthritis in six (55%) and two (18%), respectively.

Conclusion.—This study showed a high frequency of osteolysis in medium-term followup after the AES ankle replacement. The outcome was not sufficiently beneficial and we have discontinued use of this prosthesis.

▶ The orthopedic patient and surgeon alike continue to await word that the final joint has been solved. Total ankle replacement continues to lag behind the other joint replacements in being amenable to prosthetic replacement. This article describes osteolysis after the Ankle Evolutive System replacement (Fig 2a in the original article), which occurred with sufficient frequency (Fig 5 in the original article) to result in discontinuation of this device. The authors are to be commended for their analysis and offering insights as to the failure mode, in hopes that it can be avoided in subsequent designs.

B. F. Morrey, MD

Reconstruction of the Symptomatic Idiopathic Flatfoot in Adolescents and Young Adults

Oh I, Williams BR, Ellis SJ, et al (Hosp for Special Surgery, NY; et al)
Foot Ankle Int 32:225-232, 2011

Background.—The surgical indications, timing, and procedure for flexible flatfoot reconstruction in young patients remains controversial. This retrospective study reports the clinical results of reconstruction of flexible, idiopathic, symptomatic flatfoot in adolescent and young adults indicated for surgery by persistent pain and functional limitations. The hypothesis was that the results of these procedures allow patients to return to sports activities with minimal discomfort or pain.

Materials and Methods.—Sixteen consecutive idiopathic flatfeet in ten patients with a mean age of 15.6 years at the time of surgery (range, 10 to 22) were assessed at a final followup visit at average of 5.2 (range, 2 to

10) years. Reconstruction included combined medializing calcaneal osteotomy and lateral column lengthening in all 16 patients. Flexor digitorum longus transfer (nine), medial column stabilization (eight), and gastrocnemius recession (eight) were carried out as needed. The AOFAS, SF-36, and FAOS questionnaires were completed. Sports activity and patient satisfaction were also assessed. Standard preoperative and postoperative radiographic parameters were measured.

Results.—The mean AOFAS score increased on average from 49.1 to 93.4. Only one patient reported a postoperative restriction in sports. The satisfaction level was excellent in 15 feet and good in one foot. Significant improvement in radiographic parameters was noted for the AP talonavicular coverage angle ($p < 0.001$) and lateral talar-first metatarsal angle ($p < 0.001$).

Conclusion.—Flexible flatfoot reconstruction in a cohort of symptomatic adolescent and young adult patients achieved a reduction of pain and improved functional outcome including the ability to participate in sporting activities (Table 1).

▶ This study addresses a controversial area of foot surgery: can and should the flexible flatfoot be surgically corrected? This assessment of 16 patients with excellent objective and subjective results in 15 of 16 would seem to answer

TABLE 1.—Patient Demographics

Case	Age	Sex	Side	Physis	Procedures	Bone Graft
1	19	F	L	Closed	PTTR, FDL, MCO, LCL, EAN	Autograft
2	20	F	R	Closed	MCO, LCL	Autograft
3	16	F	R	Closed	MCO, LCL, Lapidus, GR	Autograft
4	13	M	R	Open	PTTR, FDL, MCO, LCL, EAN, Cotton, GR	Allograft
5	14	M	L	Open	PTTR, FDL, MCO, LCL, EAN, Cotton, GR	Allograft
6	20	F	R	Closed	PTTR, FDL, MCO, LCL, EAN, Cotton, GR	Allograft
7	21	M	L	Closed	PTTR, FDL, MCO, LCL, Lapidus, GR	Autograft
8	22	M	R	Closed	PTTR, FDL, MCO, LCL, Lapidus, GR	Autograft
9	16	M	R	Closed	PTTR, FDL, MCO, LCL, Lapidus, GR	Autograft
10	18	F	L	Closed	PTTR, FDL, MCO, LCL, Cotton, GR	Autograft
11	10	M	L	Open	MCO, LCL	Autograft
12	10	M	R	Open	MCO, LCL	Autograft
13	12	F	L	Open	PTTR, MCO, LCL, EAN	Autograft
14	12	F	R	Open	PTTR, MCO, LCL, EAN	Autograft
15	12	M	L	Open	MCO, LCL	Autograft
16	14	M	R	Open	MCO, LCL,	Autograft
Average	16	7 F / 9 M	7 L / 9 R	8 Open / 8 Closed	—	3 Allograft / 13 Autograft

LCL, lateral column lengthening; PTTR, posterior tibial tendon reconstruction; MCO, medializing calcaneal osteotomy; FDL, flexor digitorum longus; GR, gastrocnemius recession. EAN, excision of accessory navicular.

in the affirmative. My difficulty with this experience is that the exclusion criteria are clear, but the inclusion criteria are less so; specifically, the physical and radiographic basis of a surgical decision are lacking. Furthermore, the surgical plan and features of the intervention are not uniform (Table 1). So is the message that anything works on anyone who wants the surgery? Regardless, this experience does at least indicate that surgery is effective, short term, on the adolescent with the symptomatic flatfoot. This is good to know.

B. F. Morrey, MD

10 Forearm, Wrist, and Hand

Introduction

This year's selections continue the trend of refinement of clinical research on various topics that will be encountered commonly in practice. Collectively, these articles further our knowledge base and strengthen information that appears to be distilling down to accepted standards of care, including operative treatment of distal radius fractures and scaphoid fractures. We have also included selections that provide us with updated information regarding bone health and osteoporosis, the use of injectable collagenase for Dupuytren's contracture, and emerging uses of botulinum neurotoxin A for treatment of injured muscle-tendon units. In addition, we have included selections that refine or simplify surgical treatments of common wrist and hand injuries.

Stephen D. Trigg, MD

Evaluation and Diagnosis

Accuracy of In-Office Nerve Conduction Studies for Median Neuropathy: A Meta-Analysis

Strickland JW, Gozani SN (Reconstructive Hand Surgeons of Indiana, Carmel; Indiana Univ School of Medicine, Indianapolis; NeuroMetrix, Inc., Waltham, MA)
J Hand Surg 36A:52-60, 2011

Purpose.—Carpal tunnel syndrome is the most common focal neuropathy. It is typically diagnosed clinically and confirmed by abnormal median nerve conduction across the wrist (median neuropathy [MN]). In-office nerve conduction testing devices facilitate performance of nerve conduction studies (NCS) and are used by hand surgeons in the evaluation of patients with upper extremity symptoms. The purpose of this meta-analysis was to determine the diagnostic accuracy of this testing method for MN in symptomatic patients.

Methods.—We searched the MEDLINE database for prospective cohort studies that evaluated the diagnostic accuracy of in-office NCS for MN in symptomatic patients with traditional electrodiagnostic laboratories as reference standards. We assessed included studies for quality and heterogeneity in diagnostic performance and determined pooled statistical outcome measures when appropriate.

Results.—We identified 5 studies with a total of 448 symptomatic hands. The pooled sensitivity and specificity were 0.88 (95% confidence interval [CI], 0.83−0.91) and 0.93 (95% CI, 0.88−0.96), respectively. Specificities exhibited heterogeneity. The diagnostic odds ratios were homogeneous, with a pooled value of 62.0 (95% CI, 30.1−127).

Conclusions.—This meta-analysis showed that in-office NCS detects MN with clinically relevant accuracy. Performance was similar to inter-examiner agreement for MN within a traditional electrodiagnostic laboratory. There was some variation in diagnostic operating characteristics. Therefore, physicians using this technology should interpret test results within a clinical context and with attention to the pretest probability of MN, rather than in absolute terms.

▶ Carpal tunnel syndrome (CTS) describes a symptom complex involving the distribution of the median nerve and is diagnosed by specific findings on physical examination and by delayed median nerve conduction velocities across the wrist. Patient-reported symptoms of abnormal sensation, paresthesias, and frequent pain in the median nerve distribution along with recognition of provocative positioning or activity add to the clinical diagnosis. A diagnosis of CTS can in most cases be made by clinical examination, and the need for routine confirmatory electrodiagnostic study has been challenged. Moreover, routine, formal, confirmatory, laboratory-based electrodiagnostic studies are expensive and can lead to delays in treatment. This latter point, no doubt, has led to the marketing of a number of in-office nerve conduction study devices in recent years. Some, but not all, of these devices have been studied with some scientific rigor in comparison with reference to electrodiagnostic laboratory data on a limited basis. This is the first systematic meta-analysis to review the diagnostic accuracy of these in-office devices and provides us with meaningful data for their consideration and use.

S. D. Trigg, MD

Comparison of CT and MRI for Diagnosis of Suspected Scaphoid Fractures
Mallee W, Doornberg JN, Ring D, et al (Academic Med Ctr of Amsterdam, The Netherlands)
J Bone Joint Surg Am 93:20-28, 2011

Background.—There is no consensus on the optimum imaging method to use to confirm the diagnosis of true scaphoid fractures among patients with suspected scaphoid fractures. This study tested the null hypothesis that computed tomography (CT) and magnetic resonance imaging (MRI) have the same diagnostic performance characteristics for the diagnosis of scaphoid fractures.

Methods.—Thirty-four consecutive patients with a suspected scaphoid fracture (tenderness of the scaphoid and normal radiographic findings after a fall on the outstretched hand) underwent CT and MRI within ten days after a wrist injury. The reference standard for a true fracture of the scaphoid was six-week follow-up radiographs in four views. A panel including surgeons and radiologists came to a consensus diagnosis for each type of imaging. The images were considered in a randomly ordered, blinded fashion, independent of the other types of imaging. We calculated sensitivity, specificity, and accuracy as well as positive and negative predictive values.

Results.—The reference standard revealed six true fractures of the scaphoid (prevalence, 18%). CT demonstrated a fracture in five patients (15%), with one false-positive, two false-negative, and four true-positive results. MRI demonstrated a fracture in seven patients (21%), with three false-positive, two false-negative, and four true-positive results. The sensitivity, specificity, and accuracy were 67%, 96%, and 91%, respectively, for CT and 67%, 89%, and 85%, respectively, for MRI. According to the McNemar test for paired binary data, these differences were not significant. The positive predictive value with use of the Bayes formula was 0.76 for CT and 0.54 for MRI. The negative predictive value was 0.94 for CT and 0.93 for MRI.

TABLE 1.—CT Versus MRI

	6-Wk Follow-up Radiographs (Reference Standard)	CT		MRI	
		Scaphoid Fracture	No Scaphoid Fracture	Scaphoid Fracture	No Scaphoid Fracture
Scaphoid fracture	6	4	2	4	2
No scaphoid fracture	28	1	27	3	25
Totals	34	5	29	7	27
Diagnostic performance characteristics					
Sensitivity		$4/4 + 2 = 67\%$*		$4/4 + 2 = 67\%$*	
Specificity		$27/1 + 27 = 96\%$†		$25/3 + 25 = 89\%$†	
Accuracy		$4 + 27/4 + 2 + 1 + 27 = 91\%$‡		$4 + 25/4 + 2 + 3 + 25 = 85\%$‡	
Positive predictive value (PPV)		$4/4 + 1 = 80\%$§		$4/4 + 3 = 57\%$§	
PPV accounting for prevalence and incidence		76%		54%	
Negative predictive value (NPV)		$27/27 + 2 = 93\%$#		$25/25 + 2 = 93\%$#	
NPV accounting for prevalence and incidence		94%		93%	

*The proportion of patients who had a scaphoid fracture according to the reference standard and who were classified as having a positive MRI (true-positive).
†The proportion of patients who had no scaphoid fracture according to the reference standard and who were classified as having a negative CT/MRI (true-negative).
‡The proportion of patients who were correctly classified by CT/MRI.
§The probability that a patient with a positive CT/MRI has a scaphoid fracture.
#The probability that a patient with a negative CT/MRI does not have a fracture.

Conclusions.—CT and MRI had comparable diagnostic characteristics. Both were better at excluding scaphoid fractures than they were at confirming them, and both were subject to false-positive and false-negative interpretations. The best reference standard is debatable, but it is now unclear whether or not bone edema on MRI and small unicortical lines on CT represent a true fracture (Table 1).

▶ Clinical suspicion for the possibility of an occult scaphoid fracture in postinjury patients presenting with radial-sided wrist and/or anatomic snuffbox pain with negative plain radiographs is generally widely known among orthopedic surgeons and emergency room and primary care physicians alike. A standard treatment algorithm includes precautionary immobilization and follow-up imaging. Moreover, it is also generally accepted that follow-up plain radiographs may not show a fracture for several weeks, thus requiring continued cast immobilization and with it potential loss of productivity weighed against the costs of ordering more sensitive imaging studies in patients with a suspected scaphoid fracture. Despite numerous studies that show the increased sensitivity and specificity of both MRI and CT scanning for imaging an occult scaphoid fracture, there is no consensus among radiologists on which is the optimum imaging method. This study brings forth new information on the diagnostic performance of CT and MRI and study methods for the diagnosis of suspected scaphoid fracture, which warrants our review.

S. D. Trigg, MD

Osteoporosis as a Risk Factor for Distal Radial Fractures: A Case-Control Study
Øyen J, Brudvik C, Gjesdal CG, et al (Univ of Bergen, Norway; Haukeland Univ Hosp, Bergen, Norway)
J Bone Joint Surg Am 93:348-356, 2011

Background.—Distal radial fractures occur earlier in life than hip and spinal fractures and may be the first sign of osteoporosis. The aims of this case-control study were to compare the prevalence of osteopenia and osteoporosis between female and male patients with low-energy distal radial fractures and matched controls and to investigate whether observed differences in bone mineral density between patients and controls could be explained by potential confounders.

Methods.—Six hundred and sixty-four female and eighty-five male patients who sustained a distal radial fracture, and 554 female and fifty-four male controls, were included in the study. All distal radial fractures were radiographically confirmed. Bone mineral density was assessed with use of dual x-ray absorptiometry at the femoral neck, total hip (femoral neck, trochanter, and intertrochanteric area), and lumbar spine (L2-L4). A self-administered questionnaire provided information on health and lifestyle factors.

Results.—The prevalence of osteoporosis was 34% in female patients and 10% in female controls. The corresponding values were 17% in male patients and 13% in male controls. In the age group of fifty to fifty-nine years, 18% of female patients and 5% of female controls had osteoporosis. In the age group of sixty to sixty-nine years, the corresponding values were 25% and 7%, respectively. In adjusted conditional logistic regression analyses, osteopenia and osteoporosis were significantly associated with distal radial fractures in women. Osteoporosis was significantly associated with distal radial fractures in men.

Conclusions.—The prevalence of osteoporosis in patients with distal radial fractures is high compared with that in control subjects, and osteoporosis is a risk factor for distal radial fractures in both women and men. Thus, patients of both sexes with an age of fifty years or older who have a distal radial fracture should be evaluated with bone densitometry for the possible treatment of osteoporosis.

▶ This is an important study. The association of hip fractures in patients with osteoporosis with increased mortality is well known. Early detection and treatment of osteopenia and osteoporosis prior to fracture is one of the more challenging public health initiatives. The authors of this study have shown that the prevalence of osteoporosis and osteopenia is greater in both female and male patients who are 50 years and older who sustained low-energy distal radius fractures compared with controls in this region of Norway. Distal radius fractures are among the most common of all adult fractures and have been shown to occur generally earlier in life than hip fractures. And with this recognition, low-energy distal radius fractures could serve as an important bellwether for subsequent screening and longitudinal monitoring of potential at-risk patients. The findings of this large study should be known by anyone who treats distal radius fractures.

S. D. Trigg, MD

The Distal Radius, the Most Frequent Fracture Localization in Humans: A Histomorphometric Analysis of the Microarchitecture of 60 Human Distal Radii and Its Changes in Aging

Beil FT, Barvencik F, Gebauer M, et al (Univ Med Ctr Hamburg-Eppendorf, Germany)

J Trauma 70:154-158, 2011

Background.—The distal radius is the most frequent fracture localization in humans. Although younger patients receive a distal radius fracture after an adequate trauma, elderly patients suffer fractures through low-energy mechanisms. Low-energy fractures are hallmarks of osteoporosis. Osteoporotic changes of the distal radius are well described by DXA and peripheral quantitative computed tomography measurements. However, to date, the effects of aging on the microarchitecture of the distal radius have not been investigated.

Methods.—To investigate whether the microarchitecture of the human distal radius shows osteoporotic changes in bone mass and structure during aging, we dissected out 60 complete human distal radii from 30 age- and gender-matched patients at autopsy. Each of the three different age groups (group I: 20—40 years, group II: 41—60 years, group III: 61—80 years) was represented by 10 autopsy cases and 20 specimens (double-sided extraction), respectively. The specimens were analyzed by peripheral quantitative computed tomography, contact-radiography, and histomorphometry.

Results.—We observed a significant age-related decrease in bone mass, bone mineral density and an increase in typical osteoporotic changes of the bone microarchitecture in female distal radius specimens. Comparable observations of age-related changes have not been made in male specimens.

Conclusions.—The distal radius is a location of osteoporosis-specific bone changes. Our data provide evidence for the occurrence of typical osteoporotic changes, especially postmenopausal osteoporotic changes, in the distal radius during aging.

▶ There is emerging evidence to show that fractures of the distal radius are the most common human fractures. No doubt, owing to the increased mortality associated with osteoporotic fragility fractures of the hip, there has been quite rightly a more robust body of research directed toward the recognition, prevention, and surgical methods of treatment of hip fractures in the larger context of a public health concern compared with fractures of the distal radius. From a surgical perspective, the science behind the development of improved implants for treatment of hip fractures can be traced in large part to an understanding of age-related bone histologic changes of the trabecular and cortical bone about the proximal femur. This is a landmark study that analyzes the age-related changes in bone microarchitecture of the distal radius, which well deserves your review.

S. D. Trigg, MD

Ulnomeniscal Homologue of the Wrist: Correlation of Anatomic and MR Imaging Findings
Buck FM, Gheno R, Nico MAC, et al (Veterans Affairs San Diego Healthcare System, CA)
Radiology 253:771-779, 2009

Purpose.—To evaluate the anatomy of the ulnar side of the wrist in the region of the triangular fibrocartilage (TFC) complex, with special focus on the ulnomeniscal homologue (UMH) and its relationship to surrounding structures.

Materials and Methods.—Institutional review board approval and informed consent were not required. Ten upper extremities were harvested from the nonembalmed cadavers of four women and six men (age range at

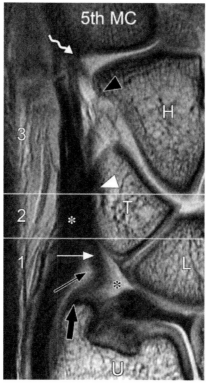

FIGURE 1.—Coronal intermediate-weighted MR image of the UMH at the level of the tip of the ulnar styloid process (thick black arrow). The styloid component (region *1*), collateral component (region *2*), and distal insertion (region *3*) are visible (separated with horizontal lines). The styloid component is recognized between the entrance to the prestyloid recess (black asterisk) and the ECU tendon (white asterisk). It can be divided into a more fibrous part (straight white arrow) and a highly vascular part with interspersed fat tissue (thin black arrow). Next to the prestyloid recess, the styloid component attaches to the ulnar styloid process. At the level of the collateral component, there is no high signal intensity (highly vascular tissue) between the ECU tendon and the UMH. The main part of the distal insertion attaches to the ulnar aspect of the triquetrum (*T*, white arrowhead). It also attaches to the hamate bone (*H*, black arrowhead) and the fifth metacarpal bone (*5th MC*, wavy arrow). *L* = lunate bone, *U* = ulna. (Reprinted from Buck FM, Gheno R, Nico MAC, et al. Ulnomeniscal homologue of the wrist: correlation of anatomic and MR imaging findings. *Radiology.* 2009;253:771-779. Copyright by the Radiological Society of North America.)

death, 56—97 years; mean age at death, 83 years) and used according to institutional guidelines. Magnetic resonance (MR) imaging and MR arthrography of the wrist were performed with the wrist in neutral position, maximal ulnar deviation, and maximal radial deviation by using intermediate-weighted sequences. The specimens were cut into 4-mm-thick sections that corresponded to the MR imaging planes. The gross anatomic features of the UMH and its relationship to adjacent structures were evaluated and compared with imaging findings. UMH variants, as described in previous articles on purely anatomic studies, were sought on MR images. MR findings of the wrist in neutral position were compared with those of the wrist in maximal ulnar and radial

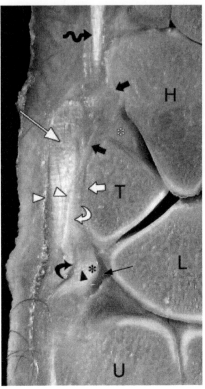

FIGURE 4.—Gross specimen shows anatomic features of the UMH in the coronal plane at the level of the tip of the ulnar styloid process. The styloid component of the UMH is seen at the tip of the ulnar styloid process. It is composed of a white ligamentous part (black asterisk) on the radial side and a more fatty, slightly yellow part (black arrowhead) next to the ulnar collateral ligament and the ECU tendon sheath (curved black arrow). The entrance to the prestyloid recess (long straight black arrow) lies between the UMH and the TFC. The opening to the prestyloid recess is the narrow type. More distally, the collateral part of the UMH, the ECU tendon sheath, and the ulnar collateral ligament merge into one structure (curved white arrow). The UMH attaches distally to the ulnar aspect of the triquetrum (T, short white arrow)and to the ulnar facet of the hamate bone (H, short black arrows), where it fuses with the joint capsule and a meniscus-shaped fatty fringe (white asterisk) between the hamate bone and the triquetrum. Wavy black arrow points to extensor digiti minimi tendon, long white arrow points to ECU tendon, white arrow heads also point to ECU tendon sheath. L = lunate bone, U = ulna. For interpretation of the references to color in this figure legend, the reader is referred to web version of this article. (Reprinted from Buck FM, Gheno R, Nico MAC, et al. Ulnomeniscal homologue of the wrist: correlation of anatomic and MR imaging findings. *Radiology.* 2009;253:771-779. Copyright by the Radiological Society of North America.)

deviations. Histologic examination was used to further elucidate the structure of the UMH.

Results.—The UMH displayed complex anatomic features because of its obliquely oriented course. However, it could be divided into styloid, radioulnar, and collateral components and a distal insertion. The UMH variants described in previously published studies could be identified, but evaluation results were highly dependent on the wrist position at imaging.

Conclusion.—The anatomy of the UMH is complex. For assessment of the UMH and the ulnar side of the TFC complex, coronal MR arthrography with the wrist in neutral position or radial deviation might be superior to standard MR imaging (Figs 1 and 4).

▶ Correctly and reliably diagnosing the anatomic locations and pathology of ulnar-sided wrist pain by physical examination is challenging even for the most seasoned examiner. The majority of the literature dealing with soft tissue injury about the ulnar side of the wrist has focused on the anatomy and patterns of injury to the triangular fibrocartilage complex (TFCC) and to a lesser extent the lunotriquetral interosseous ligament. Recently, there have been advances in the imaging techniques of CT and MR arthrograms that have significantly improved the sensitivity and specificity in the diagnosis of TFCC tears as correlated to the standards of wrist arthroscopy. However, comparatively little has been written about the imaging of the ulnomeniscal homologue or about this structure as a possible source of wrist pain following injury. Only portions of the ulnomeniscal homologue can be visualized arthroscopically, and therefore, we must rely on MRI should we suspect an injury not related to the TFCC. This study significantly furthers our knowledge and understanding of this structure and its variations and provides us with benchmark techniques to optimize imaging.

S. D. Trigg, MD

Forearm and Wrist

Wrist function recovers more rapidly after volar locked plating than after external fixation but the outcomes are similar after 1 year: A randomized study of 63 patients with a dorsally displaced fracture of the distal radius
Wilcke MKT, Abbaszadegan H, Adolphson PY (Danderyd Hosp, Stockholm, Sweden)
Acta Orthop 82:76-81, 2011

Background and Purpose.—Promising results have been reported after volar locked plating of unstable dorsally displaced distal radius fractures. We investigated whether volar locked plating results in better patient-perceived, objective functional and radiographic outcomes compared to the less invasive external fixation.

Patients and Methods.—63 patients under 70 years of age, with an unstable extra-articular or non-comminuted intra-articular dorsally displaced distal radius fracture, were randomized to volar locked plating (n = 33) or bridging external fixation. Patient-perceived outcome was assessed with the Disability of the Arm, Shoulder, and Hand (DASH) questionnaire and the Patient-Rated Wrist Evaluation (PRWE) questionnaire.

Results.—At 3 and 6 months, the volar plate group had better DASH and PRWE scores but at 12 months the scores were similar. Objective function, measured as grip strength and range of movement, was superior in the volar plate group but the differences diminished and were small at 12 months. Axial length and volar tilt were retained slightly better in the volar plate group.

Interpretation.—Volar plate fixation is more advantageous than external fixation, in the early rehabilitation period.

▶ Left in the wake of the large wave that volar locked plating has created in recent years in the ocean of treatment of unstable distal radius fractures are the comparatively smaller ripples left from other methods, including dorsal plating and external fixation. To be sure, volar locked plating of these fractures has been shown to be a preferred method for treatment of perhaps a majority of these fractures over a wide age range in the short and medium terms with respect to early range of motion recovery and patient-reported outcomes. Volar locked plating is not without complications, however, and the advances in plate design, technique, and outcomes are a rapidly moving and evolving target. External fixation of unstable distal radius fractures has a proven track record holding up under the weight of longer-term scrutiny, with advantages, complications, and treatment pearls and pitfalls generally well known. This comparative study furthers our knowledge on treatment of these common fractures and adds to our knowledge on 2 fronts, further earmarking advantages of volar locking plate treatment in the near term, while supporting continued relevance of external fixation as a treatment alternative.

S. D. Trigg, MD

Comparison of united and nonunited fractures of the ulnar styloid following volar-plate fixation of distal radius fractures

Kim JK, Yun Y-H, Kim DJ, et al (Ewha Womans Univ, Seoul, South Korea)
Injury 42:371-375, 2011

Introduction.—The purpose of this study was to determine whether associated nonunion of ulnar styloid fracture following plate-and-screw fixation of a distal radius fracture (DRF) has any effect on wrist functional outcomes, ulnar-sided wrist pain or distal radioulnar joint (DRUJ) instability.

Materials and Methods.—A total of 91 consecutive patients with a DRF and an accompanying ulnar styloid fracture treated by open reduction and volar locking plate fixation were included in this study. In the first part of the analysis, the 91 study subjects were subdivided according to the presence or not of ulnar styloid union (20 and 71, respectively) by radiography at final follow-up (average 23 months). These two cohorts were compared with respect to wrist functions at 3 months postoperatively and the final follow-up visit, and ulnar-sided wrist pain and DRUJ instability at the final follow-up visit and ulnar styloid length as determined radiographically at final follow-up. In the second part of the analysis, 49 of the 91 study subjects with an ulnar styloid base fracture were subdivided according to the presence or not of ulnar styloid base fracture union (12 and 37, respectively) at final follow-up by radiography. These two groups were also compared with respect to the above-mentioned parameters.

Results.—Ulnar styloid fractures united in 20 (22%) of the 91 patients at final follow-up visit (average 23 months). No significant differences were found at any time during follow-up between patients who achieved or did not achieve ulnar styloid fracture union or ulnar styloid base fracture union.

Conclusion.—Ulnar styloid nonunion does not appear to affect wrist functional outcomes, ulnar-sided wrist pain or DRUJ stability, at least when a DRF is treated by open reduction and volar plate fixation.

▶ Ulnar-sided wrist pain is a frequent complaint in patients who have been treated for unstable distal radius fractures with volar locking plates (similar to those treated by other methods). The pain may persist for weeks or months. The presence of an associated ulnar styloid fracture nonunion has been implicated as a source of lingering ulnar-sided wrist pain, but this has not been studied as extensively as the presence of styloid fractures and distal radioulnar joint instability. This is one of the largest studies to date with longer-term follow-up that investigates associated ulnar styloid nonunions compared with united fractures following volar locking plate fixation of distal radius fractures. The study's data are important and have clinical implications regarding treatment decisions and patient discussion.

S. D. Trigg, MD

Volar Locking Plate Implant Prominence and Flexor Tendon Rupture
Soong M, Earp BE, Bishop G, et al (Lahey Clinic, Burlington, MA; Brigham and Women's Hosp, Boston, MA)
J Bone Joint Surg Am 93:328-335, 2011

Background.—Flexor tendon injury is a recognized complication of volar plate fixation of distal radial fractures. A suspected contributing factor is implant prominence at the watershed line, where the flexor tendons lie closest to the plate.

Methods.—Two parallel series of patients who underwent volar locked plating of distal radial fractures from 2005 to 2008 and with at least six months of follow-up were retrospectively reviewed. Group 1 included seventy-three distal radial fractures that were treated by three orthopaedic hand surgeons with use of a single plate design at one institution, and Group 2 included ninety-five distal radial fractures that were treated by four orthopaedic hand surgeons with use of a different plate design at another institution. On the postoperative lateral radiographs, a line was drawn tangential to the most volar extent of the volar rim, parallel to the volar cortical bone of the radial shaft. Plates that did not extend volar to this line were recorded as Grade 0. Plates volar to the line, but proximal to the volar rim, were recorded as Grade 1. Plates directly on or distal to the volar rim were recorded as Grade 2.

Results.—In Group 1, the average duration of follow-up was thirteen months (range, six to forty-nine months). Three cases of flexor tendon

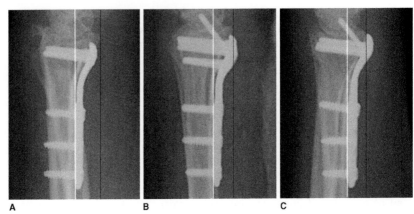

A **B** **C**

FIGURE 5.—Lateral radiographs of a distal radial fracture treated with an Acu-Loc plate demonstrating (A) Grade-0 prominence (dorsal to critical line), (B) Grade-1 prominence (volar to critical line, proximal to volar rim), and (C) Grade-2 prominence (volar to critical line, at volar rim). (Reprinted from Soong M, Earp BE, Bishop G, et al. Volar locking plate implant prominence and flexor tendon rupture. *J Bone Joint Surg Am.* 2011;93:328-335, with permission from the Journal of Bone and Joint Surgery, Inc.)

rupture were identified among seventy-three plated radii (prevalence, 4%). Grade-2 plate prominence was found in two of the three cases with rupture and in forty-six cases (63%) overall. In Group 2, the average duration of follow-up was fifteen months (range, six to fifty-six months). There were no cases of flexor tendon rupture and no plates with Grade-2 prominence among ninety-five plated radii.

Conclusions.—Flexor tendon rupture after volar plating of the distal part of the radius is an infrequent but serious complication. The plate used in Group 1 is prominent at the watershed line of the distal part of the radius, which may increase the risk of tendon injury. We found no ruptures in Group 2, perhaps as a result of the lower profile of the plate. Further studies are needed before recommending one plate over another. Regardless of plate selection, surgeons should avoid implant prominence in this area (Fig 5).

▶ Use of volar locking plate fixation for the treatment of distal radial fractures continues to grow at a rapid pace worldwide. One of the driving factors for the increased use of volar plates was to avoid tendon irritation and ruptures that were more frequently associated with dorsal plate fixation. Much of the recent literature reporting complications from volar plate fixation has focused on the necessity for understanding that multiple intraoperative fluoroscopic views are necessary to avoid intra-articular screw placement or dorsal screw prominence and less frequently on flexor tendon ruptures. This study provides us with important information about intraoperative plate positioning on the distal radius to avoid plate prominence. This information should also help us critically scrutinize current and future plate designs as their use becomes more widespread going forward.

S. D. Trigg, MD

Joint Leveling for Advanced Kienböck's Disease

Calfee RP, Van Steyn MO, Gyuricza C, et al (Washington Univ School of Medicine at Barnes-Jewish Hosp, St Louis, MO; Hosp for Special Surgery, NY)
J Hand Surg 35A:1947-1954, 2010

Purpose.—The use of joint leveling procedures to treat Kienböck's disease have been limited by the degree of disease advancement. This study was designed to compare clinical and radiographic outcomes of wrists with more advanced (stage IIIB) Kienböck's disease with those of wrists with less advanced (stage II/IIIA) disease following radius-shortening osteotomy.

Methods.—This retrospective study enrolled 31 adult wrists (30 patients; mean age, 39 y), treated with radius-shortening osteotomy at 2 institutions for either stage IIIB (n = 14) or stage II/IIIA (n = 17) disease. Evaluation was performed at a mean of 74 months (IIIB, 77 mo; II/IIIA, 72 mo). Radiographic assessment determined disease progression. Clinical outcomes were determined by validated patient-based and objective measures.

Results.—Patient-based outcome ratings of wrists treated for stage IIIB were similar to those with stage II/IIIA (shortened Disabilities of the Arm, Shoulder, and Hand score, 15 vs 12; modified Mayo wrist score, 84 vs 87; visual analog scale pain score, 1.2 vs 1.7; visual analog scale function score, 2.6 vs 2.1). The average flexion/extension arc was 102° for wrists with stage IIIB and 106° for wrists with stage II/IIIA Kienböck's Grip strength was 77% of the opposite side for stage IIIB wrists versus 85% for stage II/IIIA. Postoperative carpal height ratio and radioscaphoid angle were worse for wrists treated for stage IIIB (0.46 and 65°, respectively) than stage II/IIIA (0.53 and 53°, respectively) disease. Radiographic disease progression occurred in 7 wrists (6 stage II/IIIA, 1 stage IIIB). The one stage IIIB wrist that progressed underwent wrist arthrodesis.

Conclusions.—In this limited series, clinical outcomes of radius shortening using validated, patient-based assessment instruments and objective measures failed to demonstrate predicted clinically relevant differences between stage II/IIIA and IIIB Kienböck's disease. Given the high percentage of successful clinical outcomes in this case series of 14 stage IIIB wrists, we believe that static carpal malalignment does not preclude radius-shortening osteotomy.

Type of Study/Level of Evidence.—Therapeutic IV.

▶ Kienböck's disease is a rare disorder, therefore effectively prohibiting prospective investigation. Retrospective clinical studies of joint-leveling procedures in patients with Lichtman stages II and IIIA have shown generally favorable clinical results. These clinical data, coupled with biomechanical data showing that joint leveling by radial shortening can be effective in unloading the lunate, has led to the acceptance that these procedures are a standard method of treatment for Kienböck's disease without carpal collapse (stages I, II, and IIA). As noted in this study, the experience of joint leveling for more advanced stage IIIB is scant. Furthermore, there is a lack of meaningful data from validated patient-based outcome scoring. Although retrospective, this study significantly adds to our knowledge base about joint-leveling procedures in stages II and IIIA compared with stage IIIB and is deserving of your review.

S. D. Trigg, MD

Three-point index in predicting redisplacement of extra-articular distal radial fractures in adults

Alemdaroğlu KB, İltar S, Aydoğan NH, et al (Ankara Training and Res Hosp, Turkey; et al)
Injury 41:197-203, 2010

Introduction.—In distal radial fractures in adults, factors affecting instability have been investigated in many studies in an effort to shorten the preoperative waiting period for the fractures requiring surgery. Numerous factors, aside from the alignment-related indices, have been searched to predict redisplacement. Unlike as in paediatric counterparts, the casting technique and casting-related indices have not been appropriately considered in

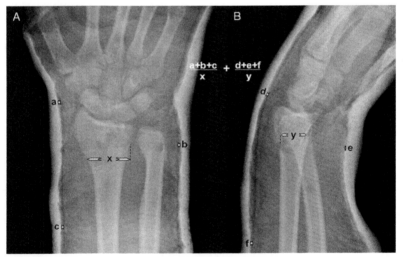

FIGURE 1.—(A and B) The formula for the three-point index is $[(a + b + c)/x] + [(d + e + f)/y]$. (A) On the anteroposterior radiograph, "a" is the narrowest distal side gap at the level of radiocarpal or proximal carpal joint, "b" is the narrowest ulnar-side gap at the level of the fracture (within 1 cm of the fracture line), and "c" is the narrowest proximal radial side gap within the area between 3 and 7 cm proximal to the fracture site. "x" is the projection of the contact length between the proximal and distal fragments in the horizontal plane on the anteroposterior radiograph. (B) On the lateral radiograph of an extension-type fracture, "d" is the narrowest distal dorsal-side gap at the level of the radiocarpal joint or proximal carpal bones, "e" is the narrowest volar-side gap within 1 cm of the level of the fracture line, and "f" is the narrowest proximal dorsal-side gap within the area between 3 and 7 cm of the fracture site. "y" is the projection of the contact length between the proximal and distal fragments in the sagittal plane on the lateral radiograph. For this example, the calculation was $[(2 + 2 + 2)/26] + [(1 + 0 + 1.5)/17] = (6/26) + (2.5/17) = 0.23 + 0.15 = 0.38$, showing the casting technique was adequate. (Reprinted from Alemdaroğlu KB, İltar S, Aydoğan NH, et al. Three-point index in predicting redisplacement of extra-articular distal radial fractures in adults. *Injury.* 2010;41:197-203, with permission from Elsevier.)

adults. The aim of this study was to determine the impact of the various previously investigated factors in addition to casting technique-related indices such as three-point index, cast index, padding index and gap index, in predicting the risk of redisplacement of extra-articular distal radial fractures in adults and the presence of the ulnar deviation of the cast.

Patients and Methods.—Seventy-five patients over 18 years who were treated with a cast in our emergency department within 24 h after a displaced distal radial fracture, were recruited into the study. Age, alignment-related indices, cast-related indices, extent of the ulnar deviation of the cast, having a non-anatomical reduction, co-existing ulnar fracture, dorsal comminution and obliquity of the fracture line were investigated. Casting technique according to three-point index, obliquity of the fracture line, degree of the ulnar deviation of the cast, and reduction accuracy were the significant factors affecting redisplacement.

Results.—The three-point index had a sensitivity of 95.8%, specificity of 96.1%, positive predictive value of 92%, and negative predictive value of 98% in predicting redisplacement. Logistic regression revealed that having an inadequate cast according to the three-point index ($p < 0.001$), degree of obliquity of the fracture line ($p = 0.018$), decreased ulnar deviation of the cast ($p = 0.002$), and having a non-anatomical reduction ($p = 0.029$) were the significant predictive factors in redisplacement.

TABLE 1.—The Formula of Each Index and Cut-Off Values

	Formula $[(a + b + c)/x] + [d + e + f)/y]^a$		Cut-off
Three-point index	In A-P radiograph a: the narrowest distal radial side gap between the skin and the cast, at the level of the radiocarpal joint or proximal carpal bones b: the narrowest ulnar-side gap within 1 cm of the fracture line c: the narrowest proximal radial side gap within the area between 3 and 7 cm proximal to the fracture site x: The projection of the contact length between the proximal and distal fragments in the horizontal plane on the A-P radiograph	In lateral radiograph d: the narrowest distal dorsal-side gap between the skin and the cast, at the level of the radiocarpal joint or proximal carpal bones e: the narrowest volar-side gap within 1 cm of the fracture line f: the narrowest proximal dorsal-side gap within the area between 3 and 7 cm of the fracture site y: The projection of the contact length between the proximal and distal fragments in the sagittal plane on the lateral radiograph	0.8
Cast index	Inner diameter of the cast in lateral radiograph/inner diameter of the cast in A-P radiograph at f.s.		0.8
Pad index	Dorsal f.s. gap/maximum interosseous length on A-P radiograph[a]		0.3
Canterbury index	Cast index + pad index		1.1
Gap index	[(Radial f.s. gap + ulnar f.s. gap)/inner diameter of the cast in A-P plane] + [(dorsal f.s. gap + volar f.s. gap)/inner diameter of the cast in lateral plane]		0.15

[a]Please see Fig 1. A-P: anteroposterior. f.s.: fracture site.

Conclusions.—Our results suggest that the casting technique plays a major role in the success of conservative treatment, which can best be examined with the three-point index. Ulnar deviation of the cast and fracture obliquity are the other dominant factors affecting redisplacement (Fig 1, Table 1).

▶ Witnessing the surge of published investigations on the operative treatment of adult distal radius fractures, one could easily lose sight of the importance of meticulous closed reduction techniques and casting methods for fractures without intra-articular displacement. Perhaps not said is that we have become all too accustomed to falling back upon our growing familiarity of operative treatment when we see a closed reduced fracture redisplace following initial cast placement. While good casting technique would seem intuitive and a core skill, this is among the very few reports in the adult orthopedic literature that objectively investigates cast technique and what principles lead to a radiographically favorable outcome. This study is a good read and worthy of your review.

S. D. Trigg, MD

The Unstable Nonunited Scaphoid Waist Fracture: Results of Treatment by Open Reduction, Anterior Wedge Grafting, and Internal Fixation by Volar Buttress Plate
Ghoneim A (Suez Canal Univ, Ismailia, Egypt)
J Hand Surg 36A:17-24, 2011

Purpose.—The purpose of this study is to evaluate the results of treatment of unstable nonunited scaphoid waist fracture by anterior wedge graft and internal fixation with the use of volar buttress plate and screws.

Methods.—Fourteen adult male patients with unstable nonunited scaphoid waist fracture with a humpback deformity were treated by reduction of the collapse deformity, insertion of anterior wedge graft, and internal fixation with the use of volar buttress plate and screws. The mean patient age was 26 years, and the mean duration of the nonunion before surgery was 16.5 months. The follow-up time ranged from 9 to 19 months (mean, 11 mo). Thirteen of the fourteen nonunions healed with sound radiographic union. Pre-existing avascular necrosis was a major adverse factor for achievement of union in one patient, even after a second bone-grafting procedure.

Results.—Union was achieved in a mean of 3.8 months. Most of the patients had satisfactory correction of scaphoid deformity and the associated dorsal intercalated segment instability. Postoperatively, improvements were seen in the range of wrist flexion and extension, grip strength, and degree of dorsal intercalated segment instability.

Conclusions.—The results of the series suggest that the method of anterior wedge graft and internal fixation with the use of volar buttress plate and screws is effective for the treatment of unstable nonunited scaphoid waist fractures.

Type of Study/Level of Evidence.—Therapeutic IV.

▶ Correction of scaphoid waist fracture nonunions that have collapsed into flexion or humpback deformity with resultant carpal malalignment by anterior interpositional corticocancellous wedge-shaped bone graft has become an accepted standard method of treatment of these challenging injuries. A crucial component for successful union and correction of the scaphoid collapse and carpal malalignment hinges upon stable internal fixation of the often complex shape of the wedge-shaped bone graft within the body of the scaphoid. A majority of the studies reporting on methods of fixation have centered on investigating various headless compression screw designs and their optimum trajectory of placement to maximize bone purchase and stabilization by compression. Even for seasoned wrist surgeons, correct screw placement can prove difficult in some cases even with the newer cannulated designs where guide wire aids in optimum trajectory prior to drilling. Anterior graft placement requires clear visualization of the volar aspect of the scaphoid, and it is perhaps interesting that so many of implant design initiatives have been directed toward compression screws and not many at all toward volar plating. This study should be considered as preliminary but nonetheless compares favorably with other smaller but accepted studies purporting the merits of a given compression screw technique, and the author suggests several advantages to this method of fixation, which will likely foster further clinical evaluative and biomechanical investigations.

S. D. Trigg, MD

Color-Aided Visualization of Dorsal Wrist Ganglion Stalks Aids in Complete Arthroscopic Excision
Yao J, Trindade MCD (Stanford Univ Med Ctr, CA)
Arthroscopy 27:425-429, 2011

Dorsal wrist ganglia are the most common mass of the upper extremity. Treatment modalities include benign neglect, aspiration, and surgical excision. Arthroscopic excision is a less invasive surgical alternative to open resection with the benefit of visualizing and treating other intra-articular pathology, fewer potential complications, earlier return to activities, and possibly, a more complete resection. This may lead to a lower rate of recurrence, although this has not been proven in the literature. Recurrence depends in part on adequate ganglion stalk visualization and resection. This is often difficult in open and arthroscopic ganglionectomy. This work describes a new technique with improved arthroscopic stalk visualization and ganglion resection using intralesional injection of an inert dye (Fig 1).

▶ Dorsal wrist ganglion cysts are among the most common of all soft tissue masses of the upper extremity. Aspiration is variably successful, and recurrences

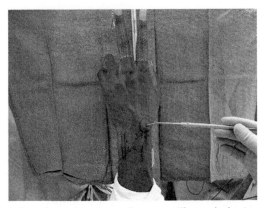

FIGURE 1.—Setup for arthroscopic wrist ganglionectomy. The standard wrist arthroscopy tower is used with 10 to 15 lb of longitudinal traction placed on the index and long fingers. Marking of the ganglion on the skin before surgery is useful, because it is often difficult to visualize and palpate once the surgery has begun. (Reprinted from Yao J, Trindade MCD. Color-aided visualization of dorsal wrist ganglion stalks aids in complete arthroscopic excision. *Arthroscopy.* 2011;27:425-429. Copyright 2011, with permission from the Arthroscopy Association of North America.)

following open excision are known to have recurrence rates as high as 40% in older studies. Moreover, many patients will require postoperative hand therapy and several weeks off work following open ganglionectomy, adding to the total expense of the procedure. There have been several reports in the literature in recent years that show that arthroscopic excision of dorsal wrist ganglion cysts compares favorably with more recent open excision reports with respect to recurrence but indicate more favorable range of motion and grip strength outcomes while allowing for direct inspection of the wrist for other pathology. However, arthroscopic visualization of the ganglion cyst is often difficult. This dye injection technique is brilliantly simple. The technique may prove to be an easy but important adjunct toward improved visualization of the ganglion stalk among experienced wrist arthroscopists and no doubt should shorten the learning curve for those who are less familiar with the technique.

S. D. Trigg, MD

The International Registry on Hand and Composite Tissue Transplantation
Petruzzo P, Lanzetta M, Dubernard J-M, et al (Hopital Edouard Herriot, Lyon, France; Italian Inst of Hand Surgery, Monza, Italy; et al)
Transplantation 90:1590-1594, 2010

Background.—The International Registry on Hand and Composite Tissue Transplantation was founded in May 2002, and the analysis of all cases with follow-up information up to July 2010 is presented here.

Methods.—From September 1998 to July 2010, 49 hands (17 unilateral and 16 bilateral hand transplantations, including 1 case of bilateral arm transplantation) have been reported, for a total of 33 patients. They were 31 men and 2 women (median age 32 years). Time since hand loss ranged from 2 months to 34 years, and in 46% of cases, the level of amputation was at wrist. Immunosuppressive therapy included tacrolimus, mycophenolate mofetil, sirolimus, and steroids; polyclonal or monoclonal antibodies were used for induction. Topical immunosuppression was also used in several cases. Follow-up ranges from 1 month to 11 years.

Results.—One patient died on day 65. Three patients transplanted in the Western countries have lost their graft, whereas until September 2009, seven hand grafts were removed for noncompliance to the immunosuppressive therapy in China. Eighty-five percent of recipients experienced at least one episode of acute rejection within the first year, and they were reversible when promptly treated. Side effects included opportunistic infections, metabolic complications, and malignancies. All patients developed protective sensibility, 90% of them developed tactile sensibility, and 82.3% also developed a discriminative sensibility. Motor recovery enabled patients to perform most daily activities.

Conclusions.—Hand transplantation is a complex procedure, and its success is based on patient's compliance and his or her careful evaluation before and after transplantation.

▶ This article speaks for itself. Hand and upper extremity composite transplantation has garnered a significant amount of press in the general media for its human interest intrigue. The early successes of limb survival and promising functional advances of individual cases highlight the very limits of what is currently possible in the field of allotransplantation pertinent to musculoskeletal surgery. Quite rightly, these procedures have led to a necessary discussion of the medical ethics for continuance, which draws on experience from the field of transplantation medicine. This article succinctly reports what is currently known about the numbers, survival, and complications of the composite hand and upper limb transplantation.

S. D. Trigg, MD

Chemical Denervation with Botulinum Neurotoxin A Improves the Surgical Manipulation of the Muscle–Tendon Unit: An Experimental Study in an Animal Model
Mannava S, Callahan MF, Trach SM, et al (Wake Forest Univ School of Medicine, Winston-Salem, NC; Wake Forest Univ Graduate School of Arts and Sciences, Winston-Salem, NC)
J Hand Surg 36A:222-231, 2011

Purpose.—The chemical denervation that results from botulinum neurotoxin A (BoNT-A) causes a temporary, reversible paresis that can result in easier surgical manipulation of the muscle–tendon unit in the context of tendon rupture and repair. The purpose of the study was to determine whether BoNT-A injections can be used to temporarily and reversibly modulate active and passive skeletal muscle properties.

Methods.—Male CD1 mice weighing 40—50g were divided into a 1-week postinjection group (n = 13: n = 5 saline and n = 8 BoNT-A) and a 2-week postinjection group (n = 17: n = 7 saline and n = 10 BoNT-A). The animals had *in vivo* muscle force testing and *in vivo* biomechanical evaluation.

Results.—There was a substantial decline in the maximal single twitch amplitude (p < .05) and tetanic amplitude (p < .05) at one week and at 2 weeks after BoNT-A injection, when compared to saline-injected controls. BoNT-A injection significantly reduced the peak passive properties of the muscle—tendon unit as a function of displacement at one week (p < .05). Specifically, the stiffness of the BoNT-A injected muscle—tendon unit was 0.417 N/mm compared to the control saline injected group, which was 0.634 N/mm, a 35% reduction in stiffness (p < .05).

Conclusions.—Presurgical treatment with BoNT-A might improve the surgical manipulation of the muscle—tendon unit, thus improving surgical outcomes. The results implicate neural tone as a substantial contributor to the passive repair tension of the muscle—tendon unit. The modulation of neural tone through temporary, reversible paresis is a novel approach that might improve intraoperative and postoperative passive muscle properties, allowing for progressive rehabilitation while protecting the surgical repair site.

▶ This article is chosen for your review, as it potentially points a way forward for applicability across a wide range of orthopedic and hand traumatic and reconstructive surgical procedures. Botulinum neurotoxin A, when injected intramuscularly, temporarily and reversibly denervates skeletal muscle, resulting in muscle paresis/paralysis. Most studies of botulinum neurotoxin A in musculoskeletal science have been centered on its effect on active muscle contraction and not on its ability to also modulate the passive stiffness of a muscle-tendon unit, which is the focus of this study. Reducing the stiffness of a contracted muscle-tendon unit, as well as temporarily weakening it, as noted by the investigators, may have significant future clinical importance in treatment of ruptured rotator cuff, biceps tendon, and flexor tendon repairs.

S. D. Trigg, MD

Hand

Injectable Collagenase Clostridium Histolyticum: A New Nonsurgical Treatment for Dupuytren's Disease

Gilpin D, Coleman S, Hall S, et al (Brisbane Hand and Upper Limb Clinic, Queensland; Rivercity Private Hosp, Auchenflower, Queensland; Emeritus Res, Malvern, Victoria, Australia; et al)
J Hand Surg 35A:2027-2038, 2010

Purpose.—The Collagenase Option for the Reduction of Dupuytren's (CORD) II study investigated the efficacy and safety of injectable Xiaflex (collagenase clostridium histolyticum), in patients with Dupuytren's contracture.

Methods.—This was a prospective, randomized, placebo-controlled trial with 90-day double-blind and 9-month open-label phases. We randomized patients with contractures affecting metacarpophalangeal (MCP) or proximal interphalangeal (PIP) joints 2 to 1 to collagenase (0.58 mg) or placebo. Cords received a maximum of 3 injections. Cord disruption was attempted the day after injection using a standardized finger extension procedure. Primary end point was reduction in contracture to 0° to 5° of normal 30 days after the last injection.

Results.—We enrolled 66 patients; 45 cords (20 MCP to 25 PIP joints) received collagenase and 21 cords (11 MCP to 10 PIP joints) received placebo in the double-blind phase. Statistically significantly more cords injected with collagenase than placebo met the primary end point (44.4% vs 4.8%; p < .001). The mean percentage decrease in degree of joint contracture from baseline to 30 days after last injection was 70.5% ± 29.2% in the collagenase group and 13.6% ± 26.1% in the placebo group (p < .001). The mean increase in range of motion was significantly greater in the collagenase (35.4° ± 17.8°) than in the placebo (7.6° ± 14.9°; p < .001) group. Efficacy after open-label treatment was similar to that after the double-blind phase: 50.7% of all joints achieved 0° to 5° of normal. More patients were satisfied with collagenase (p < .001). No joint had recurrence of contracture. One patient had a flexion pulley rupture and one patient underwent routine fasciectomy to address cord proliferation and sensory abnormality. No tendon ruptures or systemic allergic reactions were reported. Most adverse events were related to the injection or finger extension procedure.

Conclusions.—Collagenase clostridium histolyticum is the first Food and Drug Administration—approved, nonsurgical treatment option for adult Dupuytren's contracture patients with a palpable cord that is highly effective and well tolerated.

Type of Study/Level of Evidence.—Therapeutic I.

▶ Open fasciectomy and fasciotomy have been the benchmark surgical treatments for Dupuytren contracture for decades. The literature is replete with a multitude of study data reporting the efficacy, complications, and costs following open surgical treatment. More recently, percutaneous needle aponeurotomy has been proposed as a less-invasive surgical procedure, but to date, there are limited published data reporting the safety, efficacy, or complications from this procedure. Any surgeons with experience in the surgical treatment of Dupuytren contracture, especially from dealing with postoperative complications, have no doubt been intrigued with the prospect of adding an office-based nonsurgical treatment to their armamentarium. Collagenase *Clostridium histolyticum* injection is the first such treatment that has been shown to have evidence of safety and efficacy in the short term.[1] This prospective, randomized, double-blinded, placebo-controlled study (labeled Collagenase Option for the Reduction of Dupuytren [CORD] II) builds on the shorter-term outcome data of the first study (CORD I) over a longer 12-month study period. Collagenase *C histolyticum* injections have been among the most heavily marketed treatments, and no doubt, many treating surgeon readers here have been bombarded by information from the manufacturer's representatives promoting the benefits of this treatment as the panacea for the treatment of this disease going forward. The results of this study further our knowledge and show that many patients with Dupuytren contracture could be considered as candidates for collagenase injection treatment. This article is a must read.

S. D. Trigg, MD

Reference

1. Hurst LC, Badalamente MA, Hentz VR, et al. Injectable collagenase clostridium histolyticum for Dupuytren's contracture. *N Engl J Med.* 2009;361:968-969.

A Prospective Trial on the Use of Antibiotics in Hand Surgery
Aydın N, Uraloğlu M, Burhanoğlu ADY, et al (Ankara Numune Training and Res Hosp, Turkey)
Plast Reconstr Surg 126:1617-1623, 2010

Background.—Postoperative infection is a disastrous complication in the discipline of hand surgery, as it is in any field of surgery in which infection can compromise wound healing and lead to subsequent functional impairment despite the best attempts. Different results with antibiotic use by different authors have been reported. This study was planned to put forth the place of antibiotic use in hand surgery procedures.

Methods.—This prospective, randomized, double-blind study included 1340 patients who were placed in one of four groups according to the components of their hands that were injured. Half of each group received antibiotics, and the other half received placebo.

Results.—Infections among the placebo- and antibiotic-administered patients did not display significant importance ($p = 0.759$). Infections among the four groups were not statistically significant either ($p = 0.947$). Statistical significance was not found between elective and emergency procedures ($p = 0.552$). Operations longer than 2 hours had 2.5 percent infection rates in placebo patients and 3.8 percent in antibiotic patients, which was not statistically significant ($p = 0.7$). In crush/dirty wounds there was no statistical significance in development of infections between placebo and antibiotic use ($p = 1$), nor was there any statistically significant difference between crush and dirty wounds ($p = 0.929$).

Conclusions.—The authors do not support the use of antibiotic prophylaxis for surgery of the hand. Its use should be preserved for specific infections or for patients with certain types of risk factors for infection.

▶ The use and current recommendations of perioperative prophylactic antibiotics for the prevention of bacterial contamination of clean orthopedic surgical wounds has largely been driven by data derived from total joint arthroplasty, spine surgery, and open long-bone fracture studies. The extrapolation of the use of prophylactic antibiotics in clean hand surgical cases remains controversial, and the common practice for their use may be for litigious concerns trumping cost or effectiveness reasoning. Moreover, there is limited evidence-based information on the role of prophylactic antibiotics in open hand fractures and complex soft tissue injuries, which are, by definition, contaminated wounds. This prospective, randomized, double-blinded placebo-controlled study is one of the largest to date, and its findings and conclusions add significantly to our knowledge base on this subject. Perhaps of particular interest is that antibiotic administration did not show any superiority in preventing postoperative infections over placebo patients in the dirtiest machinery-caused injury subset of patients.

S. D. Trigg, MD

Avoiding Flexor Tendon Repair Rupture with Intraoperative Total Active Movement Examination
Higgins A, Lalonde DH, Bell M, et al (Dalhousie Univ, Saint John, NB; Ottawa Univ, Ontario, Canada)
Plast Reconstr Surg 126:941-945, 2010

Background.—Wide-awake flexor tendon repair in tourniquet-free unsedated patients permits intraoperative Total Active Movement examination (iTAMe) of the freshly repaired flexor tendon. This technique has permitted the intraoperative observation of tendon repair gapping induced by active movement when the core suture is tied too loosely. The gap can be repaired intraoperatively to decrease postoperative tendon repair rupture rates. The authors record their rupture rate in the first 15 years of experience with iTAMe.

Methods.—This was a retrospective chart review of 102 consecutive patients with wide-awake flexor tendon repair (no tourniquet, no sedation, and pure locally injected lidocaine with epinephrine anesthesia) in which iTAMe was performed by two hand surgeons in two Canadian cities between 1998 and 2008. Intraoperative gapping and postoperative rupture were analyzed.

Results.—The authors observed intraoperative bunching and gap formation with active movement in flexor tendon repair testing (iTAMe) in seven patients. In all seven cases, they redid the repair and repeated iTAMe to confirm gapping was eliminated before closing the skin, and those seven patients did not rupture postoperatively. In 68 patients with known outcomes, four of 122 tendons ruptured (tendon rupture rate, 3.3 percent) in three of 68 patients (patient rupture rate, 4.4 percent). All three patients who ruptured had accidental jerk forced rupture. All those patients who did what we asked them did not rupture.

Conclusions.—Tendons can gap with active movement if the core suture is tied too loosely. Gapping can be recognized intraoperatively with iTAMe and repaired to decrease postoperative rupture.

▶ To be perfectly frank, this retrospective chart review study was not selected for its scientific rigor. It was selected for its novel approach and advancement in the science of pursuing optimum results for repairing the lacerated human flexor tendon. Each year, the hand surgical literature is rather weighty with many in vitro studies comparing the strength and gap formation of proposed suturing methods with those of other published techniques. Many of these investigated in vitro suturing methods in all practicality will never see the light of day in clinical practice, owing to their complexity and difficulty to perform in the real world of the operating room. Nonetheless, what has been learned from the body of in vitro work is that gap formation leads to a weakened repair and that a symmetrical, smooth, strong repair allows the potential for a safe postoperative active range of motion protocol, the holy grail for optimizing clinical outcomes while minimizing the risk for repair ruptures. One of the authors (D.H.L.) has been an ardent crusader for implementing nonsedated, tourniquet-free, local with epinephrine anesthesia only surgery for many commonly performed outpatient hand surgical procedures. This study presents their 15-year experience with tourniquet-free local-only flexor tendon repairs and proposes why this method, which allows in vivo operating room examination/testing of the efficacy of flexor tendon repair for tendon gliding impingement and gap formation by allowing active patient-repaired digit flexion and extension, may prove to be a significant step forward toward finding the repaired lacerated flexor tendon grail.

S. D. Trigg, MD

Composite Grafting for Traumatic Fingertip Amputation in Adults: Technique Reinforcement and Experience in 31 Digits

Chen S-Y, Wang C-H, Fu J-P, et al (Natl Defense Med Ctr, Taipei, Taiwan)
J Trauma 70:148-153, 2011

Background.—Composite grafting is used to treat nonreplantable fingertip amputations. This procedure has a high success rate and good results in treating fingertip amputations in children, but a lower success rate in adults.

Methods.—From July 2007 to December 2008, 27 patients with 31 injured fingertips were admitted because of traumatic fingertip amputation at the emergency department of Tri-Service General Hospital, National Defense Medical Center, Taipei, Taiwan. All 31 injured fingers had a non-replantable distal amputated fingertip and underwent composite grafting. We refined the surgical technique by excising the bony segment, defatting, deepithelialization, tie-over suturing, and finger splinting to increase the graft survival. The patients' age, mechanism of damage, lesion size, surgical result, and postoperative complications were recorded.

Results.—The mean age of the patients was 40.5 years (range, 20–65 years). The average lesion size was 2.4 cm^2. Twenty-one fingers (67.7%) had been injured by crushing injury and the other 10 fingers (32.3%) by cutting injury. The overall graft survival rate was 93.5% (29 of 31). The average 2-point discrimination was 6.3 mm in the sixth month after the operation. The esthetic outcome evaluated by self-report questionnaire was 93.1% satisfied, and 86.2% of the patients could use their injured finger normally in daily work.

Conclusions.—This easily performed and one-stage surgical procedure provided a reliable method for treating microsurgically nonreplantable fingertip amputations caused by hand trauma. The high overall success rate, satisfactory esthetic outcome, and good functional preservation helped patients return quickly to their daily life.

▶ Fingertip amputation injuries are among the most common finger injuries presenting to the emergency department, exclusive of lacerations and fractures. Most experienced emergency room physicians are adept at treating many of these injuries with wound care, suturing, and even minor bone shortening for the distal-most amputations involving pulp tissue loss, with minimum involvement of distal phalanx and nail bed sterile matrix. Moreover, many patients will arrive without their amputated fingertip. In those patients who arrive with their amputated fingertip part that is not a candidate for microvascular replantation (most), one is presented with several options, including various advancement flaps and composite grafting. Composite grafting is arguably a much simpler procedure than advancement flaps to perform in many emergency room conditions without the need for specialty equipment or when operating room availability is limited. The procedure also is a burn no bridges salvage technique that does not preclude other reconstructive procedures should the graft fail or later sensory deficits or pain require consideration for additional surgery. The investigators of this study suggest several refinements of the technique, which the authors propose as integral to their increased graft survival. Anyone who treats finger injuries must have several options in their treatment armamentarium, and you may find this technique a viable alternative in certain injuries.

S. D. Trigg, MD

Arthrodesis as a Salvage for Failed Proximal Interphalangeal Joint Arthroplasty
Jones DB Jr, Ackerman DB, Sammer DM, et al (Mayo Clinic, Rochester, MN)
J Hand Surg 36A:259-264, 2011

Purpose.—To review the rate of fusion, complications, and subjective outcome measures of proximal interphalangeal joint arthrodesis after failed implant arthroplasty.

Methods.—We conducted a retrospective review identifying patients from 1990 to 2009 who underwent proximal interphalangeal joint arthrodesis for implant arthroplasty failure. All types of implants were included. We reviewed clinical notes and radiographs identifying patient history, implant type, revisions before arthrodesis, method of arthrodesis, rate of union, time to union, and complications. We used the Michigan Hand Outcomes Questionnaire to assess patients' function and perceived clinical outcome.

Results.—A total of 13 joints in 8 patients (6 female, 2 male) identified with an average clinical follow-up of 6.5 years (range, 1.0–12.3 y) were available for study. The average time from joint replacement to salvage for all implant types was 9.3 years (range, 1.6–32.2 y). Eight of the 13 fingers achieved union. The average time to union was 5.8 months (range, 1–11 mo). Eight of 13 fingers underwent removal of K-wires, tension band, or both. Excluding hardware-related problems, there were 4 additional complications in 4 patients.

Conclusions.—Salvage of failed proximal interphalangeal joint arthroplasty remains a challenging clinical problem. Although achieving solid fusion with arthrodesis is not completely reliable or without complication, patients' subjective and functional outcomes demonstrate fair to good results.

Type of Study/Level of Evidence.—Therapeutic IV.

▶ The difficulties of salvage of a failed proximal interphalangeal joint arthroplasty with successful arthrodesis are a sobering business. This is a small retrospective study inclusive of heterogeneous implants and arthrodesis techniques, but it clearly points out the pitfalls and technical challenges that we all face when performing these procedures. Despite the limitations of the study, the authors present important information that one should share with prospective patients in preoperative discussions.

S. D. Trigg, MD

Nerve

Scope-Assisted Release of the Cubital Tunnel
Mirza A, Reinhart MK, Bove J, et al (St Catherine of Siena Med Ctr, Smithtown, NY; Stony Brook Univ, NY; the New York College of Osteopathic Medicine, Old Westbury)
J Hand Surg 36A:147-151, 2011

We report on a technique of endoscopic release of the cubital tunnel, which is a modification of Bruno and Tsai's technique. This article covers the history, complications, indications, and postoperative management of ulnar nerve entrapments treated endoscopically, with a special focus on our technique. This minimally invasive alternative to transposition requires no mobilization of the ulnar nerve, which could potentially reduce iatrogenic trauma to the nerve and its vascularity.

▶ Cubital tunnel syndrome is the second most common nerve entrapment syndrome of the upper extremity behind carpal tunnel syndrome. Despite the commonality of this neuropathy, the optimum method of treatment remains controversial, with decompression in situ, anterior transposition, and medial epicondylectomy all yielding equivalent outcomes. Anyone who performs any of these procedures with regularity has realized that lingering medial elbow and proximal medial forearm pain or incision scar tenderness can become a nagging postoperative problem in some, often persisting for months. Development of a less invasive yet effective procedure, therefore, has considerable appeal, there is growing interest in endoscopic cubital tunnel release, and new equipment technology is emerging. The authors of this technique-based study report their experience and refinements of previous techniques and equipments. Interestingly, their stated opinion is that from a technical standpoint, the learning curve for performing endoscopic cubital tunnel release using their method is less steep than that for endoscopic carpal tunnel release. For those interested in learning this procedure, this article is a good starting point.

S. D. Trigg, MD

Very Distal Sensory Nerve Transfers in High Median Nerve Lesions

Bertelli JA, Ghizoni MF (Governador Celso Ramos Hosp, Florianópolis, Brazil; Univ of Southern Santa Catarina (Unisul), Tubarão, Brazil)
J Hand Surg 36A:387-393, 2011

Purpose.—We report on the results of reconstruction of fingertip sensation by very distal nerve transfer in 8 patients with high median nerve lesions.

Methods.—Before surgery, patients underwent sensory testing of the hand using Semmes-Weinstein monofilaments. All patients had surgery within 1 year of trauma. For sensory reconstruction, branches of the radial nerve on the proximal phalanx of the index and thumb were sutured to the ulnar proper digital nerve of the thumb and radial proper digital nerve of the index finger. Patients were followed up for 12 months.

Results.—After median nerve lesions, zones of lost protective sensation were confined to the middle and index finger and the thumb. Sensation on the palm of the hand and proximal phalanx was preserved. Radial nerve transfer to palmar nerves restored protective or better sensation to the fingertips in all patients. Better results were observed for the thumb. Locognosia was acquired in all thumbs, and in 4 of 8 index fingers. Good results were detected even in patients who had undergone surgery later than 6 months after injury.

Conclusions.—Fingertip sensation can be restored by very distal nerve transfer of radial nerve branches to palmar nerves at the level of the proximal phalanx. This method of reconstruction appears useful in high median nerve lesions. In chronic lesions of the median nerve at the wrist and lesions in older patients, very distal nerve transfers might be adjunct to nerve grafting (Fig 2).

▶ This is an interesting method for restoration of sensation of the thumb and index finger following high median nerve injuries. Proximal repair and grafting have yielded mixed results, owing to the distance from the repair site to the distal target sensory receptors. Distal nerve transfers more closely approximate

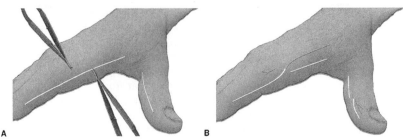

FIGURE 2.—Schematic representation of the surgical procedure for transferring dorsal sensory branches of the radial nerve to proper digital nerves in the index finger and thumb. **A** Note that the dorsal sensory branch of the radial nerve to the index finger is sectioned distally, whereas the proper digital nerve of the index is sectioned proximally. Distal section of the donor nerve and proximal section of the recipient nerve also are performed in the thumb. **B** Because of redundancy on the length of the nerve stumps, the coaptation of the dorsal sensory branch of the radial nerve with the proper digital nerve in the thumb and in the index finger is performed without tension. (Reprinted from Bertelli JA, Ghizoni MF. Very distal sensory nerve transfers in high median nerve lesions. *J. Hand Surg.* 2011;36A:387-393, Copyright 2011, with permission from the American Society for Surgery of the Hand.)

the site of the repair to the sensory receptors. This transfer is very distal indeed, and the anatomy is straightforward, thus making this an intriguing procedure to consider. While their series is limited in number, most reports on distal nerve transfers generally are. The sensory recovery is, however, acceptable even in more chronic cases.

S. D. Trigg, MD

Clinical Outcomes Following Median to Radial Nerve Transfers
Ray WZ, Mackinnon SE (Washington Univ, St Louis, MO)
J Hand Surg 36A:201-208, 2011

Purpose.—To evaluate the clinical outcomes in patients with radial nerve palsy who underwent nerve transfers using redundant fascicles of median nerve (innervating the flexor digitorum superficialis and flexor carpi radialis muscles) to the posterior interosseous nerve and the nerve to the extensor carpi radialis brevis.

Methods.—This was a retrospective review of the clinical records of 19 patients with radial nerve injuries who underwent nerve transfer procedures using the median nerve as a donor nerve. All patients were evaluated using the Medical Research Council (MRC) grading system. The mean age of patients was 41 years (range, 17–78 y). All patients received at least 12 months of follow-up (range, 20.3 ± 5.8 mo). Surgery was performed at a mean of 5.7 ± 1.9 months postinjury.

Results.—Postoperative functional evaluation was graded according to the following scale: grades MRC 0/5 to MRC 2/5 were considered poor outcomes, whereas an MRC grade of 3/5 was a fair result, 4/5 was a good result, and 4+/5 was an excellent outcome. Postoperatively, all patients except one had good to excellent recovery of wrist extension.

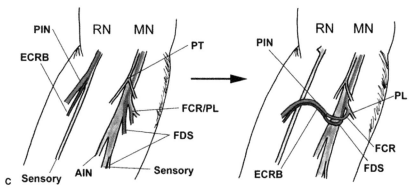

FIGURE 1.—C Illustration of our current preferred technique: FDS nerve to ECRB nerve and FCR nerve to PIN. (Reprinted from Ray WZ, Mackinnon SE. Clinical outcomes following median to radial nerve transfers. *J Hand Surg.* 2011;36A:201-208. Copyright 2011, with permission from the American Society for Surgery of the Hand.)

A total of 12 patients recovered good to excellent finger and thumb extension, 2 had fair recovery, and 5 had poor recovery.

Conclusions.—The radial nerve is commonly injured, causing severe morbidity in affected patients. The median nerve provides a reliable source of donor nerve fascicles for radial nerve reinnervation. The important nuances of both surgical technique and motor reeducation critical for the success of this transfer have been identified and are discussed.

Type of Study/Level of Evidence.—Therapeutic IV (Fig 1C).

▶ Nerve transfer surgery has substantially changed the treatment of traumatic and birth-related brachial plexus injuries over the past decade. The successes of these proximal nerve procedures have led to an emerging practice of distal nerve transfers. The senior author of this article (S.E.M.) is one of the pioneers in distal nerve transfer surgery and in median to radial nerve transfers in particular for radial nerve injuries. Tendon transfer for established radial nerve palsies is arguably one of the more successful of all tendon transfer procedures in the upper extremity but is not applicable in all patients. The authors of this study report their experience of median to radial nerve transfers over a 10-year period and give us insight as to their recommendations for this procedure over a consideration for nerve grafting following radial nerve injuries. Unfortunately, the radial nerve is the most frequently injured nerve of the upper extremity following orthopedic trauma. This article proposes new information that is worthy of review.

S. D. Trigg, MD

11 Orthopedic Oncology

Introduction

The orthopedic oncology chapter this year covers a wide variety of pathologic entities. The articles I have chosen cover the topics of biopsy, reconstructive techniques, treatment, radiation therapy, and a few articles of general interest.

The section on reconstructive techniques contains some interesting results on the durability and long-term results of endoprosthetic replacement of tumor defects of the lower extremity. The results are from the work out of UCLA. While the short-term and midterm results are good, we need a more durable reconstruction for the long-term survivors. The fact that the results continue to get better in terms of longevity is encouraging. The results of total femoral replacement were also reported to be very satisfactory. While this sounds to be a drastic procedure, the long-term performance is surprisingly good.

The topic of unplanned excision for soft tissue sarcomas is again included this year. This topic and errors related to the execution of the biopsy continue to be a problem that plagues the management of patients with malignant musculoskeletal tumors.

Christopher P. Beauchamp, MD

Biopsy

A Comparison of Fine-needle Aspiration, Core Biopsy, and Surgical Biopsy in the Diagnosis of Extremity Soft Tissue Masses
Kasraeian S, Allison DC, Ahlmann ER, et al (Univ of Southern California + Los Angeles County Med Ctr)
Clin Orthop Relat Res 468:2992-3002, 2010

Background.—Biopsy tissue can be obtained through a fine needle, a wider coring needle, or through an open surgical incision. Though much literature exists regarding the diagnostic yield of these techniques individually, none compare accuracy of diagnosis in the same mass.

Questions/Purposes.—We asked how the diagnostic accuracy of fine-needle aspiration, core biopsy, and open surgical biopsy compare in regard to identifying malignancy, establishing the exact diagnosis, and guiding the appropriate treatment of soft tissue masses.

271

Patients and Methods.—We prospectively studied 57 patients with palpable extremity soft tissue masses, performing fine-needle aspiration, followed by core biopsy, followed by surgical biopsy of the same mass.

Results.—Open surgical biopsy was 100% accurate on all accounts. With regard to determining malignancy, fine-needle aspiration and core biopsy had 79.17% and 79.2% sensitivity, 72.7% and 81.8% specificity, 67.9% and 76% positive predictive value, 82.8% and 84.4% negative predictive value, and an overall accuracy of 75.4% and 80.7%, respectively. In regard to determining exact diagnosis, fine-needle aspiration had a 33.3% accuracy and core biopsy had a 45.6% accuracy. With regard to eventual treatment, fine-needle aspiration was 38.6% accurate and core biopsy was 49.1% accurate.

Conclusions.—In soft tissue mass diagnosis, core biopsy is more accurate than fine-needle aspiration on all accounts, and open biopsy is more accurate than both in determining malignancy, establishing the exact diagnosis, and the guiding appropriate treatment.

▶ I chose this article because it is a well-done prospective study evaluating 47 patients with soft tissue masses. Although the number of patients in this study is small, it still provides quite valuable information regarding the various techniques of obtaining biopsy material for diagnosis. This topic is a subject of continued debate. There are strong proponents of each method used. This study again confirms the reliability of open biopsy and reaffirms it as the gold standard. Those of us who use other methods realize that nondiagnostic biopsy warrants further tissue sampling. This is particularly true with fine needle biopsies, as they are notoriously known for nondiagnostic diagnoses. It must be emphasized that an experienced pathologist is crucial to the success of any biopsy method. Some pathologists are very comfortable with fine needle aspirates. Minimally invasive biopsy methods are certainly more convenient for the surgeon and the patient. It must be understood that an open biopsy may be necessary when other methods are inconclusive. This article contains a very good summary of all the literature on this topic.

C. P. Beauchamp, MD

Analysis of Nondiagnostic Results after Image-guided Needle Biopsies of Musculoskeletal Lesions
Yang J, Frassica FJ, Fayad L, et al (Washington Univ Dept of Orthopaedic Surgery, St Louis, MO; Johns Hopkins Dept of Orthopaedic Surgery, Baltimore, MD; Johns Hopkins Dept of Radiology and Radiological Science, Baltimore, MD; et al)
Clin Orthop Relat Res 468:3103-3111, 2010

Background/Rationale.—Image-guided needle biopsies are commonly used to diagnose musculoskeletal tumors, but nondiagnostic (ND) results can delay diagnosis and treatment. It is important to understand which

TABLE 1.—Diagnostic Rates for Categorical Diagnosis

Category	Clinically Useful	Nondiagnostic	Incorrect	Total
Malignant bone tumors	70 (82%)	12 (14%)	3 (4%)	85
Benign bone tumors	63 (83%)	13 (17%)	0 (0%)	76
Malignant soft tissue tumors	56 (85%)	4 (6%)	6 (9%)	66
Benign soft tissue tumors	102 (96%)	4 (4%)	0 (0%)	106
Metastasis	48 (89%)	5 (9%)	1 (2%)	54
Nonneoplastic lesions	114 (94%)	7 (6%)	0 (0%)	121
All biopsies	453 (89%)	45 (9%)	10 (2%)	508

factors or diagnoses predispose to a ND result so that appropriate patient education or a possible change in the clinical plan can be made. Currently it is unclear which factors or specific lesions are more likely to lead to a ND result after image-guided needle biopsy.

Questions/Purposes.—We therefore identified specific factors and diagnoses most likely to yield ND results. We also asked whether an image-guided needle biopsy of bone and soft tissue lesions is an accurate and clinically useful tool.

Methods.—We retrospectively reviewed data from a prospectively collected database for a case-control study of 508 image-guided needle biopsies of patients with suspected musculoskeletal tumors between 2003 and 2008.

Results.—The interpretations of 453 of the 508 (89%) needle biopsies were accurate and clinically useful. Forty-five biopsies (9%) were ND and 10 (2%) were incorrect (IC). Bone lesions had a higher ND rate than soft tissue lesions (13% vs. 4%). The specific diagnosis with the highest ND rate was histiocytosis. Elbow and forearm locations had higher ND rates than average. Malignant tumors had a higher IC rate than benign tumors (5% vs. 0%); fibromyxoid sarcoma and rare subtypes of osteosarcoma had higher IC rates than other diagnoses. Repeat needle or open biopsies were performed in 71 (14%) patients. Bone lesions were more likely than soft tissue lesions to require repeat biopsies (18% vs. 9%).

Conclusions.—A high rate of accuracy and clinical usefulness is possible with image-guided needle biopsies of musculoskeletal lesions. We believe these biopsies appropriate in selected circumstances but a key factor for appropriate use is an experienced musculoskeletal tumor team with frequent communication to correlate clinical, radiographic, and histologic information for each patient (Table 1).

▶ This article was selected to emphasize evaluating image-guided needle biopsies provided to patient care. This large group of patients was treated at a large experienced medical center providing orthopedic oncology services. That there is success with CT or ultrasound-guided biopsies emphasizes the usefulness and accuracy of this technique. In those patients in whom a nondiagnostic biopsy was obtained, further attempts at either repeat biopsy or open biopsy are necessary. Image-guided biopsies have proven to be a tremendous benefit in my practice both to the patient and the surgeon.

C. P. Beauchamp, MD

Radiation

Elderly patients with painful bone metastases should be offered palliative radiotherapy

Campos S, Presutti R, Zhang L, et al (Univ of Toronto, Ontario, Canada)
Int J Radiat Oncol Biol Phys 76:1500-1506, 2010

Purpose.—To investigate the efficacy of palliative radiotherapy (RT) in relieving metastatic bone pain in elderly patients.

Methods and Materials.—The response to RT for palliation of metastatic bone pain was evaluated from a prospective database of 558 patients between 1999 and 2008. The pain scores and analgesic intake were used to calculate the response according to the International Bone Metastases Consensus Working Party palliative RT endpoints. Subgroup analyses for age and other demographic information were performed.

Results.—No significant difference was found in the response rate in patients aged ≥ 65, ≥ 70, and ≥ 75 years compared with younger patients at 1, 2, or 3 months after RT. The response was found to be significantly related to the performance status.

Conclusion.—Age alone did not affect the response to palliative RT for bone metastases. Elderly patients should be referred for palliative RT for their painful bone metastases, regardless of age, because they receive equal benefit from the treatment.

▶ This is a Canadian study of patients treated with palliative radiation therapy for metastatic bone disease. There was a perception by the authors that there is a reluctance to prescribe palliative radiation therapy to elderly patients for fear of either ineffectiveness or potential toxic side effects. This results in fewer elderly patients receiving palliative radiation therapy to relieve bone pain originating from bone metastases. This reluctance is occurring at the referring physician level. Patients in Canada cannot self-refer to a radiation oncologist. The authors have demonstrated quite clearly that palliative radiation therapy is extremely effective in the elderly patient population. There is no reason why palliative radiation therapy should be withheld based solely on the patient's age.

C. P. Beauchamp, MD

Radiology

Comparative study of whole-body MRI and bone scintigraphy for the detection of bone metastases

Balliu E, Boada M, Peláez I, et al (Hospital Universitari de Girona Dr Josep Trueta, Spain; et al)
Clin Radiol 65:989-996, 2010

Aim.—To assess and compare the diagnostic accuracy of whole-body magnetic resonance imaging (MRI) and bone scintigraphy in the detection of metastases to bone.

Material and Methods.—Forty randomly selected patients with known malignant tumours were prospectively studied using bone scintigraphy and whole-body MRI. Two patients were excluded. Symptoms of bone metastasis were present in 29 (76%) patients and absent in nine (24%). Findings were classified into four categories according to the probability of bone metastasis: (1) negative, (2) probably negative, (3) probably positive, and (4) positive. Diagnostic accuracy was determined according to the area under the receiver operating characteristic (ROC) curve. The definitive diagnosis was reached using other imaging techniques, biopsy, or 12 months clinical follow-up.

Results.—Metastases were present in 18 patients. The sensitivity, specificity, and diagnostic accuracy were 94, 90, and 92%, respectively, for whole-body MRI and 72, 75, and 74%, respectively, for bone scintigraphy. Diagnostic accuracy measured by the area under the ROC curve was significantly higher for whole-body MRI (96%) than for bone scintigraphy (77%; $p<0.05$). Interobserver agreement measured by the kappa index was significantly higher for whole-body MRI (0.895) than for bone scintigraphy (0.524; $p<0.05$). Whole-body MRI detected lesions in tissues other than bone in 17 (45%) patients.

Conclusions.—Whole-body MRI is more accurate and more objective than bone scintigraphy for the detection of bone metastases. Whole-body MRI can also detect lesions in tissues other than bone.

▶ This study compares whole-body MRI with bone scintigraphy for the detection of bone metastasis. It is widely known that bone scans can be unreliable in the detection of some types of metastatic bone disease. Multiple myeloma, for example, is notoriously known to be unreliable when detected by conventional bone scans. Also, aggressive metastatic carcinoma can sometimes be missed because of the rapid growth within the bone such that the bone does not have time to respond to the destructive process. MRI is far more sensitive in the detection of bone and soft tissue neoplasms. The authors have demonstrated that whole-body imaging is far more sensitive than bone scanning. The use of whole-body MRI is not very practical and is extremely expensive, but in some certain circumstances, it may be necessary to localize difficult neoplastic lesions. A good example of this is a patient who presents with osteomalacia secondary to a phosphaturic mesenchymal tumor.

C. P. Beauchamp, MD

Joint Space Widening in Synovial Chondromatosis of the Hip

Yoon PW, Yoo JJ, Koo K-H, et al (Seoul Natl Univ College of Medicine, Republic of Korea)

J Bone Joint Surg Am 93:303-310, 2011

Background.—One of the radiographic findings in synovial chondromatosis of the hip is widening of the joint space between the femoral head and the acetabulum, although the cause and sequelae of the widening are unclear.

Methods.—Between May 1991 and June 2005, twenty-one patients with synovial chondromatosis of the hip were treated with open synovectomy and removal of osteochondral fragments. Joint space widening was assessed on radiographs made preoperatively, immediately after surgery, and at the time of follow-up. The changes of the radiographic joint space width were evaluated during the mean follow-up period of 5.9 years (range, 2.3 to 12.3 years).

Results.—Twelve patients had joint space widening on preoperative radiographs of the hip. Medial joint space widening was seen in three patients, and both medial and superior joint space widening was evident in nine patients. Compared with the medial and superior joint spaces in the unaffected, contralateral hip, those in the affected hip were wider by an average of 44.7% and 35.9%, respectively. The medial joint space widths of the affected hip decreased slightly during the early postoperative period; however, widened joint spaces were persistent at the final follow-up visit, without other important changes. The superior joint space widths did not show substantial changes throughout the postoperative follow-up period.

Conclusions.—Joint space widening is a recognized radiographic finding in primary synovial chondromatosis of the hip. Although there was persistence of joint space widening after synovectomy in all patients, this joint space widening did not influence the clinical results at the time of follow-up.

▶ Synovial chondromatosis is a rare disorder. While some of the patients would today be treated with a joint replacement, all of the patients in this series were treated with an open synovectomy. The observation of joint space widening is new. This is not a feature of osteochondromatosis that I was aware of before. This radiographic sign can be helpful in the early detection of this unusual entity when it first presents. The ready availability of MRI eliminates the delay in diagnosis of this disorder.

C. P. Beauchamp, MD

Reconstruction Techniques

Endoprosthetic reconstruction of the distal tibia and ankle joint after resection of primary bone tumours
Shekkeris AS, Hanna SA, Sewell MD, et al (Royal Natl Orthopaedic Hosp, Stanmore, Middlesex, England)
J Bone Joint Surg [Br] 91-B:1378-1382, 2009

Endoprosthetic replacement of the distal tibia and ankle joint for a primary bone tumour is a rarely attempted and technically challenging procedure. We report the outcome of six patients treated between 1981 and 2007. There were four males and two females, with a mean age of 43.5 years (15 to 75), and a mean follow-up of 9.6 years (1 to 27). No patient developed a local recurrence or metastasis. Two of the six went on to have a below-knee amputation for persistent infection after a mean 16 months (1 to 31). The four patients who retained their endoprosthesis had a mean musculoskeletal tumour society score of 70% and a mean Toronto extremity salvage score of 71%. All were pain free and able to perform most activities of daily living in comfort.

A custom-made endoprosthetic replacement of the distal tibia and ankle joint is a viable treatment option for carefully selected patients with a primary bone tumour. Patients should, however, be informed of the risk of infection and the potential need for amputation if this cannot be controlled.

▶ Most tumors of the distal tibia and ankle joint are treated with limb ablation. It is difficult to reconstruct distal tibial defects primarily because of the poor soft tissue envelope in the area. Large allografts and large metallic components are prone to deep infections because of the high risk of wound healing complications. Hence, limb salvage is infrequently attempted in this area. This article reports on the results from a very experienced tumor center using a custom-made endoprosthesis. As expected, one-third of patients were converted to a below-knee amputation because of infection. Those patients who were able to retain their prosthesis had a very acceptable result. Tumors in this location are fortunately rare, and attempts at limb salvage can be recovered with a below-knee amputation if carefully planned limb salvage does not burn any bridges. In this study, it would have been interesting to compare the functional results of the 4 patients who successfully underwent limb salvage with a matched group of patients with a below-knee amputation.

C. P. Beauchamp, MD

Custom-made endoprostheses for the femoral amputation stump: An alternative to hip disarticulation in tumour surgery
Kalson NS, Gikas PD, Aston W, et al (Royal Natl Orthopaedic Hosp, Stanmore, UK)
J Bone Joint Surg [Br] 92-B:1134-1137, 2010

Disarticulation of the hip in patients with high-grade tumours in the upper thigh results in significant morbidity. In patients with no disease of the proximal soft tissue a femoral stump may be preserved, leaving a fulcrum for movement and weight-bearing. We reviewed nine patients in whom the oncological decision would normally be to disarticulate, but who were treated by implantation of an endoprosthesis in order to create a functioning femoral stump. The surgery was undertaken for chondrosarcoma in four patients, pleomorphic sarcoma in three, osteosarcoma in one and fibrous dysplasia in one. At follow-up at a mean of 80 months (34 to 132), seven patients were alive and free from disease, one had died from lung metastases and another from a myocardial infarction. The mean functional outcome assessment was 50 (musculoskeletal tumor society), 50 and 60 (physical and mental Shortform 36 scores).

Implantation of an endoprosthesis into the stump in carefully selected patients allows fitting of an above-knee prosthesis and improves wellbeing and the functional outcome.

▶ I have used this technique on a few occasions. Any time there is an opportunity to preserve length in an amputation setting, this technique should be considered. I have used conventional modular components to preserve length, but the problem I have encountered is soft tissue motion occurring around the prosthesis to which there is no soft tissue attachment. I have also had problems with the component eroding through the skin. The authors use a custom-made implant, and many of the problems I have encountered are addressed by the use of this implant. The addition of a porous coating would help with soft tissue attachment.

C. P. Beauchamp, MD

Intercalary Allograft Reconstructions Using a Compressible Intramedullary Nail: A Preliminary Report
Miller BJ, Virkus WW (Rush Univ Med Ctr, Chicago, IL)
Clin Orthop Relat Res 468:2507-2513, 2010

Background.—Although intercalary allograft reconstructions are commonly performed using intramedullary devices, they cannot generate compression across host-allograft junctions. Therefore, they sometimes are associated with gap formation and suboptimal healing conditions.

Questions/Purposes.—We describe a new technique and present preliminary results for intercalary allograft reconstructions for tumors using a compressible intramedullary nail.

Patients and Methods.—We retrospectively reviewed 10 patients (19 host-allograft junctions) who underwent intercalary allograft reconstruction using the compression nailing technique. Two patients were excluded as they had additional vascularized fibular autografts, leaving 15 junctions in eight patients for analysis. Three of the intercalary reconstructions had supplemental plate fixation at one junction. All patients received host bone reamings and cancellous allograft and one had bone marrow aspirate and demineralized bone matrix in addition to the cancellous allograft. The minimum followup was 3 months (mean, 18 months; range, 3–39 months).

Results.—Thirteen of 15 junctions healed without additional surgery. Two diaphyseal-diaphyseal junctions did not unite after allograft arthrodeses. One patient underwent revision for nonunion 8 months after the initial procedure, with subsequent healing. The second patient had no evidence of union at 6 months, after which he was lost to followup. There were no allograft fractures or infections in any reconstruction. One patient died of metastatic renal cell carcinoma, and one patient had multicentric local soft tissue recurrences of a periosteal osteosarcoma requiring resection.

Conclusions.—Our early observations indicate newer compressible intramedullary nails reliably address junctional gap formation, providing for a high rate of union while retaining the long-term benefits of intramedullary stabilization.

Level of Evidence.—Level IV, case series. See Guidelines for Authors for a complete description of levels of evidence.

▶ Use of allograft is probably the most common method chosen to reconstruct intercalary defects. One of the more common technical problems associated with this technique is achieving a tight graft-host junction under compression. The graft can be held in place with either a plate or plates or an intramedullary rod plus or minus plates. None of these methods provide the predictable rigid fixation necessary for allograft healing. This article reports on the experience using a new-generation intramedullary rod capable of providing compressive forces. In this series, high union rates were achieved using this device. The problem of grafting and accurate graft-host junction still remains, as the effect of inserting the rod ultimately determines the fit between the allograft and the host bone. It is difficult to adjust this junction with an intramedullary device in place. More work is still needed to perfect the technical aspects of this reconstruction.

C. P. Beauchamp, MD

Computer-assisted Navigation in Bone Tumor Surgery: Seamless Workflow Model and Evolution of Technique
So TYC, Lam Y-L, Mak K-L (Queen Elizabeth Hosp, Hong Kong, SAR, China)
Clin Orthop Relat Res 468:2985-2991, 2010

Background.—Computer-assisted navigation was recently introduced to aid the resection of musculoskeletal tumors. However, it has not always been possible to directly navigate the osteotomy with real-time manipulation of available surgical tools. Registration techniques vary, although most existing systems use some form of surface matching.

Questions/Purposes.—We developed and evaluated a workflow model of computer-assisted bone tumor surgery and evaluated (1) the applicability of currently available software to different bones; (2) the accuracy of the navigated excision; and (3) the accuracy of a new registration technique of fluoro-CT matching.

Methods.—Our workflow involved detailed preoperative planning with CT-MRI image fusion, three-dimensional mapping of the tumor, and planning of the resection plane. Using the workflow model, we reviewed 15 navigation procedures in 12 patients, including four with joint-saving resections and three with custom implant reconstructions. Intraoperatively, registration was performed with either paired points and surface matching (Group 1, n = 10) or a new technique of fluoro-CT image matching (Group 2, n = 5). All osteotomies were performed under direct computer navigation. Postoperatively, each case was evaluated for histologic margin and gross measurement of the achieved surgical margin.

Results.—The margins were free from tumor in all resected specimens. In the Group 1 procedures, the correlation between preoperative planned margins and actual achieved margins was 0.631, whereas in Group 2 procedures (fluoro-CT matching), the correlation was 0.985.

Conclusions.—Our findings suggest computer-assisted navigation is accurate and useful for bone tumor surgery. The new registration technique using fluoro-CT matching may allow more accurate resection of margins.

▶ I have attempted to use a computer-assisted navigation for tumor resections. I have found this to be a rather frustrating exercise. It is critical, however, particularly in difficult pelvic resections or juxta-articular resections to be extremely precise when we are at the limits of our limb-sparing capabilities. The authors provide some good technical tips to improve the value of computer navigation. For those interested in using this method, this article provides useful and helpful information.

C. P. Beauchamp, MD

How Long Do Endoprosthetic Reconstructions for Proximal Femoral Tumors Last?
Bernthal NM, Schwartz AJ, Oakes DA, et al (Univ of California Los Angeles Med Ctr, Santa Monica; et al)
Clin Orthop Relat Res 468:2867-2874, 2010

Background.—As the life expectancy of patients with musculoskeletal tumors improves, long-term studies of endoprosthetic reconstructions are necessary to establish realistic expectations for the implants and compare them to other reconstruction approaches.

Questions/Purposes.—(1) What is the long-term survival of cemented bipolar proximal femoral replacements? (2) How does prosthesis survival compare to patient survival among patients with Stage I, II, and III disease? (3) Do modular implants outperform custom-built prostheses? (4) Do some proximal femoral replacements require conversion to THA?

Patients and Methods.—We retrospectively reviewed all 86 proximal femoral replacements used for tumor reconstruction from 1982 to 2008. Primary diagnoses were 43 high-grade tumors (IIA/IIB), 20 low-grade tumors (IA/IB or benign), and 23 with metastatic disease. We reviewed prosthesis survival, patient survival, complication rates, functional outcomes, and rates of conversion to THA.

Results.—Five of 86 patients (5.8%) required revision of the femoral component. Five-, 10-and 20-year implant survivorships were 93%, 84%, and 56%, respectively. All patients with low-grade disease survived; the 5-year survival rate for patients with metastatic disease was 16%; the 5-, 10-, and 20-year survival for IIA/IIB patients was 54%, 50%, and 44%, respectively. Five of 86 patients (5.8%) underwent conversion to THA for groin pain.

Conclusions.—Cemented bipolar proximal femoral replacements after tumor resection proved a durable reconstruction technique. The implants outlived patients with metastatic disease and high-grade localized disease while patients with low-grade disease outlived their implants. The survival of modular prostheses was comparable to that of older, one-piece custom designs.

▶ There are a number of different options available to reconstruct proximal femoral deficiencies following tumor resections. In general, if the abductor mechanism can be preserved or reconstructed, allograft-prosthetic composite is generally the preferred method of reconstruction. Most other defects are reconstructed with an endoprosthesis, which often is in conjunction with a bipolar acetabular reconstruction. This article reviews the results from perhaps the most experienced center using endoprosthetic reconstructions. A cemented bipolar proximal femoral replacement provides a durable result. Surprisingly, only a small number of patients required conversion to a total hip replacement because of problems related to the bipolar prosthesis. Loosening requiring revision in this population of patients was very low. A cemented proximal femoral replacement in combination with a bipolar acetabular reconstruction is a predictable reconstructive technique and a prescription to patients.

C. P. Beauchamp, MD

Cemented Endoprosthetic Reconstruction of the Proximal Tibia: How Long Do They Last?

Schwartz AJ, Kabo JM, Eilber FC, et al (Univ of California Los Angeles Med Ctr, Santa Monica; California State Univ, Northridge)
Clin Orthop Relat Res 468:2875-2884, 2010

Background.—The few available studies documenting the long-term survival of cemented proximal tibial endoprostheses for musculoskeletal tumors do not differentiate between stem designs or patient diagnosis. There is wide variation in survival rates reported, possibly a result of this heterogeneity in patient population and implant design.

Questions/Purposes.—We therefore asked: (1) How long do proximal tibial endoprostheses last? (2) What is the typical long-term functional result after proximal tibial replacement? And (3) what are the short- and long-term complications associated with endoprosthetic reconstruction of the proximal tibia, particularly with respect to the soft tissue reconstruction?

Patients and Methods.—We retrospectively reviewed 52 patients with 52 proximal tibial endoprosthetic reconstructions for a tumor-related diagnosis. Kaplan-Meier survivorship analysis was performed using revision of the stemmed components for any reason as an endpoint for implants, and death due to disease progression for patients. Function was assessed using the MSTS scoring system. The minimum followup was 1 month (mean, 96 months: range, 1–284 months; median, 69 months).

Results.—Using revision of the stemmed components for any reason as an end point, overall prosthesis survival at 5, 10, 15, and 20 years was 94%, 86%, 66%, and 37%, respectively. The 29 modular implants demonstrated a trend toward improved survival compared to the 23 custom-designed components, with a 15-year survivorship of 88% versus 63%. The mean postoperative Musculoskeletal Tumor Society score at most recent followup was 82% of normal function (mean raw score, 24.6; range, 4–29).

Conclusions.—Cemented endoprosthetic reconstruction of the proximal tibia provides a reliable method of reconstruction following tumor resection.

▶ This is a large series from a very experienced musculoskeletal tumor center. They have reported extremely encouraging long-term results in patients treated for tumors of the proximal tibia. It has become clear that we are going to be seeing an ever-increasing number of patients who are long-term survivors of their disease who present with failed reconstructions. Revision of endoprosthetic devices will become an ever-increasing challenge in the future. Revision of these implants should include the skills of a revision arthroplasty surgeon.

C. P. Beauchamp, MD

Local Recurrence, Survival and Function After Total Femur Resection and Megaprosthetic Reconstruction for Bone Sarcomas
Ruggieri P, Bosco G, Pala E, et al (Univ of Bologna, Italy)
Clin Orthop Relat Res 468:2860-2866, 2010

Background.—The choices of treatment for patients with extensive tumors of the femur include total femur megaprosthesis or large allograft-prosthetic composites. Previous reports suggest variable survival ranging from 60—70% at 1 to 2 years. However, these studies described earlier prostheses and techniques.

Questions/Purposes.—To confirm previous reports we determined (1) risk of local recurrence; (2) overall survivorship; and (3) function in patients with total femur reconstructions for tumors.

Methods.—We retrospectively reviewed 23 patients with total femur megaprostheses implanted between 1987 and 2006 after resection of bone tumors. Two patients lost at followup were excluded; the remaining 21 included 15 males and six females with a mean age of 21 years. The mean followup was 48 months (range, 1 month 17 years). Function was assessed according to the MSTS System II.

Results.—No patient developed a local recurrence during followup. At last followup, six patients were continuously disease-free at a mean of 148 months, one patient had no evidence of disease after treatment of a recurrence, one patient was alive with disease, and 13 patients died of their disease at a mean time of 17 months. In 15 patients evaluated with the MSTS score, the mean score was 66%; four patients had over 75%, eight from 51% to 75%, three from 26% to 50%. Four patients (19%) had complications requiring further surgery in absence of trauma. A fifth patient had a posttraumatic periprosthetic fracture.

Conclusions.—A total femur prosthesis allows a limb-preserving procedure in tumors with extensive femoral involvement or in the presence of a skip lesion along the femur. The prognosis of these tumors is poor, but this reconstruction provides function with a relatively low rate of major complications.

▶ Resection of the entire femur is rarely required. When it is performed, the subsequent reconstruction is technically quite simple. This report from Bologna, Italy, describes a large series of patients treated with a total femur megaprosthesis. These patients obviously have extensive disease; many of them have skip lesions dictating the need for total femoral resection. As a group, therefore, they have a poor prognosis because of this. This point is reflected in their results. The ability to achieve a satisfactory functional result in this group of patients is gratifying considering the magnitude of the resection. The repair or reconstruction of the soft tissue envelope surrounding the prosthesis is critical to the success and avoidance of complications. Careful attention to the capsular repair of the hip and knee is necessary to avoid instability of the reconstruction.

This technique results in dependable maintenance of function with a relatively low complication rate.

C. P. Beauchamp, MD

Tumor General

A Comparative Study of F-18 FDG PET and ^{201}Tl Scintigraphy for Detection of Primary Malignant Bone and Soft-Tissue Tumors

Yamamoto Y, Kawaguchi Y, Kawase Y, et al (Kagawa Univ, Japan)
Clin Nucl Med 36:290-294, 2011

Purpose.—The purpose of this study was to compare 2-[F-18]fluoro-2-deoxy-D-glucose (FDG) positron emission tomography (PET) and Tl-201 chloride (Tl) scintigraphy for detection of primary malignant bone and soft-tissue tumors.

Materials and Methods.—A total of 40 patients with suspicion of malignant bone and soft-tissue tumors were examined. FDG PET imaging was performed at 1-hour post-FDG injection. Tl planar and single photon emission computed tomography images were acquired 10 minutes (early) and 2 hours (delayed) after injection of Tl. We evaluated FDG and Tl uptake visually and semiquantitatively using standardized uptake value and tumor to contralateral normal tissue ratio on planar images, respectively.

Results.—Of the 33 patients with malignant tumors, all but 2 liposarcomas showed positive accumulation on FDG PET. However, all 7 benign lesions were also positive on FDG PET. Both early and delayed Tl images were positive for 27 of the 33 malignant tumors. Of the 6 false-negative cases on Tl images, 5 were liposarcomas. Both early and delayed Tl images were negative for 5 of the 7 benign lesions. The sensitivity of FDG PET for detection of primary malignant bone and soft-tissue tumors was 94% and the specificity, 0%. The corresponding values for Tl scintigraphy were 82% and 71%. The mean FDG standardized uptake value in malignant tumors was higher than that in benign lesions, but this difference was not statistically significant. Statistically significant differences were observed between malignant and benign lesions for both early and delayed tumor to contralateral normal tissue ratios.

Conclusions.—FDG PET was found to be more sensitive than Tl scintigraphy for primary malignant bone and soft-tissue tumors, although it was less specific.

▶ We are continuing to look at new techniques to evaluate patients with primary malignant bone and soft tissue tumors. Positron emission tomographic scans and thallium scans are both useful tools to assist us in the staging of these bone and soft tissue sarcomas. These are expensive tests and sometimes are denied by insurance providers. This study provides us useful information to document the effectiveness of these techniques in the staging of our patients. Both of these techniques provide value to our ability to accurately predict the biologic behavior of bone and soft tissue sarcomas, but neither of these studies is absolute. Both of these may provide complementary information regarding patients. It is clear that both of these nuclear medicine tests are tools that are clearly scientifically proven to benefit our patients.

C. P. Beauchamp, MD

Local Recurrence After Initial Multidisciplinary Management of Soft Tissue Sarcoma: Is there a Way Out?
Abatzoglou S, Turcotte RE, Adoubali A, et al (McGill Univ Health Centre, Montreal, Quebec, Canada; Maisonneuve-Rosemont Hosp, Montreal, Quebec, Canada)
Clin Orthop Relat Res 468:3012-3018, 2010

Background.—Multimodality treatment of primary soft tissue sarcoma by expert teams reportedly affords a low incidence of local recurrence. Despite advances, treatment of local recurrence remains difficult and is not standardized.

Questions/Purposes.—We (1) determined the incidence of local recurrence from soft tissue sarcoma; (2) compared characteristics of the recurrent tumors with those of the primary ones; (3) evaluated local recurrences, metastases and death according to treatments; and (4) explored the relationship between the diagnosis of local recurrence and the occurrence of metastases.

Methods.—From our prospective database, we identified 618 soft tissue sarcomas. Thirty-seven of the 618 patients (6%) had local recurrence. Leiomyosarcoma was the most frequent diagnosis (eight of 37). The mean delay from original surgery was 22 months (range, 2—75 months). Mean size was 4.8 cm (range, 0.4—28.0 cm). Median followup after local recurrence was 16 months (range, 0—98 months).

Results.—Recurrent tumors had a tendency toward becoming deeper seated and higher graded. Nineteen of the 37 patients with recurrence underwent limb salvage (nine free flaps) and six had an amputation. Twenty-two (59%) had metastases, including 10 occurring after the local recurrence event at an average delay of 21 months (range, 1—34 months). Six patients developed additional local recurrences, with no apparent difference in risk between amputation (two of six) and limb salvage (four of 19).

Conclusions.—Patients with a local recurrence of a soft tissue sarcoma have a poor prognosis. Limb salvage and additional radiotherapy remain possible but with substantial complications. Amputation did not prevent additional local recurrence or death (Fig 1).

▶ We continue to struggle with patients receiving inappropriate or poorly planned management of soft tissue sarcomas. This problem is not going to go away. The consequences of these situations result in patients being at higher risk for local recurrence. Even when thoughtfully planned and properly executed treatments are provided for these patients, they are still at risk for

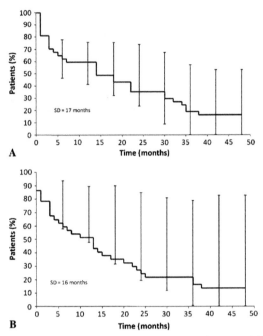

FIGURE 1.—(A) Kaplan-Meier analysis of survival and (B) disease-free survival following local recurrence from soft-tissue sarcoma are shown. (With kind permission from Springer Science+Business Media: Abatzoglou S, Turcotte RE, Adoubali A, et al. Local recurrence after initial multidisciplinary management of soft tissue sarcoma: is there a way out? *Clin Orthop Relat Res.* 2010;468:3012-3018.)

a local recurrence. This report is made by a very experienced group of musculoskeletal oncologists. With careful planning, their recurrence rate is 6%. This group of patients did not do well. It emphasizes the significant effect a local recurrence has on prognosis. It is probably correct to emphasize that in this setting, the effect of local recurrence is worse even when a patient is managed by an experienced team.

C. P. Beauchamp, MD

Clinicopathologic Prognostic Factors of Pure Myxoid Liposarcoma of the Extremities and Trunk Wall

Nishida Y, Tsukushi S, Nakashima H, et al (Nagoya Univ Graduate School and School of Medicine, Japan; Aichi Cancer Ctr Aichi Hosp, Japan)
Clin Orthop Relat Res 468:3041-3046, 2010

Background.—Myxoid liposarcoma is generally considered a low grade tumor but the presence of areas of round cells exceeding 5% is reportedly associated with a worse prognosis. Whether "pure" tumors without round cells are low grade has not been confirmed. While radiotherapy has been used for patients' myxoid liposarcoma it is unclear whether it reduces local recurrences.

Questions/Purposes.—We therefore determined the survival, roles of radiotherapy for local control, and prognostic factors of pure myxoid liposarcoma of the extremities and trunk wall.

Methods.—We retrospectively reviewed 53 patients histologically diagnosed with pure myxoid liposarcoma arising in extremities and the trunk wall. Nine patients of the 53 received radiotherapy for primary tumors. Clinical features and prognosis were determined, and various factors were analyzed as to their usefulness as prognostic factors (age, gender, location, size, depth, surgical margin, and adjuvant radiotherapy). The minimum followup was 12 months (mean, 60 months; range, 12−226 months).

Results.—Seven (13%) and 6 (11%) patients developed a local recurrence and distant metastasis, respectively. The 5- and 10-year disease-specific and disease-free survival rates were 90% and 83% and 77% and 77%, respectively. Radiotherapy had no impact on either overall or disease free survival. Age (older than 60 years) independently predicted worse overall and disease-free survival.

Conclusions.—In pure myxoid liposarcoma located in the extremities and trunk wall, relatively few patients developed distant metastasis suggesting the tumor is generally low grade. Local control could be achieved with wide surgical margins without radiotherapy. Age was associated with

TABLE 2.—Overall (OAS) (53 Patients) and Disease Free (DFS) (53 Patients) Survival at 5 Years

Variable	OAS (%)	DFS (%)
All	90.3	76.5
Gender		
Male	82.8	77.5
Female	85.7	74.1
Age		
>60	77.3	57.4
<60	96.6	84.7
Depth		
Superficial	100	77.8
Deep	85.4	69.5
Size		
10≤	86.9	66.0
5−10	88.0	85.1
<5	100	77.1
Location		
Trunk	87.5	64.9
Upper Extrem.	80.0	68.6
Lower Extrem.	93.3	81.0
Surgical margin		
Wide	88.3	80.2
Marginal	50.0	66.7
Radiotherapy		
(+)	83.3	76.2
(−)	91.8	76.9
Local recurrence		
(+)	75.0	
(−)	92.1	

lower survival but size and depth were not. Myxoid liposarcoma in older patients requires special consideration for treatment and followup (Table 2).

▶ A true myxoid liposarcoma is a low-grade neoplasm. The presence of round cells is an ominous finding. This neoplasm is different from a pure myxoid liposarcoma. This article describes the outcome of treatment of pure myxoid liposarcoma. Treatment with a wide surgical margin without adjuvant therapy is adequate for the management of this lesion. Local control and long-term survival can be achieved with wide surgical margins. Radiation therapy did not provide an increased rate of local control. Metastatic disease is rare with this tumor, and it is important to separate this lesion from a myxoid liposarcoma with round cell presence.

C. P. Beauchamp, MD

Tumor Reconstruction

Extracorporeally Irradiated Autograft-prosthetic Composite Arthroplasty With Vascular Reconstruction for Primary Bone Tumor of the Proximal Tibia
Emori M, Hashimoto N, Hamada K-I, et al (Osaka Med Ctr for Cancer and Cardiovascular Diseases, Japan; Osaka Univ Graduate School of Medicine, Japan)
Ann Vasc Surg 25:266.e1-266.e4, 2011

The proximal tibia is a common site for primary bone tumors. Proximal tibial tumors may invade the adjacent soft-tissue by destroying the cortex and may further invade neurovascular bundles. We treated a patient with primary bone tumor of the proximal tibia with neurovascular invasion by extracorporeally irradiated autograft-prosthetic composite arthroplasty with vascular reconstruction. In cases of concomitant allograft arthroplasty and vascular reconstruction, we recommend that vascular reconstruction be performed before arthroplasty to minimize ischemia time. Good oncological and functional outcomes were achieved 75 months after surgery. Therefore, this reconstruction technique can be considered as a good treatment option (Figs 1-3).

▶ I include an article on this topic almost yearly. This is an interesting technique to have available for situations where reconstructive options are limited. Reconstructive options for proximal tibial defects are numerous. The defect can be reconstructed with a tumor prosthesis, osteoarticular graft, allograft prosthetic composite, modified amputation or some modification of the resected tissue. The bone and surrounding soft tissues can be autoclaved, pasteurized, or irradiated. No matter what the choice, the challenge has always been how to reconstruct the extensor mechanism. Some form of a biologic reconstruction generally offers the best results. Allograft prosthetic composite reconstruction provides the best tissue to reconstruct the extensor mechanism. In areas of

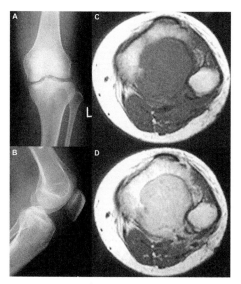

FIGURE 1.—A Anteroposterior view indicating a lytic lesion with no marginal sclerosis of the left proximal tibia. B Lateral view. C Tumor mass, homogeneous isointense to skeletal muscle, on T1-weighted axial image. D Tumor mass, heterogenous isointense and hyperintense to skeletal muscle, encompassing popliteal vascular structures on T2-weighted axial image. (Reprinted from Emori M, Hashimoto N, Hamada K-I, et al. Extracorporeally irradiated autograft-prosthetic composite arthroplasty with vascular reconstruction for primary bone tumor of the proximal tibia. *Ann Vasc Surg*. 2011;25: 266.e1-266.e4, with permission from Annals of Vascular Surgery Inc.)

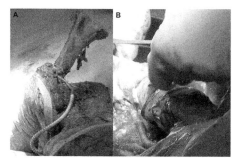

FIGURE 2.—A A long and redundant synthetic vascular prosthesis was observed after the popliteal anastomosis. B We excised the excess synthetic vascular prosthesis and repeated popliteal anastomosis. (Reprinted from Emori M, Hashimoto N, Hamada K-I, et al. Extracorporeally irradiated autograft-prosthetic composite arthroplasty with vascular reconstruction for primary bone tumor of the proximal tibia. *Ann Vasc Surg*. 2011;25:266.e1-266.e4, with permission from Annals of Vascular Surgery Inc.)

the world where allografts are not available, other biologic methods are used. In this case, the method used is extracorporal irradiation. The authors have reported a good outcome in this case report. In circumstances where an

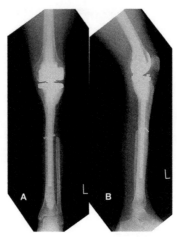

FIGURE 3.—A Anteroposterior view of the autograft-prosthetic composite. The distal tibial graft is fixed to the residual tibia with screws. B Lateral view. (Reprinted from Emori M, Hashimoto N, Hamada K-I, et al. Extracorporeally irradiated autograft-prosthetic composite arthroplasty with vascular reconstruction for primary bone tumor of the proximal tibia. *Ann Vasc Surg.* 2011;25:266.e1-266.e4, with permission from Annals of Vascular Surgery Inc.)

allograft is not an option, sterilization of the resected bone with radiation is a good technique to consider.

C. P. Beauchamp, MD

Evolution of Surgical Treatment for Sarcomas of Proximal Humerus in Children: Retrospective Review at a Single Institute Over 30 Years

Manfrini M, Tiwari A, Ham J, et al (Istituto Ortopedico Rizzoli, Bologna, Italy)
J Pediatr Orthop 31:56-64, 2011

Background.—Proximal humerus, although a common site for primary bone sarcomas, finds scant mention in literature as far as options and outcome of reconstruction in the skeletally immature skeleton are concerned. Reconstruction after resection of proximal humeral sarcomas in the immature skeleton poses specific challenges to the surgeon, and there has been a definite evolution of these techniques over the decades. We studied the evolution and compared the outcome of various techniques for such reconstruction over 3 decades at a single institution.

Methods.—All 61 children younger than 13 years of age and treated for a primary sarcoma of the proximal humerus at Department of Musculoskeletal Oncology, Rizzoli Orthopedic Institute, from 1976 to 2006 were studied for techniques of resection and reconstruction, complications, surgical procedures needed during follow up, and functional and radiologic outcomes during and at final follow-up. The functional outcomes after various procedures were compared using the Musculoskeletal Tumor Society scoring system.

Results.—A definite trend from amputation in the first decade, to the use of nonbiological reconstruction (endoprostheses, K nail cement spacer) in the second and biological reconstruction (vascular proximal fibula autograft, osteoarticular allograft, and allograft prosthesis composite) in the third decade was seen. There was a trend of improvement in the functional outcome over the 3 decades, although the complication rates and the need for repeated surgical procedures remained a major problem in all the techniques.

Conclusions.—Reconstruction of proximal humerus after resection for sarcomas is a challenging task. Although endoprostheses do have a definite role to play in reconstruction of proximal humerus in children, the use of biological techniques in well-selected patients is being carried out more often now than before, as is reflected in this series, with a potentially improved functional outcome.

Level of Evidence.—Level III—Retrospective comparative study.

▶ This is a large series from a very experienced group in Italy. Sarcoma of the proximal humerus in children is a rare occurrence. The authors have shared their extensive experience with 61 children with primary sarcoma in the proximal humerus. A variety of reconstructive techniques ranging from amputation to nonbiologic and biologic reconstructions were seen. Patients' survival and functional outcome have consistently improved over the years. Although there are many different ways to reconstruct the skeletal defects following resection, we are gradually evolving toward biologic reconstructions whenever possible. Age of the patient, the presence or absence of metastatic disease, and the status of the rotator cuff determine the reconstructive options.

C. P. Beauchamp, MD

Is Humeral Segmental Defect Replacement Device A Stronger Construct than Locked IM Nailing?

Heck R, Marinescu R, Janda H, et al (InMotion Musculoskeletal Inst, Memphis, TN)
Clin Orthop Relat Res 468:252-258, 2010

Intramedullary (IM) nailing is currently the most common method for treating patients with impending pathologic humeral fractures; however, this treatment is associated with known complications primarily owing to violation of the rotator cuff during insertion. A better option is needed. To determine if a humeral segmental replacement prosthesis would provide a stronger construct compared with an IM nail in this setting, we compared the mechanical properties of these two devices in a cadaver model simulating an impending pathologic fracture. In each of nine matched pairs of fresh human humeri one was randomly selected to undergo a 50% lateral middiaphyseal defect simulating an impending pathologic fracture and subsequent fixation with an IM nail and bone cement. The contralateral humerus underwent fixation using a humeral segmental defect prosthesis. We determined T-scores using DEXA. Each specimen subsequently was tested in torsion to failure. Peak torque and peak rotation at failure were greater for the prosthesis specimens whereas torsional stiffness was greater for the IM nail specimens. We found a linear relationship between peak torque and T-score for each device with the slopes of the lines suggesting the construct with the prosthesis can withstand greater forces than the IM nail and the differences between devices were greater in weaker bones.

▶ Metastatic bone disease involving the humerus is a common condition. There are various different ways of managing impending pathologic fractures. The usual debate is between intramedullary and plate fixation. In situations where there is a large segmental defect, plate fixation, unless the defect is small and shortening of the limb and intramedullary fixation are unattractive choices for stability, is difficult to obtain. In this situation, an intercalary prosthesis is the best choice. This study evaluates the strength of an intramedullary nail under fairly good conditions compared with a segmental reconstruction. It shows the superiority of an intercalary prosthesis. There is a limit to the use of this device, however; lesions close to either end of the humerus ultimately obtain inferior fixation with an intercalary reconstruction because the stems are short. Our preference is plate fixation and cementation whenever possible and intercalary prosthetic reconstructions for diaphyseal segmental defects. We rarely use intramedullary devices.

C. P. Beauchamp, MD

Femoral diaphyseal endoprosthetic reconstruction after segmental resection of primary bone tumours
Hanna SA, Sewell MD, Aston WJS, et al (Royal Natl Orthopaedic Hosp, Stanmore, England)
J Bone Joint Surg [Br] 92-B:867-874, 2010

Segmental resection of malignant bone disease in the femoral diaphysis with subsequent limb reconstruction is a major undertaking. This is a retrospective review of 23 patients who had undergone limb salvage by endoprosthetic replacement of the femoral diaphysis for a primary bone tumour between 1989 and 2005.

There were 16 males and seven females, with a mean age of 41.3 years (10 to 68). The mean overall follow-up was for 97 months (3 to 240), and 120 months (42 to 240) for the living patients. The cumulative patient survival was 77% (95% confidence interval 63% to 95%) at ten years. Survival of the implant, with failure of the endoprosthesis as an endpoint, was 85% at five years and 68% (95% confidence interval 42% to 92%) at ten years. The revision rate was 22% and the overall rate of re-operation was 26%. Complications included deep infection (4%), breakage of the prosthesis (8%), periprosthetic fracture (4%), aseptic loosening (4%), local recurrence (4%) and metastases (17%). The 16 patients who retained their diaphyseal endoprosthesis had a mean Musculoskeletal Tumour Society score of 87% (67% to 93%). They were all able to comfortably perform most activities of daily living.

Femoral diaphyseal endoprosthetic replacement is a viable option for reconstruction following segmental resection of malignant bone disease. It allows immediate weight-bearing, is associated with a good long-term functional outcome, has an acceptable complication and revision rate and, most importantly, does not appear to compromise patient survival.

▶ Intercalary defects of the femur can be reconstructed in a variety of ways. Most commonly, an allograft with or without a vascularized fibula is used. When successful and healed without infection, the results are excellent. In fact, the best results of allograft reconstructions are seen with intercalary defect reconstructions. Intercalary endoprosthetic reconstruction has some appeal in its technical ease and immediate return of function. This large series from a large tumor center reports results similar to allograft reconstructions but with different complications and reasons for revision surgery. One of the problems with intercalary devices is when the tumor resection extends into the metaphysis of the femur. This makes fixation difficult, as the stems have to be short. Some of the technical concerns regarding this implant could be addressed with compressive osseointegration technology.

C. P. Beauchamp, MD

Joint-sparing or Physeal-sparing Diaphyseal Resections: The Challenge of Holding Small Fragments
Agarwal M, Puri A, Gulia A, et al (Tata Memorial Centre, Mumbai, India)
Clin Orthop Relat Res 468:2924-2932, 2010

Background.—Joint-sparing or physeal-sparing diaphyseal resections are technically challenging when only a small length of bone is available for implant purchase.

Questions/Purposes.—We describe a series of cases with the aim of generating some guidelines as to the choice of reconstruction method and the implant used.

Methods.—We retrospectively reviewed 25 patients with diaphyseal resections in which the remaining epiphyseal or metaphyseal segment provided 3 cm or less of purchase. Reconstruction was performed with bone (allograft, extracorporeally radiated autograft, or vascularized fibula) in 19 cases or a custom diaphyseal implant (CDI) in six. The implants used for holding the bone construct varied from standard plates to custom plates. The presence of union, function, complications, and disease status at last followup was recorded.

Results.—Sixteen of the 25 patients are disease-free and alive with the original construct at a median followup of 34 months (range, 12–66 months). Implant-related complications such as plate breakage (four) and angulation (three) happened more frequently when weak plates such as reconstruction plates were used. Local recurrence with pulmonary metastases occurred in two cases. The two deep infections required an amputation or rotationplasty for control. Custom plates were successful in three of four patients.

Conclusions.—Weak plates such as reconstruction plates are best avoided for these reconstructions. Custom plates allow secure fixation with technical ease. CDIs allow immediate weightbearing and ability to lengthen with predictable good functional short-term outcome.

▶ The best results of limb-sparing reconstructions are seen with those patients who have undergone an intercalary resection and reconstruction. The extremes of intercalary resections result in very short lengths of bone available for fixation. This is particularly an issue in patients with open epiphyses. Obtaining fixation in this group of patients can be very difficult. The authors share their experience with a variety of different devices and describe the use of a custom implant. Many of these reconstructions exceed the limits of conventional fixation plates. Further work is needed in this area to provide a device that provides predictable, durable long-term fixation.

C. P. Beauchamp, MD

Late Complications and Survival of Endoprosthetic Reconstruction after Resection of Bone Tumors
Shehadeh A, Noveau J, Malawer M, et al (Washington Cancer Inst at Washington Hosp Ctr, DC)
Clin Orthop Relat Res 468:2885-2895, 2010

Background.—While complications following massive endoprosthetic reconstruction have been previously described, the incidence and effects of these complications over extended periods of time have not been well characterized in large series.

Questions/Purposes.—We therefore determined: (1) incidence and types of complications; (2) relative risk of complications; (3) likelihood of secondary complications; (4) whether modularity altered such complications; (5) implant failure and limb salvage rates and (6) implant survival over extended followup.

Methods.—We retrospectively reviewed 232 patients (241 implants: 50 custom, 191 modular) who underwent endoprosthetic reconstruction for malignant and aggressive bone tumors between 1980 and 2002. Complications were classified as infection, mechanical, superficial soft tissue, deep soft tissue, or dislocation. Survival was determined by Kaplan-Meier analysis. Minimum followup was 5 years (mean: 10 years; range: 5–27 years).

Results.—One hundred thirty-seven of 232 patients (59%) underwent a single reconstruction. Ninety-five patients had 242 additional procedures. Forty-four revised patients retained their original prosthesis. Limb salvage rate was 90%; implant failure (removal of the cemented part) was seen in 29% (70/241) with a median survival of 190 months. Twenty-five of 50 custom implants failed (8 then failed again) while 30/180 modular implants failed (7 then failed again). Of 70 instances of implant failure, 38/70 were mechanical, 27/70 infectious. Risk of infection increased 30% after a second procedure; 16 of 24 amputations were performed because of infection.

Conclusions.—Mechanical complications were the most common cause of implant failure. Infection was the leading cause of both complication and amputation; risk of infection increased substantially with revision surgery. Modular implants had fewer mechanical complications, thus leading to fewer revisions and subsequent infections.

▶ This is a large series of patients from an oncology group with extensive experience using endoprosthetic reconstructions for musculoskeletal tumor defects. Endoprosthetic reconstruction has become the method of choice for tumor reconstruction. More and more patients are surviving their malignancy, resulting in more patients returning with complications related to their reconstruction. Most of these patients are seen by their original orthopedic oncologist. Subsequent corrective surgery is now becoming an expanding problem. Complex revision surgery is challenging, and many orthopedic oncologists do not have experience with revision arthroplasty. Most of the mechanical problems, broken axles, worn bushings, etc, are quite straightforward to revise. Revision of a loose long-stem cemented femur is far more difficult. Revision of this type of problem may benefit from the assistance of a revision arthroplasty surgeon.

We need to continue to work toward implants that are more durable than our current devices. Permanent durable fixation to the patient and parts that are resistant to breakage are the necessary requirements of the endoprosthesis of the future. Work is currently going on in methods and techniques to reduce the incidence of infection. Avoidance of complications is the only way to ensure long-term survival of endoprosthetic reconstruction.

C. P. Beauchamp, MD

Extraarticular Knee Resection for Sarcomas with Preservation of the Extensor Mechanism: Surgical Technique and Review of Cases
Zwolak P, Kühnel SP, Fuchs B (Univ of Zurich, Switzerland)
Clin Orthop Relat Res 469:251-256, 2011

Background.—Sarcomas in or contaminating the knee are rare but extremely challenging to treat. Complete resection of the joint is necessary, and often the entire extensor mechanism is removed as well. Reconstruction of the knee is challenging, and the resulting function may be compromised.

Description of Technique.—We describe a surgical technique of extraarticular resection of the knee while preserving the extensor mechanism combined with prosthetic reconstruction. The medial and lateral retinaculum is prepared such that it allows extraarticular placement of K-wires that are driven through the patella and the proximal tibia, serving as in situ guides for the osteotomies.

Patients and Methods.—We retrospectively reviewed 11 patients with sarcomas contaminating the knee. The minimum followup was 14 months (mean, 38 months; range, 14–80 months).

Results.—At last followup patients had a mean flexion of 88° (range, 65°–120°). We observed no complications related to the extensor mechanism, and there was one local recurrence.

Conclusions.—We believe extraarticular resection of the knee with preservation of the extensor mechanism is a reasonable treatment option for intraarticular sarcomas with functional scores comparable to those for patients having intraarticular resections.

Level of Evidence.—Level IV, therapeutic study. See the Guidelines for Authors for a complete description of levels of evidence.

▶ I chose this article because this comes up yearly. I follow with interest the results of patients treated with reconstructions involving a radiated autologous tissue. Reconstruction of defects of the proximal tibia can be challenging in their many options. The defect can be reconstructed with an endoprosthesis, osteoarticular allograft, an allograft prosthetic composite, some form of amputation, or using the resected tissue biologically, modified either with heat or radiation. In the review seen, the resected specimen has a number of advantages. The graft-host junction is perfect, and the graft size is ideal in all the soft tissues present. In situations in which allograft tissue is not available, the radiated resected host bone solves a number of problems. While I have not used this type of reconstruction, it is something I consider especially in situations in which it is technically difficult to fit an allograft accurately.

C. P. Beauchamp, MD

Tumor Treatment

Disparity in limb-salvage surgery among sarcoma patients
Downing S, Ahuja N, Oyetunji TA, et al (Howard Univ College of Medicine, Washington, DC; Johns Hopkins Univ School of Medicine, Baltimore, MD)
Am J Surg 199:549-553, 2010

Background.—Recent studies have shown that aggressive preoperative radiation increases the likelihood of limb salvage in sarcoma patients.

Method.—The Surveillance, Epidemiology and End Results database was used to run an adjusted logistic regression for the receipt of cancer-directed treatment modalities.

Results.—Of patients with specific surgical procedures recorded (n = 2,104), 86.0% had undergone a limb-sparing procedure. On bivariate analysis, African American patients were less likely to receive a limb-sparing procedure than white patients (80.4% vs 86.9%; $P = .02$). On multivariate analysis, African Americans were significantly more likely to receive preoperative radiation (odds ratio [OR], 2.31; 95% confidence interval [CI], 1.22–4.40; $P = .011$), yet this did not translate into an increase in limb salvage (OR, .67; 95% CI, .42–1.08; $P = .10$). Limb salvage significantly increased for all groups in 2001 and after (OR, 2.75; 95% CI, 1.55–4.88; $P = .001$) without a decrease in survival. For those with tumors greater than 4 cm, there was a trend away from limb salvage for African Americans (OR, .59; 95% CI, .32–1.07; $P = .08$).

Conclusions.—Our results of an increase in limb-salvage surgeries after 2001 without a decrease in survival support previous studies. The trend away from limb salvage for African Americans cannot be answered by this study.

▶ The Surveillance, Epidemiology, and End Results database contains information on the incidence, prevalence, and survival of cancer from 17 geographic regions in the United States. These data are collected retrospectively. This database is a powerful source of information on a wide variety of cancers. The authors reviewed data from the years 1973 to 2003. The data review was done during a period when sarcoma care in extremities was evolving. With this in mind and the fact that it was a retrospective review, it is difficult to make definitive conclusions regarding this group of patients. The authors noted African American patients and patients with more extensive disease had a worse survival rate. Excessive emphasis was placed on the role of radiation therapy in this study. The group of diseases encompassed by this review included entities that would not include radiation therapy as a component of their care. This article emphasizes the important role of databases in our understanding of disease processes and the effect our treatment has on them.

C. P. Beauchamp, MD

Factors Predicting Local Recurrence, Metastasis, and Survival in Pediatric Soft Tissue Sarcoma in Extremities
Sawamura C, Springfield DS, Marcus KJ, et al (Harvard School of Public Health, Boston, MA; Massachusetts General Hosp, Boston; Children's Hosp, Boston, MA)
Clin Orthop Relat Res 468:3019-3027, 2010

Background.—Pediatric soft tissue sarcomas are rare and differ from those in adults regarding the spectrum of diagnoses and treatment. Sarcomas in extremities may have different prognoses from those located elsewhere.

Questions/Purposes.—We sought risk factors predicting local recurrence, metastasis, and overall survival and asked whether radiation and chemotherapy influenced local recurrence, metastasis, and overall survival.

Methods.—We retrospectively reviewed all 98 patients aged 18 years or younger diagnosed with soft tissue sarcomas in extremities from 1990 to 2008. Age, tumor size, depth, location, bone or neurovascular involvement, histologic subtypes, unplanned excision, surgical margins, metastasis at diagnosis, and adjuvant treatments were reviewed for each patient. We determined the effect of each prognostic variable on local recurrence, metastasis, and overall survival.

Results.—Ninety-four patients underwent surgical excision and seven patients had local recurrence at a median time of 18.6 months. Radiation therapy reduced the rate of local recurrence. Fourteen patients had metastasis at diagnosis and seven patients later developed metastasis. The median time to metastasis was 20.9 months. Six patients died and the median time to death was 28.0 months. Metastasis at diagnosis was a predictive factor for death.

Conclusions.—When limited to extremities, radiation therapy reduced the rate of local recurrence in pediatric soft tissue sarcomas. Metastases at diagnosis predict death.

▶ Soft tissue sarcomas are rare in children. The authors have accumulated a large group of patients in this series. They had an astonishing nearly 50% rate of unplanned excisions. Surprisingly, this did not have an effect on tumor behavior. This population of patients has been shown to benefit from radiation therapy. Radiation therapy can be challenging to apply in children because of growth issues, but the authors have confirmed its benefit. Newer, more precise radiotherapy offers promise in extending its application to this age group.

C. P. Beauchamp, MD

Clinical and Treatment Outcomes of Planned and Unplanned Excisions of Soft Tissue Sarcomas
Arai E, Nishida Y, Tsukushi S, et al (Nagoya Univ Graduate School and School of Medicine, Japan)
Clin Orthop Relat Res 468:3028-3034, 2010

Background.—Soft tissue sarcomas are often inappropriately excised without adequate preoperative planning. Inappropriate (unplanned) excisions may adversely affect local recurrence, distant metastasis, patient survival, and /or postoperative function once properly evaluated.

Questions/Purposes.—We asked whether the clinical and treatment characteristics, survival (overall, local recurrence-free, distant metastasis-free), and functional scores of patients with unplanned excisions differ from those with a planned excision.

Methods.—We retrospectively reviewed 128 patients with planned excisions and 63 patients with unplanned excisions at prereferral hospitals followed by additional reexcisions. We determined whether age, gender, tumor size, depth, histologic grade, operative duration, blood loss, survival, or functional scores differed between the two groups. The minimum followup was 6 months (mean, 55 months; range, 6−275 months).

Results.—The tumor was larger and its location deeper in the planned excision group. Overall, metastasis-free, and local recurrence-free survival were similar in the two groups: 86%, 71%, and 85% in the planned excision group and 96%, 86%, and 92% in the unplanned excision group, respectively. However, additional soft tissue reconstruction was more often necessary for patients with unplanned excisions. No difference in postoperative function was observed.

Conclusions.—The data suggest an adequate additional wide excision may improve the local control and survival in patients with an unplanned excision as well as the patients with a planned excision. While patients with unplanned excisions had superficial and smaller tumors, survival and postoperative function were similar to those with planned excisions.

▶ Managing the patient with a poorly planned excision of a soft tissue sarcoma continues to be a problem encountered by all orthopedic oncologists. This problem will never go away. It is reassuring, though, to see that when this problem is dealt by further more extensive surgery, local control can be achieved with satisfactory results. These patients unfortunately require more extensive surgery than was originally required. The real challenge is the patient who underwent a shell-out procedure of a large deep soft tissue sarcoma. The patient unfortunately continued to present to the orthopedic oncologist for management. Only with continued education can we help reduce the number of patients we encounter with this problem. But as I have stated, this problem is not going to go away.

C. P. Beauchamp, MD

Double Ray Amputation for Tumors of the Hand
Puhaindran ME, Athanasian EA (Memorial Sloan-Kettering Cancer Ctr (Affiliated with Weill Med College of Cornell Univ), NY)
Clin Orthop Relat Res 468:2976-2979, 2010

Background.—Partial hand amputations for malignant tumors allow tumor resection with negative resection margins, which is associated with lower local recurrence rates and improved overall survival while preserving native tissue, which improves functional outcome.

Questions/Purposes.—We conducted this study to assess the functional outcome of double ray amputations of the hand.

Methods.—We retrospectively reviewed the records of five patients who underwent double ray amputations at our center over 12 years: four amputations of the fourth and fifth rays and one amputation of the second and third rays. Mean age at surgery was 34 years (range, 10—45 years), and minimum followup was 64 months (mean, 98 months; range, 64—136 months). All five patients had high-grade soft tissue sarcomas of the hand, two synovial sarcomas, two malignant peripheral nerve sheath tumors, and one undifferentiated sarcoma. No patients had detectable metastases at surgery.

Results.—Four of the five patients were completely disease-free at latest followup. One patient was alive with lung metastases detected 32 months after surgery. No patients developed local tumor recurrence. Functional assessment showed a mean Musculoskeletal Tumor Society score of 24 (range, 19—28) and mean grip strength 24% of the contralateral side (range, 17%—35%).

Conclusions.—Although double ray amputation results in worse functional outcome than single ray, good key, tip, and tripod pinch can be preserved when the deep motor branch of the ulnar nerve is preserved, and this hand can still assist in bimanual hand activities. Our observations suggest double ray amputation is an acceptable hand-preserving procedure.

▶ The management of patients with sarcomas of the hand can be difficult. It is common for patients to have unintentional poorly planned surgical intervention prior to the diagnosis of a sarcoma. Limb salvage surgery under these circumstances can be difficult or impossible without an amputation. Wide excision without some form of partial hand amputation is usually not possible. Resections involving more than 1 ray can still result in acceptable hand function. It is important to emphasize that sarcomas of the hand and foot continue to be a source of misadventure with partial marginal surgery. Obtaining a diagnosis with a biopsy prior to surgical intervention needs to be continually emphasized.

C. P. Beauchamp, MD

Chondrosarcoma of Bone: Lessons From 46 Operated Cases in a Single Institution
de Camargo OP, Baptista AM, Atanásio MJ, et al (Univ of São Paulo, Brazil; Univ of São Paulo Med School, Brazil)
Clin Orthop Relat Res 468:2969-2975, 2010

Background.—Bone chondrosarcomas are rare malignant tumors that have variable biologic behavior, and their treatment is controversial. For low-grade tumors, there is no consensus on whether intralesional en bloc resections are the best treatment.

Questions/Purposes.—We therefore compared patients with Grade 1 and Grade 2 primary central chondrosarcomas to (1) determine difference in survival and (2) local recurrence rates; and (3) determine any association of histological grade with some clinical and demographic characteristics.

Methods.—We retrospectively reviewed 46 patients with grade 1 and 2 chondrosarcomas. There were 25 men and 21 women with a mean age of 43 years (range, 17—79 years). Minimum followup was 32 months (mean, 99 months; range, 32—312 months) for the patients who remained alive in the end of the study. Twenty-three of the tumors were intracompartmental (Enneking A); of these, 19 were Grade 1 and 4 were Grade 2. Twenty-three tumors were extracompartmental (Enneking B); of these, 4 were Grade 1 and 19 were Grade 2. Twenty-five patients underwent intralesional resection, 18 had wide resection, and three had amputations.

Results.—The overall survival rate was 94% and the disease-free survival rate was 90%. Among the 23 Grade 1 tumors, we observed six local recurrences and none of these patients died; among the 23 Grade 2 tumors, 10 recurred and two patients died. Local recurrence negatively influenced survival.

Conclusions.—For lesions with radiographic characteristics of intra-compartmental Grade 1 chondrosarcoma, we believe intralesional resection followed by electrocauterization and cement is the best treatment. When the imaging suggests aggressive (Grade 2 or 3) chondrosarcoma, then wide resection is promptly indicated.

▶ I chose this article because it reaffirms the safety of intralesional resection of grade 1 chondrosarcomas. The authors note that it is sometimes difficult to differentiate between an enchondroma and a low-grade chondrosarcoma. The indication for surgery in such a situation was progression of the radiographic appearance of the lesion. Their results are similar to those of other authors who have reported success in treating low-grade chondrosarcomas with intralesional curettage and adjuvant agents.

C. P. Beauchamp, MD

Cemented Distal Femoral Endoprostheses for Musculoskeletal Tumor: Improved Survival of Modular versus Custom Implants
Schwartz AJ, Kabo JM, Eilber FC, et al (Univ of California Los Angeles Med Ctr, Santa Monica; California State Univ, Northridge)
Clin Orthop Relat Res 468:2198-2210, 2010

Background.—Advocates of newer implant designs cite high rates of aseptic loosening and failure as reasons to abandon traditional cemented endoprosthetic reconstruction of the distal femur.

Questions/Purposes.—We asked whether newer, modular distal femoral components had improved survivorship compared with older, custom-casted designs.

Patients and Methods.—We retrospectively reviewed 254 patients who underwent distal femoral endoprosthetic reconstruction. We excluded two patients with cementless implants, 27 with expandable prostheses, and 39 who had a nontumor diagnosis. This left 186 patients: 101 with older custom implants and 85 with contemporary modular implants. The minimum followup was 1 month (mean, 96.0 months; range, 1–336 months). The tumor was classified as Stage IIA/IIB in 122 patients, Stage IA/IB or benign in 43, and Stage III or metastatic in 21.

Results.—Kaplan-Meier analysis revealed overall 10-, 20-, and 25-year implant survival rates of 77%, 58%, and 50%, respectively, using revision of the stemmed components as an end point. The 85 modular components had a greater 15-year survivorship than the 101 custom-designed implants: 93.7% versus 51.7%, respectively. Thirty-five stemmed components (18.8%) were revised for aseptic loosening in 22 patients, implant fatigue fracture in 10, infection in two, and local recurrence in one.

Conclusions.—Cemented modular rotating-hinge distal femoral endoprostheses demonstrated improved survivorship compared with custom-casted implants during this three-decade experience. Patients with low-grade disease and long-term survivors of high-grade localized disease should expect at least one or more revision procedures in their lifetime.

Level of Evidence.—Level IV, therapeutic study. See the Guidelines for Authors for a complete description of levels of evidence.

▶ This is a very large series reflecting the lifetime experience of a pioneer in musculoskeletal oncology. Many of the great advances in endoprosthetic reconstructions can be attributed to the work of Dr Jeffrey Eckardt. One of our greatest challenges, as patients are surviving their life-threatening malignancies, is how we are going to improve the durability of nonbiologic tumor implants. It is encouraging to see the benefits of improved technology as it is applied to cemented femoral fixation. But we have an ever-growing population of young active adults with endoprosthetic reconstructions, and we are going to see an increasing population of patients' failed implants. We need to not only provide even slightly better initial fixation but also predictable and durable methods of revision surgery.

C. P. Beauchamp, MD

MFH of Bone and Osteosarcoma Show Similar Survival and Chemosensitivity
Jeon D-G, Song WS, Kong C-B, et al (Korea Cancer Ctr Hosp, Nowon-gu, Seoul; et al)
Clin Orthop Relat Res 469:584-590, 2011

Background.—Patients with malignant fibrous histiocytoma of bone (MFH-B) and osteosarcoma reportedly have comparable survival rates, despite the lesser chemosensitivity of patients with MFH-B compared with those with osteosarcoma.

Questions/Purposes.—We therefore asked (1) whether there is a difference in the initial tumor volume, histologic response, and survival between cohorts with MFH-B and osteosarcoma, and (2) whether histologic responses and survival rates differed between two groups even after matching for volume and age.

Patients and Methods.—We retrospectively compared 27 patients with Stage IIB MFH-B with 389 patients with localized osteosarcoma for initial tumor volume, age, histologic response, and survival. We compared histologic response and survival between 27 patients with MFH-B and 54 patients with osteosarcoma matched for tumor volume and age.

Results.—MFH-B occurred more frequently in older patients and they presented with a smaller mean tumor volume and more frequent osteolytic pattern when compared with patients with osteosarcoma. The 5-year metastasis-free survival rates of the MFH-B and osteosarcoma groups were similar: 61.2% ± 9.7% and 61.3% ± 2.5%, respectively. We observed similar proportions of good responders to chemotherapy in the two groups, and the 5-year metastasis-free survival rates were 61.2% ± 9.7% and 70.4% ± 6.2%, respectively.

Conclusions.—Patients with MFH-B and osteosarcoma have similar survival rates and histologic responses to chemotherapy. Although MFH-B and osteosarcoma differ in clinical presentation, their response pattern to contemporary therapy is similar.

Level of Evidence.—Level III, prognostic study. See the Guidelines for Authors for a complete description of levels of evidence.

▶ This is a well-designed study. Patients with malignant fibrous histiocytoma (MFH) of bone were matched with those with osteosarcoma of bone. Volume and age were used to match the patient groups. Both groups had similar histological responses, and the 5-year metastasis-free survival rates were similar. While there was a slight advantage to osteosarcoma, this was not significant. We have been treating MFH of bone in the same manner as osteosarcoma for years. This article adds support for this treatment protocol. It is encouraging to see that survival rates in older patients can come close to younger patients, as it is more challenging to administer chemotherapy in older populations.

C. P. Beauchamp, MD

Does Increased Rate of Limb-sparing Surgery Affect Survival in Osteosarcoma?
Ayerza MA, Farfalli GL, Aponte-Tinao L, et al (Italian Hosp of Buenos Aires, Potosí, Argentina)
Clin Orthop Relat Res 468:2854-2859, 2010

Background.—The emergence of limb salvage surgery as an option for patients with osteosarcoma is attributable to preoperative chemotherapy and advancements in musculoskeletal imaging and surgical technique. While the indications for limb salvage have greatly expanded it is unclear whether limb salvage affects overall survival.

Questions/Purposes.—We asked whether over the past three decades limb-sparing procedures in high-grade osteosarcoma had increased, and whether this affected survival and ultimate amputation.

Methods.—We retrospectively reviewed 251 patients with high-grade osteosarcoma treated from 1980 to 2004 with a multidisciplinary approach, including neoadjuvant chemotherapy. We compared survival rates, limb-salvage treatment, and amputation after limb-sparing procedure during three different periods of time. Fifty-three patients were treated from 1980 to 1989, 97 from 1990 to 1999, and 101 from 2000 to 2004. Thirty-seven patients were treated with primary amputations and 214 with primary limb salvage.

Results.—The 5-year survival rate in the first period was 36%, whereas in the 1990s, it was 60% and 67% from 2000–2004. Limb salvage surgery rate in the 1980s was 53% (28 of 53), whereas in the 1990s, it was 91% (88 of 97) and 97% from 2000–2004 (98 of 101). In the limb salvage group, 22 of the 214 patients (10%) required secondary amputation; the final limb salvage rate in the first period was 36% (19 of 53), whereas in the 1990s, it was 81% (79 of 97) and 93% from 2000–2004 (94 of 101).

Conclusions.—Patients with osteosarcoma treated in the last two periods had higher rates of limb salvage treatment and survival, with lower secondary amputation.

▶ These results are reported by a very experienced oncologic group. We have been debating and continuously evaluating this topic for the last 30 years. We have all been concerned that in our zeal to perform limb-sparing surgery, we would adversely affect survival. Thus far, we have not seen an adverse consequence of limb-sparing surgery in terms of survival or local recurrence. The authors' tremendous experience confirms this, and today it is almost universal that patients with osteosarcoma can be offered limb-sparing surgery with safety.

C. P. Beauchamp, MD

Curettage and Graft Alleviates Athletic-Limiting Pain in Benign Lytic Bone Lesions

Moretti VM, Slotcavage RL, Crawford EA, et al (Univ of Pennsylvania, Philadelphia; et al)
Clin Orthop Relat Res 469:283-288, 2011

Background.—Solitary bone cysts (SBC), nonossifying fibromas (NOF), and fibrous dysplasia (FD) create benign intramedullary lytic bone lesions. They are typically asymptomatic and treated conservatively. We present a series of lesions that caused performance-limiting pain in young athletes, a symptom phenomenon and possible treatment indication that has been poorly described in the literature.

Questions/Purposes.—We asked whether intralesional curettage and defect grafting of these lesions would alleviate pain in young athletes and permit their return to unrestricted athletic activities.

Patients and Methods.—We retrospectively identified 29 patients (30 lesions) who underwent curettage and grafting for SBC (12 patients), NOF (nine), or FD (eight). All patients had pain predominantly with athletic involvement. The mean age of the patients was 18 years (range, 12—31 years). Tumor locations were the femur (eight lesions), humerus (seven), tibia (six), fibula (five), pubic ramus (two), ulna (one), and calcaneus (one). Signs/symptoms were pain alone (24 patients) and pain plus fracture (five). Surgery involved curettage and packing with allograft cancellous chips, bone substitute, or demineralized bone matrix. Two patients required internal fixation. The mean followup was 21 months (range, 2—114 months).

Results.—Twenty-four patients had no pain and five had occasional mild pain at last followup. All patients resumed full activity at a mean of 3.3 months (range, 1.5—8.3 months), excluding two who required repeat surgery.

Conclusions.—Our observations suggest curettage and packing with bone graft/substitute can provide pain relief and allow full athletic recovery for young athletes with benign lytic bone lesions.

Level of Evidence.—Level IV, therapeutic study. See Guidelines for Authors for a complete description of levels of evidence.

▶ There are many benign bone tumors that are often found incidentally. Solitary bone cysts, fibrous dysplasia, and nonossifying fibromas are some of the more common lesions seen in adolescents and young adults. These lesions often require no surgical intervention. The authors share their experience with young high-level athletes who presented with symptomatic benign bone lesions. These lesions would normally be asymptomatic in less-active individuals. All patients underwent curettage and bone grafting. Surgical management of these lesions enabled the patients to return to their former level of activity.

C. P. Beauchamp, MD

Endoscopic Surgery for Young Athletes With Symptomatic Unicameral Bone Cyst of the Calcaneus
Innami K, Takao M, Miyamoto W, et al (Teikyo Univ School of Medicine, Tokyo, Japan; et al)
Am J Sports Med 39:575-581, 2011

Background.—Open curettage with bone graft has been the traditional surgical treatment for symptomatic unicameral calcaneal bone cyst. Endoscopic procedures have recently provided less invasive techniques with shorter postoperative morbidity.

Hypothesis.—The authors' endoscopic procedure is effective for young athletes with symptomatic calcaneal bone cyst.

Study Design.—Case series; Level of evidence, 4.

Methods.—Of 16 young athletes with symptomatic calcaneal bone cyst, 13 underwent endoscopic curettage and percutaneous injection of bone substitute under the new method. Three patients were excluded because of short-term follow-up, less than 24 months. For the remaining 10 patients, with a mean preoperative 3-dimensional size of 23 × 31 × 35 mm as calculated by computed tomography, clinical evaluation was made with the American Orthopaedic Foot and Ankle Society Ankle-Hindfoot Scale just before surgery and at the most recent follow-up (mean, 36.2 months; range, 24-51 months), and radiologic assessment was performed at the most recent follow-up, to discover any recurrence or pathologic fracture. Furthermore, the 10 patients—all of whom returned to sports activities—were asked how long it took to return to initial sports activity level after surgery.

Results.—Mean ankle-hindfoot scale score improved from preoperative 78.7 ± 4.7 points (range, 74-87) to postoperative 98.0 ± 4.2 points (range, 90-100) ($P < .001$). Pain and functional scores significantly improved after surgery ($P < .01$ and $P < .05$, respectively). Radiologic assessment at most recent follow-up revealed no recurrence or pathologic fracture, with retention of injected calcium phosphate cement in all cases. All patients could return to their initial levels of sports activities within 8 weeks after surgery (mean period, 7.1 weeks; range, 4-8 weeks), which was quite early as compared with past reports.

Conclusion.—Endoscopic curettage and injection of bone substitute appears to be an excellent option for young athletes with symptomatic calcaneal bone cyst for early return to sports activities, because it has the possibility to minimize the risk of postoperative pathologic fracture and local recurrence after early return to initial level of sports activities.

▶ This is a technique that I use whenever possible. Unicameral bone cyst is particularly well suited to endoscopic examination. The use of a scope allowed for complete examination of the entire cavity. Septations are easily identified, assisting in the complete obliteration of the cyst with bone graft material. The portal is small, resulting in minimal patient morbidity. This is really a surgical technique article. This technique is very helpful for the management of unicameral bone cyst.

C. P. Beauchamp, MD

Curettage and Cryosurgery for Low-grade Cartilage Tumors Is Associated with Low Recurrence and High Function
Mohler DG, Chiu R, McCall DA, et al (Stanford Univ Med Ctr, CA)
Clin Orthop Relat Res 468:2765-2773, 2010

Background.—Chondrosarcomas of bone traditionally have been treated by wide or radical excision, procedures that may result in considerable lifelong disability. Grade 1 chondrosarcomas have little or no metastatic potential and are often difficult to distinguish from painful benign enchondromas. Curettage with adjuvant cryosurgery has been proposed as an alternative therapy for Grade 1 chondrosarcomas given the generally better function after the procedure. However, because it is an intralesional procedure, curettage and cryosurgery may be associated with higher rates of recurrence.

Questions/Purposes.—We asked whether Grade 1 chondrosarcomas and enchondromas of uncertain malignant potential treated by curettage and cryosurgery are associated with low recurrence rates and high functional scores.

Patients and Methods.—We retrospectively reviewed the records of 46 patients with Grade 1 chondrosarcomas and enchondromas of uncertain malignant potential treated by curettage and cryosurgery. Forty-one patients had tumors of the long bones. Patients were followed a minimum of 18 months (average, 47.2 months; range, 18—134 months) for evidence of recurrence and for assessment of Musculoskeletal Tumor Society (MSTS) functional score.

Results.—Two of the 46 patients had recurrences in the original tumor site (4.3% recurrence rate), which subsequently were removed by wide excision, and both patients were confirmed to be disease-free 36 and 30 months, respectively, after the second surgery. The mean MSTS score was 27.2 of 30 points (median, 29 points).

Conclusions.—Our observations show curettage with cryosurgery is associated with low recurrence of Grade 1 chondrosarcoma and high functional scores. Curettage with cryosurgery is a reasonable alternative to wide or radical excision as the treatment for Grade 1 chondrosarcomas, and allows for more radical surgery in the event of local recurrence.

Level of Evidence.—Level IV, therapeutic study. See the Guidelines for Authors for a complete description of levels of evidence (Table 3).

▶ For the past few years, I have chosen articles reporting the results of treatment with intralesional curettage for grade 1 chondrosarcoma. Each oncologic group has consistently reported good results with this approach. Careful patient selection is important in ensuring a low risk of local recurrence. As always, in this group of patients there may be included patients with benign lesions. It is difficult to truly distinguish enchondromas from grade 1 chondrosarcomas in some cases. Careful patient selection, meticulous attention to detail, and

TABLE 3.—Summary of Studies of Intralesional Resections of Grade 1 Chondrosarcomas and Enchondromas

Study	Date of Publication	Treatment	Tumor Site	Sample Size (Number of Patients)	Followup (Months)	Recurrence (Number/%)	MSTS
Current study	–	Cu, Cr, Ce	47L, 2P, 2D, 1Sa	52	40 (13–134)	2 (3.8%)	27.2
Souna et al. [30]	2010	Cu, Cr	15L	15	96 (60–132)	0 (0.0%)	27.9
Donati et al. [6]	2010	Cu, Ph/Ce, Bg	15L	15	145 (81–251)	2 (13.3%)	27
Hanna et al. [14]	2009	Cu, Ce	39L	39	61 (36–104)	2 (5.1%)	28.2
Okada et al. [24]	2009	Cu, Pa, Bg	2L	2	132*	0 (0.0%)	–
Aarons et al. [1]	2009	Cu, Ca, Ph/Cr/Ce	17L	17	56 (29–130)	1 (5.9%)	29.5
van der Geest et al. [31]	2008	Cu, Cr, Ce/Bg	–	123	60 (24–119)	2 (1.6%)	28
Leerapun et al. [17]	2007	Cu, Ph, Ce/Bg	13L	13	102 (2–274)	1 (7.7%)	–
Normand et al.[23]	2007	Cu, Ce/Bg	5P	5	69 (14–142)	2 (40%)	–
Ahlmann et al. [3]	2006	Cu, Cr, Ce	7L, 2S, 1P	10	39 (24–60)	0 (0.0%)	27
Etchebehere et al. [10]	2005	Cu, Ca, Ce	11L	11	52 (24–108)	0 (0.0%)	–
Kollender et al. [16]	2003	Cu, Cr, Ce	1Sa	1	120	0 (0.0%)	–
Schreuder et al. [27]	1998	Cu, Cr, Bg	17L, 6D	23	26 (15–40)	0 (0.0%)	29
Ozaki et al. [25]	1996	Cu	1L, 1P, 1D	3	45 (24–70)	3 (100%)	–
Bauer et al. [4]	1995	Cu, Ce/Bg	45L, 1D	46	77 (36–156)	3 (6.5%)	–
Aboulafia et al. [2]	1994	Cu, Cr, Ce	1L	1	52	0 (0.0%)	30
Eriksson et al. [9]	1980	Cu, Bg	1L†	2	17†	1 (50%)	–
Marcove et al. [21]	1977	Cu, Cr	4I, 2S, 1P	7	78 (59–104)	0 (0.0%)	–

All cases involve Grade 1 chondrosarcomas or enchondromas only.
MSTS = Musculoskeletal Tumor Society mean functional score (out of 30); Cu = curettage; Cr = cryosurgery; Ce = cementation; Bg = bone graft; Ph = phenolization; Ca = cauterization; Pa = pasteurization; L = long bone; P = pelvis; D = distal (hand, feet); S = scapula; Sa = sacrum.
Editor's Note: Please refer to original journal article for full references.
*Both subjects had the same followup time.
†Information given for recurrent case only, nonrecurrent case is not described;

a restoration of bone strength will avoid complications and reduce the risk of local recurrence.

C. P. Beauchamp, MD

Is Sclerotherapy Better than Intralesional Excision for Treating Aneurysmal Bone Cysts?
Varshney MK, Rastogi S, Khan SA, et al (Lady Harding Med College and Associated Hosps, New Delhi, India; All India Inst of Med Sciences, New Delhi, India)
Clin Orthop Relat Res 468:1649-1659, 2010

Background.—Minimally invasive approaches such as sclerotherapy have been introduced to treat aneurysmal bone cysts. Sclerotherapy has been associated with reasonable healing rates during the past two decades. However, it is unclear whether sclerotherapy compares with the more traditional extended curettage and bone grafting.

Questions/Purposes.—We therefore compared the healing rates and functional scores in patients having percutaneous repetitive sclerotherapy using polidocanol (Group 1) with those with intralesional excision (extended curettage with a high-speed burr) and bone grafting (Group 2) for treatment of aneurysmal bone cyst.

Patients and Methods.—We randomly divided 94 patients into two treatment groups. We assessed healing rates (primary outcome measure), pain relief, time to healing and recurrence, hospital stay, and the Enneking functional score. Forty-five patients from Group 1 and 46 from Group 2 were available for study. The minimum followup was 3.2 years (mean, 4.4 years; range, 3.2—6.1 years).

Results.—At last followup, 93.3% in Group 1 and 84.8% in Group 2 had achieved healing. Complications in Group 1 were minor and resolved. In Group 2, three patients had deep infections and five had superficial infections, and two had growth disturbances. Although the healing rates were similar, we found higher rates of clinically important complications, worse functional outcomes, and higher hospital burden associated with intralesional excision.

Conclusions.—Repetitive sclerotherapy using polidocanol is a minimally invasive, safer method of treatment for aneurysmal bone cysts compared with intralesional excision and bone grafting. In this preliminary study, we found similar recurrence rates for the two treatment methods, however, this will require confirmation in larger studies.

Level of Evidence.—Level II, therapeutic study. See Guidelines for Authors for a complete description of levels of evidence.

▶ Treating aneurysmal bone cysts can be challenging. The ease of treatment is often determined by their location. Standard conventional management usually involves intralesional curettage and bone grafting or cementation. Nonsurgical options are often sought for treatment of lesions in difficult anatomic sites.

Sclerotherapy was introduced as a form of treatment in the 1990s. Ethibloc is the most commonly used agent and has success rates as high as 92%. Polidocanol is a popular agent used in the treatment of various vascular malformations. This well-designed study randomized patients between conventional surgery and sclerotherapy using polidocanol. This preliminary study demonstrated safety and efficacy for the use of sclerotherapy. Consideration should be given to this technique and the agent for the selective management of aneurysmal bone cysts in challenging locations. Other treatment methods, including repetitive embolization, could perhaps complement this noninvasive treatment method.

C. P. Beauchamp, MD

Giant Cell Tumor of Bone: Risk Factors for Recurrence
Klenke FM, Wenger DE, Inwards CY, et al (Mayo Clinic, Rochester, MN)
Clin Orthop Relat Res 469:591-599, 2011

Background.—Many surgeons treat giant cell tumor of bone (GCT) with intralesional curettage. Wide resection is reserved for extensive bone destruction where joint preservation is impossible or when expendable sites (eg, fibular head) are affected. Adjuvants such as polymethylmethacrylate and phenol have been recommended to reduce the risk of local recurrence after intralesional surgery. However, the best treatment of these tumors and risk factors for recurrence remain controversial.

Questions/Purposes.—We evaluated the recurrence-free survival after surgical treatment of GCT to determine the influence of the surgical approach, adjuvant treatment, local tumor presentation, and demographic factors on the risk of recurrence.

Methods.—We retrospectively reviewed 118 patients treated for benign GCT of bone between 1985 and 2005. Recurrence rates, risk factors for recurrence and the development of pulmonary metastases were determined. The minimum followup was 36 months (mean, 108.4 ± 43.7; range, 36–233 months).

Results.—Wide resection had a lower recurrence rate than intralesional surgery (5% versus 25%). Application of polymethylmethacrylate decreased the risk of local recurrence after intralesional surgery compared with bone grafting; phenol application alone had no effect on the risk of recurrence. Pulmonary metastases occurred in 4%; multidisciplinary treatment including wedge resection, chemotherapy, and radiotherapy achieved disease-free survival or stable disease in all of these patients.

Conclusion.—We recommend intralesional surgery with polymethylmethacrylate for the majority of primary GCTs. Because pulmonary metastases are rare and aggressive treatment of pulmonary metastases is usually successful, we believe the potential for metastases should not by itself create an indication for wide resection of primary tumors.

TABLE 3.—Kaplan-Meier Survival Analysis of Recurrence-Free Survival 10 Years After Surgery

Surgical Treatment	Recurrence-Free Survival	Standard Error	Mean Recurrence-Free Survival (Months)	95% Confidence Interval	p (Versus Wide Resection)	P (Versus PMMA + Phenol)
Wide resection	0.955	0.051	116	109–123	–	–
Intralesional surgery	0.747	0.045	93	84–103	0.036	–
PMMA + phenol	0.854	0.056	105	93–116	0.209	–
Bone grafting + phenol	0.656	0.084	83	66–101	0.009	0.044
No adjuvants (bone grafting)	0.682	0.099	87	67–107	0.018	0.107

*Level of Evidence.—*Level III, therapeutic study. See Guidelines for Authors for a complete description of levels of evidence (Table 3).

▶ Most will agree that intralesional curettage is the preferred method of treatment of giant cell tumors of the bone. Most will also agree that the preferred method of reconstruction is with polymethylmethacrylate. For years, adjuvant agents such as phenol have been advocated for use to reduce the risk of local recurrence. Other agents such as alcohol, hydrogen peroxide, or liquid nitrogen have been added to the cavity to assist in local tumor treatment. Whether or not these agents truly reduce the risk of local recurrence is not known. This article highlights the fact that young age is a risk factor for local recurrence. The continued use of phenol is not supported by this study. In my practice, I use 100% ethanol as an adjuvant agent; it is similar to use, probably safer than phenol, but I have no data to support its efficacy.

C. P. Beauchamp, MD

12 Spine

Introduction

Welcome to the 2011 YEAR BOOK OF ORTHOPEDICS chapter on the spine. I believe this year's selections offer an accurate reflection of the most controversial and educational articles recently available. I am hopeful they will challenge and augment your experience and elicit a strong response from our readers.

The major areas reviewed include spinal infection, practice management, degenerative and traumatic conditions, bone morphogenic protein, biomechanics, and minimally invasive surgery. Two very well-done reviews on the respective state of the art of minimally invasive surgery (MIS) and lumbar interspinous spacers will bring practitioners up to date. The latest and most insightful articles in the area of specific minimally invasive techniques and methods are reviewed, with additional papers dedicated to MIS economics, clinical trials comparing fusion rate, and clinical outcomes for head-to-head MIS versus standard techniques for lumbar spinal stenosis. Trends and complications with the use of bone morphogenic protein are included along with several articles concerning diagnosing spine implant infection and one eye-opening publication concerning its proposed treatment. The ever-important issue of adjacent segment disease is covered as well as provocative discussion on the effects of patient and physician preferences on regional variations in spine surgery. A nice companion article to the MIS studies concerns the accuracy of intraoperative imaging on pedicle screw placement, and several reports are included in the area of spinal trauma practice, outcomes measurements, thromboembolic disease, and infection prevention and treatment. A soon-to-be-classic article concerning the treatment of adult degenerative scoliosis is included, which I believe will be enjoyed by all. Also included is a discussion of the biomechanical characteristics of various lumbosacral instrumentation and fusion techniques.

I sincerely hope these reviews will enhance and augment your practice going forward this next year, and I wish you the very best!

Paul M. Huddleston III, MD

313

The Economics of Minimally Invasive Spine Surgery: The Value Perspective

Allen RT, Garfin SR (Univ of California San Diego Med Ctr)
Spine 35:S375-S382, 2010

Study Design.—Review of the literature.

Objective.—To summarize current cost and clinical efficacy data in minimally invasive spine (MIS) surgery.

Summary of Background Data.—Cost effectiveness (CE), using cost per quality-adjusted life-years gained, has been shown for lumbar discectomy, decompressive laminectomy, and for instrumented and noninstrumented lumbar fusions in several high-quality studies using conventional, open surgical procedures. Currently, comparisons of costs and clinical outcomes of MIS surgery to open (or nonoperative) approaches are rare and of lesser quality, but suggest that a potential for cost benefits exists using less-invasive surgical approaches.

Methods.—A literature review was performed using the database of the National Center for Biotechnology Information (NCBI), PUBMED/Medline.

Results.—Reports of clinical results of MIS approaches are far more common than economic evaluations. MIS techniques can be classified as endoscopic or nonendoscopic. Although endoscopic approaches decrease some approach morbidities, the high cost of instrumentation, steep learning curves, and new complication profiles introduced have prevented widespread adoption. Additionally, the high costs have not been shown to be justified by superior clinical benefits. Nonendoscopic MIS approaches, such as percutaneous posterior or lateral, and mini-open lateral and anterior approaches, use direct visualization, standard operative techniques, and report lower complication rates, reduced length of stay, and faster recovery time. For newer MIS and mini-open techniques, significantly lower acute and subacute costs were observed compared with open techniques, mainly due to lower rates of complications, shorter length of stay, and less blood loss, as well as fewer discharges to rehab. Although this suggests that certain MIS procedures produce early cost benefits, the quality of the existing data are low.

Conclusion.—Although the CE of MIS surgery is yet to be carefully studied, the few economic studies that do exist suggest that MIS has the potential to be a cost-effective intervention, but only if improved clinical outcomes are maintained (durable). Longer follow-up and better outcome and cost data are needed to determine if incremental CE exists with MIS techniques, *versus* open or nonsurgical interventions.

▶ This article brings together 2 of the most controversial topics in orthopedics, the implementation of value as an outcomes measure in health care and the idea of minimally invasive surgery as an alternative to traditional surgical approaches. This review from the University of California San Diego Medical Center is an excellent review of the current literature-based justification for minimally invasive spine (MIS) surgery with a balanced assessment of both the pros and cons. One of the most important points of the article is the concept of value in spine care. Most clinicians are not fluent in discussions of quality-adjusted life-years (QALYs) and why this might be significant. For example, a procedure performed in an MIS fashion might appear to be cheaper or more cost-effective in the short-term perspective of a hospital stay but may trail in comparison to more traditional open procedures and techniques as its benefits to the patient and society fail to prove durable over time. The authors correctly suggest that the important issues for advocates of MIS surgery to prove will be differences in infection rate, approach- and surgery-related complications, and a more rapid return to work and productivity. The point of returning to productivity can't be underestimated, as most of the costs in any calculation of QALYs in spine surgery will be dwarfed by the society costs of a patient not being at work. The calculations will then likely support the use of traditionally open techniques for patients who are retired and/or not previously employed unless rather dramatic differences can be shown in other factors with MIS techniques.

P. M. Huddleston III, MD

Trends in the Use of Bone Morphogenetic Protein as a Substitute to Autologous Iliac Crest Bone Grafting for Spinal Fusion Procedures in the United States

Lad SP, Nathan JK, Boakye M (Stanford Univ School of Medicine, CA)
Spine 36:E274-E281, 2011

Study Design.—Analysis of Nationwide Inpatient Sample (NIS) database for data related to spinal fusion procedures.

Objective.—To identify trends in the use of bone morphogenetic protein (BMP) *versus* iliac crest bone grafts in various spinal fusion procedures performed in the United States, explore stratification by patient demographics, and analyze the impact on treatment cost.

Summary of Background Data.—BMP has been shown to achieve better clinical outcomes in anterior lumbar interbody fusions procedures, which led to its Food and Drug Administration approval for this indication in 2002. Since then, significant off-label use has occurred, without a full description of the results.

Methods.—We searched the NIS for data relating to BMP administration or iliac crest bone grafting in a variety of spinal fusion procedures performed from 1993 to 2006, based on *International Classification of Diseases, Ninth Revision classification.* The NIS is the largest all-payer inpatient care database, with demographic, outcome, and cost data from approximately eight million annual patient discharges throughout the United States. Demographics among patients treated with BMP *versus* iliac crest bone graft were compared to reduce the likelihood of bias in the analysis.

Results.—BMP became applied more frequently in each type of spinal fusion procedure examined over our study period, with the exception of anterior lumbar interbody fusions. Patients receiving iliac crest bone grafts versus BMP exhibited very similar demographic characteristics, including age, socioeconomic status, and type of health care setting. Although BMP typically increased the cost of the procedure itself, it improved outcomes and shorter hospital stays often provided a net benefit.

Conclusion.—BMP is increasingly being used in spinal fusion procedures, including ones for which it is not officially approved, because of the surgical and postsurgical benefits it provides. Given the morbidity that this may entail, monitoring outcomes trends will help to inform guidelines for BMP use and ensure that its benefits continue to outweigh its costs.

▶ With continuing unanswered questions concerning the appropriate use of INFUSE (recombinant human bone morphogenetic protein-2), the authors from Stanford University School of Medicine have performed an impressive and even-handed review of the drug in the United States. Though limited by its use of a large administrative database, it probably underestimates the significance of the use of INFUSE with regard to off-label use. The paucity of non—industry-supported research into this implant critically limits the usefulness of available studies. Several elegant cost-effectiveness studies have attempted to justify the use of INFUSE by demonstrating the benefits of equivalent fusion rates with potentially shorter hospital stays and lower patient morbidity secondary to the avoidance of autologous iliac crest bone grafting.[1] I strongly support the authors' suggestion that the data be used to generate a healthy discourse on the appropriate utilization of this powerful drug to benefit both patients and society. This article should be a must read for all surgeons struggling with either the cost or safety profile of INFUSE when used in a physician-directed application.

P. M. Huddleston III, MD

Reference

1. Polly DW Jr, Ackerman SJ, Shaffrey CI, et al. A cost analysis of bone morphogenetic protein versus autogenous iliac crest bone graft in single-level anterior lumbar fusion. *Orthopedics.* 2003;26:1027-1037.

Quantifying the variability of financial disclosure information reported by authors presenting at annual spine conferences

Ju BL, Miller CP, Whang PG, et al (Yale Univ School of Medicine, New Haven, CT)

Spine J 11:1-8, 2011

Background Context.—In recent years, greater attention has been directed toward determining how potential financial conflicts of interest may affect the integrity of biomedical research. To address this issue, various disclosure policies have been adopted in an attempt to increase the transparency of this process. However, the consistency of such reporting among spine surgeons remains unknown. This study quantifies the variability in the self-reported disclosures of individual authors presenting at multiple spine conferences during the same year.

Methods.—The author disclosure information published for the 2008 North American Spine Society (NASS), Cervical Spine Research Society (CSRS), and Scoliosis Research Society (SRS), conferences were compiled into a database. We evaluated the disclosure policy for each society and compared the disclosure listings of authors who presented at more than one of these meetings.

Results.—Disclosure records were available for 1,231 authors at NASS, 550 at CSRS, and 642 at SRS. Of these individuals, 278 (NASS), 129 (CSRS), and 181 (SRS) presented at one of the other conferences and 40 presented at all three conferences. North American Spine Society and CSRS required disclosure of all financial relationships, whereas SRS only requested disclosures pertinent to authors' presentations. Of the 153 authors who presented at the NASS and CSRS meetings, 51% exhibited discrepancies in their disclosure information. In contrast, only 9% of the 205 individuals whose data was listed at both the NASS and SRS conferences demonstrated irregularities. Similarly, 18% of the 56 authors who had provided information to both CSRS and SRS were inconsistent in their reporting.

Conclusions.—These findings emphasize the significant variability that currently exists in the reporting of financial conflicts of interest by authors who presented at three major spine conferences within the past year. We believe these discrepancies are likely because of confusion regarding what relationships should be acknowledged in certain situations and the clear lack of uniformity among the disclosure policies established by these various associations.

Clinical Relevance.—This study evaluates financial conflicts of interests in clinical research (Fig 4).

▶ This article was chosen to illustrate the importance of financial disclosure and how the current reporting policies of 3 widely attended societies compare. In short, the current report in the authors' words, "one of every two authors (51%) ... exhibited contradictory information in the final programs with nearly half of them (44%) having three or more discrepancies" (Fig 4). This editor would say that you get the results the system was designed to deliver, and the current systems of the major spine societies are different enough from each other to cause a consistent widespread confusion among the reporting authors. I believe that this reporting is important and should be standardized across all the societies so that it is consistent. Additionally, I believe that it would convey more meaningful information to the audiences in journals, presentations, and meetings if the dollar amount of conflict was displayed too. Is it possible that a hypothetical audience for a presentation on the potential surgical outcomes gained by using INFUSE (recombinant human bone morphogenetic protein-2) might view the results of the study differently if

Discrepancies in disclosure reporting for authors who attended both SRS and CSRS

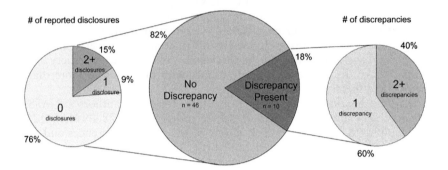

Percentage of common SRS/CSRS authors who disclosed something at SRS vs. nothing at CSRS

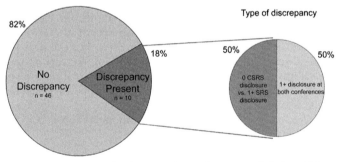

FIGURE 4.—(Top) Proportion of authors attending Scoliosis Research Society (SRS) and Cervical Spine Research Society (CSRS) who were noted to have discrepancies between their project-specific disclosures at SRS and their global disclosures at CSRS, including the number of discrepancies exhibited by individuals with inconsistencies and the number of industry relationships reported by those without any discrepancies. (Bottom) Proportion of authors attending SRS and CSRS with documented discrepancies identified no disclosures at CSRS but declared at least one conflict of interest at SRS. (Reprinted from Ju BL, Miller CP, Whang PG, et al. Quantifying the variability of financial disclosure information reported by authors presenting at annual spine conferences. *Spine J.* 2011;11:1-8, Copyright 2011, with permission from Elsevier.)

they were informed on the first slide of the presentation and the meeting handouts that the major authors had no industry conflicts to disclose versus receiving more than $1 million as consulting fees by the manufacturer of the product during that calendar year? I think so. As the funding for research from government sources becomes harder to obtain, this issue of disclosure may be the single most important question facing any clinician analyzing any published scientific endeavor.

P. M. Huddleston III, MD

Who's in the Driver's Seat? The Influence of Patient and Physician Enthusiasm on Regional Variation in Degenerative Lumbar Spinal Surgery: A Population-Based Study
Bederman SS, Coyte PC, Kreder HJ, et al (Univ of California at Irvine, Orange; Univ of Toronto, Ontario, Canada)
Spine 36:481-489, 2011

Study Design.—Cross-sectional population-based study using administrative databases, census data, and surveys of orthopedic/neurosurgeons, family physicians (FPs) and patients in Ontario, Canada.

Objective.—To determine the influence of the enthusiasm of patients, FPs, and surgeons for surgery on the regional variation in surgical rates for degenerative diseases of the lumbar spine (DDLS), such as spinal stenosis and degenerative spondylolisthesis.

Summary of Background Data.—Rates of surgery and healthcare costs for treating DDLS have been increasing. Regional variation in spinal surgical rates has been observed and it is thought that the enthusiasm of patients and physicians for surgery contributes to this variation.

Methods.—Using population-based administrative databases, we included all patients aged 50 years and older who underwent DDLS surgery (*i.e.*, decompression/laminectomy, fusion) from 2002 to 2006 and calculated standardized utilization rates across counties. We measured regional "enthusiasm for surgery" for surgeons, FPs, and patients, using responses from a province-wide survey. Small-area variation analysis and multivariate Poisson regression models were performed calculating incidence rate ratios (IRRs) controlling for county demographics, socioeconomic measures, prevalence of disease, and community resources.

Results.—We identified 10,318 DDLS surgeries (mean age 65 years, 50.6% female). Significant regional variation was observed (extremal quotient 5.0, coefficient of variation 28.0). Counties with higher rates of surgery had higher surgeon enthusiasm for surgery (IRR: 1.26, $P < 0.013$), older (IRR: 2.17, $P < 0.0001$) male patients (IRR: 1.19, $P < 0.0001$), lower income (IRR: 0.89, $P < 0.0015$), more knowledge of official languages (IRR: 1.12, $P < 0.0003$), and the presence of magnetic resonance imaging scanners (IRR: 1.30, $P < 0.004$). FP and patient enthusiasm for surgery, physician supply, and prevalence of disease were not statistically associated with higher surgical rates.

Conclusion.—Prior studies have not addressed the role of patient enthusiasm for surgery. Although patients and FPs had variable enthusiasm for surgery, surgeon enthusiasm was the dominant potentially modifiable factor influencing surgical rates. Prevalence of disease and community resources were not related to surgical rates. Strategies targeting surgeon practices may reduce regional variation in care and improve access disparities.

▶ With the costs associated with care of degenerative spine conditions skyrocketing, clinicians can be certain that there will be more frequent studies like this report from Ontario, Canada. Similar to Weinstein et al,[1] the authors demonstrate large variations in spine surgical rates. In this study, the most significant factor in the variation in spine surgery rates is the surgeon's enthusiasm for surgical treatment of degenerative disease of the lumbar spine. This might not seem surprising to most; many surgeons I know believe that surgery is their job. I would suggest a more patient-centric role and offer a word of caution from the cardiac surgeons about the perils of becoming mere technicians in a patient's care. As the adjutant of the most expensive and invasive treatments of these degenerative conditions, the surgeon should be an orthopedist first, the musculoskeletal expert in all the surgical, procedural, and nonoperative management for the axial and appendicular skeleton. This does not mean that as orthopedists, we should be antisurgery. As the authors also comment, "strategies to understand why surgeons have variable 'enthusiasm' for surgery, despite high-quality evidence for its effectiveness with specific indications (ie, spinal stenosis and degenerative spondylolisthesis) are needed." Many patients who could benefit from procedural intervention are not currently being offered the treatments. We should strive as a profession to deliver the right surgery to the right patient with the right condition or the payers will begin to dictate that for us.

P. M. Huddleston III, MD

Reference

1. Weinstein JN, Lurie JD, Olson PR, Bronner KK, Fisher ES. United States' trends and regional variations in lumbar spine surgery: 1992-2003. *Spine (Phila Pa 1976)*. 2006;31:2707-2714.

Surgical Outcomes of Decompression, Decompression with Limited Fusion, and Decompression With Full Curve Fusion for Degenerative Scoliosis With Radiculopathy
Transfeldt EE, Topp R, Mehbod AA, et al (Twin Cities Spine Ctr, Minneapolis, MN)
Spine 35:1872-1875, 2010

Study Design.—A retrospective clinical cohort study at a single spine center of patients with degenerative scoliosis and radiculopathy severe enough to require surgery.

Objective.—To evaluate the functional outcomes of 3 surgeries for degenerative scoliosis with radiculopathy; decompression alone, decompression and limited fusion, and decompression and full curve fusion.

Summary of Background Data.—Although these 3 surgical treatments have all been described for this problem, there exists little information as to what outcomes to expect.

Methods.—The study cohort consisted of 85 patients who met the inclusion criteria of degenerative scoliosis and radiculopathy, who had undergone 1 of the above 3 surgeries, who had not had any previous lumbar spine surgery, who had a minimum follow-up of at least 2 years, and who had filled out preoperative and postoperative functional evaluation forms including SF-36, Oswestry Disability Index, Roland Morris Scores, and a satisfaction questionnaire. Logistic regression analysis was conducted to predict the likelihood of success as related to decompression alone of rotatory olisthetic segments, extent of fusion, and postoperative sagittal balance. Patient demographics including curve magnitude, operative blood loss, length of hospital stay, complications, and need for revision surgeries were analyzed. The patients having decompression alone had the highest mean age (76.4 years) compared to decompression and limited fusion (70.4), and decompression and full curve fusion (62.5).

Results.—Cobb scoliosis angles remained unchanged in the 2 groups not having full curve fusion, while the full curve fusion group changed from a mean 39° before surgery to 19° at follow-up. The complication rate was highest (56%) in the full fusion group, was 40% in the limited fusion group, and 10% in the decompression alone group. The overall SF-36 analysis showed significant improvement in bodily pain, social function, role emotional, mental health, and mental composite domains. Oswestry Disability Indexes improved significantly in the decompression alone and limited fusion groups, but not in the full fusion group. In contrast, the satisfaction questionnaire showed the highest success to be in the full-curve fusion group and the lowest in the decompression-only group.

Regression analysis revealed that sacrum to curve apex fusions and positive postoperative sagittal imbalance were associated with poor outcomes.

Conclusion.—Both good and poor results were seen with each of the 3 procedures.

▶ This very interesting article from the Twin Cities Spine Center tries to answer, in a retrospective fashion, the question of "how much surgery is too much?" The clinical question is one that I see every week: an elderly female with a degenerative scoliosis and back and leg pain is referred for surgical consultation for chronic unrelenting back and leg pain. In the clinicians' mind, the choice of a decompressive operation may address the leg pain but not stabilize the spine to prevent progression of the curve or stabilize an iatrogenic instability. The choice of a long fusion, according to the rules of King and Moe, may, indeed, be too much surgery with an unacceptable complication rate.[1] Many surgeons have tried to compromise with a combination of decompression and fusion over a limited number of motion segments. Transfeldt and colleagues have described their experience with all 3 of these interventions in a retrospective review of 85 patients collected over 6 years. Their findings suggest that patients reported improved outcomes of Oswestry Disability Index (ODI) in the decompression and decompression and limited fusion groups and poor outcomes in the long fusion group. Interestingly, patient satisfaction scores were still positive in the long fusion group, with 75% of patients saying their surgery was a success at 2-year follow-up. In the end, the decompression alone group had the lowest blood loss, fewest complications, and need for further surgery. It may be that in this case, the demonstration of their superior postoperative function, in comparison to the other groups, outweighs whatever peculiarities the patient satisfaction scores might produce.

P. M. Huddleston III, MD

Reference

1. King HA, Moe JH, Bradford DS, Winter RB. The selection of fusion levels in thoracic idiopathic scoliosis. *J Bone Joint Surg Am*. 1983;65:1302-1313.

The Current State of Minimally Invasive Spine Surgery

Kim CW, Siemionow K, Anderson DG, et al (Spine Inst of San Diego, CA; Rush Univ Med Ctr, Chicago, IL; Thomas Jefferson Univ, Philadelphia, PA)
J Bone Joint Surg Am 93:582-596, 2011

The posterior spine is dynamically stabilized by a diverse group of muscles that lie in close proximity to the vertebrae and possess multiple tendon insertion sites. In humans, stability and motion are controlled by active and passive means. The multifidus muscle is a powerful spine stabilizer as it has short and powerful fibers that enable it to produce large forces over short distances. Traditional posterior midline open approaches disrupt the function of this muscle through tendon detachment, devascularization, and crush injury. Minimally invasive spine surgery techniques were developed in an attempt to minimize surgical damage and preserve normal function. The rationale of this approach relies on limiting the surgical corridor to the minimum necessary to safely expose the surgical target site and to minimize injury to the anatomic structures necessary for normal function. The traditional use of self-retaining retractors, which can induce crush injuries to muscle, has been supplanted by table-mounted, tubular-type retractors that minimize pressure on muscles, vessels, and nerves. As minimally invasive spine surgery continues to evolve, it is important to properly evaluate the risks and benefits of various minimally invasive techniques with prospective, long-term clinical studies.

▶ While minimally invasive surgery (MIS) may have its limitations, this editor must say that there have been few developments in spine surgery over the last 10 years that have been game changers. One would be the advances in imaging, and the second the development and refinement of minimally invasive techniques. It could be said that there could not have been one without the other. I think in their modern context, they complement each other and hopefully, in the right hands, improve patient care.

This article of the American Academy of Orthopaedic Surgeons *Instructional Course Lectures* is a state-of-the-art review of the techniques and pitfalls of MIS by some of the current top advocates in the field. The figures are excellent in illustrating some of the angles and approaches so critical to this philosophy and well worth reviewing. It will be up to the evangelists in this area to continue to prove that the new procedures deliver the same or equivalent clinical results at a similar cost over time.

P. M. Huddleston III, MD

Lumbar Decompression Using a Traditional Midline Approach *Versus* **a Tubular Retractor System: Comparison of Patient-Based Clinical Outcomes**
Anderson DG, Patel A, Maltenfort M, et al (Thomas Jefferson Univ, Philadelphia, PA)
Spine 36:E320-E325, 2011

Study Design.—Retrospective analysis of matched cohorts undergoing surgery for unilateral lumbar radiculopathy using either a traditional midline or tubular retractor approach.

Objective.—To document the clinical outcome after lumbar decompression for unilateral radiculopathy, using validated, patient-based outcome measures.

Summary of Background Data.—Minimal objective data are available comparing the patient-based clinical outcomes between lumbar decompressive procedures utilizing traditional midline or tubular retractor approaches.

Methods.—A retrospective analysis was performed for two matched cohorts of patients undergoing decompressive surgery for unilateral lumbar radiculopathy: one group using a tubular retractor approach and a second group with a traditional midline approach. Demographic and surgical data were collected for each group. All patients completed preoperative and postoperative Oswestry Disability Index, Short Form-12, and visual analog scale measures of back and leg pain. The cohorts were compared to determine whether there were any differences in patient-based clinical outcomes.

Results.—At a mean follow-up of 20.2 and 24.7 months, respectively, the tubular retractor and traditional midline approach groups both achieved significant improvements in physical component scores (Short Form-12), Oswestry Disability Index, and visual analog scale for both back and leg pain compared with their preoperative statuses. Mental component scores (Short Form-12) remained largely unchanged in both groups. There were no significant differences in outcome between the surgical approaches with regards to patient-based outcome measures.

Conclusion.—Patients with unilateral radiculopathy achieved equally significant improvements in patient-based clinical outcome measures after decompressive surgery with either a traditional midline or tubular retractor approach. Surgeons should choose the surgical approach for unilateral lumbar radiculopathy on the basis of experience and preference and not on the basis of an expected difference in long-term patient outcome.

▶ While there is a growing body of literature expounding the potential benefits of minimally invasive surgical techniques over standard approaches, the metaphorical war will be won with the results of solid clinical studies. This retrospective review nicely matches 2 cohorts with unilateral lumbar radiculopathy. The authors, not surprisingly, found no difference in the outcomes of the groups at almost 2-year follow-up. I have come to believe this outcome in my practice and have reverted to the old-school treatment of an open decompression with limited unilateral exposure and a microscope-assisted visualization and decompression. All patients are treated as outpatients and close attention is placed on pre- and postoperative pain management, patient teaching, family teaching, and realistic occupational expectations. While this may avoid the additional cost of the many disposables, it won't make the preoperative evaluation and recommendations any easier for the surgeon when the patient demands a minimally invasive surgery because he or she saw the latest advertisement in the airline magazine! I agree with the authors from Thomas Jefferson University that "surgeons should choose the surgical approach for unilateral lumbar radiculopathy on the basis of experience and preference and not on the basis of an expected difference in long-term patient outcome."

P. M. Huddleston III, MD

Minimally Invasive Surgery: Lateral Approach Interbody Fusion: Results and Review
Youssef JA, McAfee PC, Patty CA, et al (Durango Orthopedic Associates, Spine Colorado; St Josephs Hosp, Townson, MD)
Spine 35:S302-S311, 2010

Study Design.—A retrospective review of patients treated at 2 institutions with anterior lumbar interbody fusion using a minimally invasive lateral retroperitoneal approach, and review of literature.

Objective.—To analyze the outcomes from historical literature and from a retrospectively compiled database of patients having undergone anterior interbody fusions performed through a lateral approach.

Summary of Background Data.—A paucity of published literature exists describing outcomes following lateral approach fusion surgery.

Methods.—Patients treated with extreme lateral interbody fusion (XLIF) were identified through retrospective chart review. Treatment variables included operating room (OR) time, estimated blood loss (EBL), length of hospital stay (LOS), complications, and fusion rate. A literature review, using the National Center for Biotechnology Information databases PubMed/MEDLINE and Google Scholar, yielded 14 peer-reviewed articles reporting outcomes scoring, complications, fusion status, long-term follow-up, and radiographic assessments related to XLIF. Published XLIF results were summarized and evaluated with current study data.

Results.—A total of 84 XLIF patients were included in the current cohort analysis. OR time, EBL, and length of hospital stay averaged 199 minutes, 155 mL, and 2.6 days, respectively, and perioperative and postoperative complication rates were 2.4% and 6.1%. Mean follow-up was 15.7 months. Sixty-eight patients showed evidence of solid arthrodesis and no subsidence on computed tomography and flexion/extension radiographs. Results were within the ranges of those in the literature. Literature review identified reports of significant improvements in clinical outcomes scores, radiographic measures, and cost effectiveness.

Conclusion.—Current data corroborates and contributes to the existing body of literature describing XLIF outcomes. Procedures are generally performed with short OR times, minimal EBL, and few complications. Patients recover quickly, requiring minimal hospital stay, although transient hip/thigh pain and/or weakness is common. Long-term outcomes are generally favorable, with maintained improvements in patient-reported pain and function scores as well as radiographic parameters, including high rates of fusion.

▶ A simplistic analysis of a new medical procedure or technique would attempt to demonstrate an equivalency with standard methods. Secondary questions might involve an exploration of similarities or differences in complication rates. More detailed and involved analyses would investigate differences in cost and value to the patient and society. Applying this line of questioning to extreme lateral interbody fusion, the investigators reported an 80% fusion rate at an average follow-up of 15 months. This is far less than reported in studies of transforaminal lumbar interbody fusion (TLIF) or circumferential lumbar fusion. Assuming the arthrodesis rates were similar, an examination in the reported literature of complication rates of direct lateral lumbar interbody fusion would demonstrate a shockingly high rate of serious problems, such as perforated bowel, major blood vessel injury, and peripheral nerve irritation.[1] Assuming the complication rates were similar, the costs of a spinal fusion composed of an extreme lateral interbody fusion procedure for the anterior spine and a posterior instrumentation would almost always be greater than a posterior procedure alone, such as a TLIF. Lastly, assuming the costs were similar, the surgeon who would have otherwise only been compensated in a pay-per-procedure model of reimbursement for a TLIF can now be paid for an anterior procedure; they otherwise would not have performed had they had to split the anterior procedure fee with an access surgeon. An oversimplistic explanation? Maybe. A provocative explanation? Probably. This editor encourages readers to follow this developing procedure closely and make their own decisions.

P. M. Huddleston III, MD

Reference

1. Tormenti MJ, Maserati MB, Bonfield CM, Okonkwo DO, Kanter AS. Complications and radiographic correction in adult scoliosis following combined transpsoas extreme lateral interbody fusion and posterior pedicle screw instrumentation. *Neurosurg Focus.* 2010;28:E7.

Percutaneous Vertebroplasty for Pain Management in Malignant Fractures of the Spine with Epidural Involvement

Saliou G, Kocheida EM, Lehmann P, et al (Hôpital Nord, Amiens, France; Hôpital Raymond Poincaré, Garches, France; et al)
Radiology 254:882-890, 2010

Purpose.—To evaluate the feasibility, efficacy, and safety of percutaneous vertebroplasty (PV) in the treatment of pathologic fractures owing to malignancy with epidural involvement, with or without neurologic symptoms of spinal cord or cauda equina compression.

Materials and Methods.—This study was approved by the local ethics committee; informed consent was obtained from all patients. This retrospective review was performed for 51 consecutive patients with metastatic disease or multiple myeloma treated by means of vertebroplasty, who presented with at least one vertebral lesion with epidural involvement, with or without clinical symptoms of spinal cord or cauda equina compression. All patients with neurologic deficit were terminally ill. A neurologic examination was performed before and after treatment in all patients. All imaging examinations and treatments were reviewed, and χ^2, Mann Whitney, or Fisher exact testing was performed for univariate analysis of variables.

Results.—A total of 74 vertebrae were treated in 51 patients, 22 women and 29 men with a mean age of 62.5 years (range, 28–85 years). Fifteen (29%) patients presented symptoms of complete or incomplete spinal cord or cauda equina compression before vertebroplasty and no further clinical deterioration was observed after treatment. The analgesic efficacy of vertebroplasty was satisfactory for 94% (48 of 51) of patients after 1 day, 86% (31 of 36) patients after 1 month, and 92% (11 of 12) patients after 1 year. One patient with no clinical neurologic deficit before treatment experienced symptoms of cauda equina compression 2 days after vertebroplasty. No other major complication was observed.

Conclusion.—The feasibility, efficacy, and safety of PV were confirmed in patients experiencing pain related to malignant spinal tumors with epidural extension, with a low complication rate. PV should become part of the palliative analgesic treatment for such patients (Fig 1).

▶ As there seems to be more and more discussion regarding the appropriate use of vertebroplasty for osteoporotic patients, I have included this article to illustrate an even edgier indication for what has become a controversial procedure. The authors, in a way, are returning to the roots of the procedure, the treatment

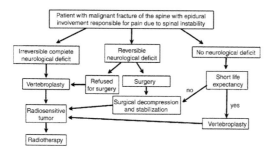

FIGURE 1.—Decision flowchart used to determine treatment. (Reprinted from Saliou G, Kocheida EM, Lehmann P, et al. Percutaneous vertebroplasty for pain management in malignant fractures of the spine with epidural involvement. *Radiology*. 2010;254:882-890. Copyright by the Radiological Society of North America.)

of pathologic lesion of the spinal vertebra that is not related to osteoporosis. In this article, the authors report a series of patients who were not otherwise candidates for standard surgical treatment of lesion in the spine with adjuvant therapy or had maxed out their capability for such treatments and received vertebroplasty for painful pathologic fractures of the spinal column. Many patients had what would otherwise have been seen as an untreatable lesion with epidural involvement or frank pressure on the spinal cord. I believe the value of the study rests in recognizing the humanity and compassion in providing pain relief to a vulnerable patient population for whom the surgeon might not otherwise have any other treatment. The enclosed figure best illustrates the authors' treatment algorithm, and the text details a well-done survival analysis depicting a significant and durable pain relief following the procedure.

P. M. Huddleston III, MD

Minimal Access *Versus* Open Transforaminal Lumbar Interbody Fusion: Meta-Analysis of Fusion Rates

Wu RH, Fraser JF, Härtl R (New York Presbyterian Hosp)
Spine 35:2273-2281, 2010

Study Design.—A quantitative meta-analysis was conducted on published studies reporting fusion rates after open or minimally invasive/mini-open transforaminal lumbar interbody fusion (TLIF) procedures for single or multilevel degenerative disease including stenosis with spondylolisthesis and degenerative disc disease.

Objectives.—The primary aim of this study was to establish benchmark fusion rates for open TLIF and minimally invasive TLIF (mTLIF) based on published studies. A secondary goal was to review complication rates for both approaches.

Summary of Background Data.—Lumbar fusion for the treatment of degenerative disease has evolved from a purely posterior noninstrumented approach to a combination of anterior and/or posterior surgery with instrumentation. The increasingly popular transforaminal approach has advanced to incorporate minimally invasive spinal techniques. There currently exist no controlled comparisons between open TLIF and mTLIF.

Methods.—A Medline search was performed to identify studies reporting fusion rate on open TLIF or mTLIF with instrumentation. A database including patient demographic information, fusion rate, and complication rate was created. Fusion and complication rates were pooled according to whether TLIF was performed with open or minimally invasive technique. Publication bias was assessed with Eggers test, and adjustments were performed using Duval and Tweedie's Trim and Fill algorithm.

Results.—Twenty-three articles were identified that fit inclusion criteria. In each of the 23 studies, TLIF was performed with pedicle fixation and fusion was evaluated using radiograph or computed tomography scan at minimum 6-month follow-up. Overall, the studies included 1028 patients, 46.8% of which were female. The mean age of all patients was 49.7 (range, 38–64.9), and mean follow-up interval for assessment of fusion was 26.6 months (range, 6–46 months). The usage of recombinant bone morphologic protein was higher in the mTLIF group (50% vs. 12%). Mean fusion rate from 16 studies (716 patients) of open TLIF was 90.9%, whereas mean fusion rate from 8 studies (312 patients) of mTLIF was 94.8%. Complication rate was 12.6% and 7.5% for open and mTLIF, respectively.

Conclusion.—Fusion rates for both open and mTLIF are relatively high and in similar ranges. Complication rates are also similar, with a trend toward mTLIF having a lower rate. This analysis provides clear benchmarks for fusion rates in open and mTLIF procedures for spine surgeons.

▶ This publication from Weill Cornell Medical College, New York, attempts to determine if there is a significant published difference in the fusion rates of open transforaminal lumbar interbody fusion (TLIF) versus minimally invasive transforaminal lumbar interbody fusion (mTLIF). On first examination, readers will probably be surprised that the authors of the study found and included only one prospective randomized study researching the difference between fusion rates of TLIF versus mTLIF and rated only that particular study as class III evidence because of methodological flaws. In short, there is very little quality head-to-head evidence justifying mTLIF versus TLIF by any metric, much less specifically examining fusion rates. The results also illuminate the need for strict definitions of what exactly constitutes a TLIF. This editor would suggest that the spectrum of this surgery can be very subtle at the margins, and that failure of the spine surgery community to coalesce around a common nomenclature will be the critical error that will prevent a valid contrast between the procedures. This editor remembers the development and initial marketing of the TLIF as an alternative to a more invasive 360° or circumferential lumbar fusion. In that example, the minimization of morbidity was in the absence of an anterior thoracolumbar retroperitoneal approach. The original technique I learned called for a subtotal discectomy through a unilateral facetectomy. The surgeon saved the facetectomy bone and any bone from a decompressive laminectomy and placed that in the interbody space dorsal to the interbody spacer and compressed the autograft through a pedicle screw/rod construct posteriorly.

The contralateral facet was decorticated, and the tip of the spinous process was removed and impacted into the joint. Any remaining bone was distributed over the decorticated contralateral lamina and the wound closed. Current techniques have de-emphasized the use of autologous or allograft bone and advocated the use of INFUSE (recombinant human bone morphogenetic protein-2) and structural supports composed of polyether ether ketone. I suspect the demonstrable acute postoperative differences between standard and mTLIF techniques may be because of variations in postoperative pain control and hospital dismissal criteria, similar to that demonstrated in 1- versus 2-incision total hip arthroplasty. With increasing governmental influence on procedural reimbursement, I suspect surgeons will begin to feel an unavoidable pressure to demonstrate added value with both TLIF and mTLIF techniques and will need to produce not only compelling evidence of both immediate benefits (decreased blood loss and length of stay and pain), but also, because of the high costs of these interventions when compared with nonoperative management.

P. M. Huddleston III, MD

Adjacent Segment Disease After Interbody Fusion and Pedicle Screw Fixations for Isolated L4–L5 Spondylolisthesis: A Minimum Five-Year Follow-up
Kim KH, Lee S-H, Shim CS, et al (Hyundae General Hosp, Namyangju, Korea; Wooridul Spine Hosp, Seoul, Korea)
Spine 35:625-634, 2010

Study Design.—A retrospective study.

Objective.—The purposes of this study are (1) to analyze prevalence of clinical and radiologic adjacent segment diseases (ASD), (2) to find precipitating factor of clinical ASD in each isthmic and degenerative spondylolisthesis groups, and (3) to compare clinical and radiologic change in isthmic and degenerative spondylolisthesis.

Summary of Background Data.—There is no clinical report regarding the use of magnetic resonance imaging (MRI) for evaluating ASD in patients who underwent 360° fusion with single-level spondylolisthesis with healthy adjacent segment.

Methods.—A total of 69 patients who underwent instrumented single-level interbody fusion at the L4–L5 level and showed no definitive degenerated disc in adjacent segments on preoperative MRI and plain radiographs were evaluated at more than 5 years after surgery. The patients were divided into 2 groups: group I was isthmic spondylolisthesis patients and group II was degenerative spondylolisthesis patients. The radiologic ASD was diagnosed by plain radiographs and MRI. Clinical ASD is defined as symptomatic spinal stenosis, intractable back pain, and subsequent sagittal or coronal imbalance with accompanying radiographic changes. Symptomatic spinal stenosis was defined as stenosis diagnosed by MRI and combined with neurologic claudication.

Results.—The prevalence of radiologic ASD on group I and group II was 72.7% and 84.0%, respectively. About 7 (15.9%) patients showed clinical ASD in group I and 6 (24.0%) patients showed clinical ASD in group II. MRI showed significant reliability for diagnosis of clinical ASD. Compared with patients with asymptomatic ASD, patients with clinical ASD showed significantly less postoperative lordotic angle at the L4–L5 level (i.e., less than 20°) in both groups.

Conclusion.—Maintaining postoperative L4–L5 segmental lordotic angle at about 20° or more is important for prevention of clinical ASD in single-level 360° fusion operation. MRI is reliable method for diagnosing clinical ASD.

▶ This very interesting article from Korea retrospectively reviewed the results of a cohort of individuals who had undergone a one-level lumbar fusion for the diagnosis of degenerative or isthmic spondylolisthesis. Although the study results may not be directly applicable to the cervical or thoracic spine, this research tries to address one of the single most controversial unanswered questions in spine surgery. The authors suggest a provocative answer that the single most important factor is not age or gender but the degree of lordosis the surgeon places the patient in postoperatively at the operated motion segment. Previous studies have acknowledged the deleterious effects of iatrogenically damaging the facet capsules of a cranial motion segment with a pedicle screw or the cervical equivalent of damaging the adjacent cervical disc with a plate or screw. This study would support abandoning the standard transforaminal lumbar interbody fusion (TLIF) procedure if a patient had a very collapsed and kyphotic motion segment, as the surgeon's ability to produce lordosis with the TLIF technique is mild to modest at best. Presented with this scenario choosing the 360° degree fusion technique or an anterior lumbar interbody fusion may be a better option to achieve the 20° of lordosis the authors found protective against adjacent segment diseases at 5-year follow-up.

P. M. Huddleston III, MD

The Effect of Sacral Decortication on Lumbosacral Fixation in a Calf Spine Model
Thomas A, Kepler CK, Meyers K, et al (Hosp for Special Surgery, NY)
Spine 36:E388-E392, 2011

Study Design.—Animal cadaveric biomechanical study.

Objective.—We hypothesized that increasing bony destabilization of a bovine cadaveric sacrum by anterior pedicle screw penetration and bilateral alar decortication would decrease the amount of load necessary for failure of the construct and result in failure through the decortication sites.

Summary of Background Data.—Fusion to the sacrum has become commonly used for treatment of neuromuscular scoliosis and fusions in osteoporotic patients. Fixation failure after attempted fusion to the sacrum may be attributed to iatrogenic causes such as S1 screw penetration and sacral ala decortication.

Methods.—Sixteen fresh-frozen 6- to 8-week-old calf spines were tested after instrumentation with pedicle screws and bilateral rods from L2 to S1 using four constructs: (1) S1 screws with posterior-only purchase; (2) S1 screws with bicortical purchase; (3) S1 screws with bicortical purchase and sacral alar decortication; and (4) S1 screws with bicortical purchase, decortication, and iliac fixation. A destructive flexural bending load was applied at L2 to each construct. Ultimate failure moment (Nm) was compared among the four groups, using a one-way analysis of variance combined with Holm-Sidak *post hoc* test.

Results.—No significant difference in failure moment was found among groups 1, 2, and 3. The addition of iliac fixation (group 4) significantly increased bending load to failure ($P < 0.01$), and iliac screw dislodgement was the dominant mechanism of failure. All specimens in group 3 failed with fractures extending through the decortication site. Groups 1 and 2 specimens failed by fracturing through the S1 body.

Conclusion.—Sacral alar decortication and anterior pedicle screw purchase did not decrease the failure moment in long instrumentation to the sacrum. Pattern of failure was affected, with alar decortication being the site of fracture in each construct in which it was performed. Iliac fixation increased the failure moment under catastrophic loading conditions even when combined with sacral alar decortication and bicortical pedicle screw purchase.

▶ It seems to me that the singular purpose of a spinal fusion surgery, to obtain an arthrodesis, often gets metaphorically lost in all the metal implants and monitoring and focus on exposures or autograft bone alternatives. While every surgeon should remain open to the ideas of innovation and attempt to minimize patient morbidity, the temporary joy for the surgeon and patient with a minimally invasive surgery (MIS) attempt will long be forgotten as they confront the physical and emotional pain of a pseudoarthrosis. The Spanish philosopher George Santayana wrote, "those who cannot remember the past are condemned to repeat it," and orthopedists are not exempt. In my spine surgery practice, I believe I am just beginning to see a large wave of patients with failed fusion attempts. Readers should read this article with interest, as it strongly suggests that, in biomechanical testing, there is no merit to the claim by some MIS surgeons that sacral alar decortication, in the manner necessary to facilitate a successful lumbosacral arthrodesis, will cause a fracture or failure secondary to iatrogenic weakening of the sacrum.

P. M. Huddleston III, MD

Acute airway obstruction associated with the use of bone-morphogenetic protein in cervical spinal fusion

Yaremchuk K, Toma M, Somers M (Henry Ford Health System, Detroit, MI; Wayne State Univ - School of Medicine, Detroit, MI)
Laryngoscope 120:S140, 2010

Objectives.—Bone morphogenetic protein (BMP) used in anterior cervical spinal fusion procedures causes an inflammatory response resulting in upper airway obstruction between postoperative days 4-7. The purpose of this study is to determine the incidence and severity of airway complications associated with use of BMP, the associated clinical outcomes, morbidities and mortalities following its use, and to create a clinical awareness of patients with acute airway obstruction associated with the use of BMP in cervical spinal fusion.

Methods.—This is a retrospective study of 260 patients who underwent cervical spinal fusion procedures with BMP from 2004-2009 and 520 patients, matched on procedure, who underwent cervical spinal fusion procedures without BMP during the same period at a tertiary care center. The two groups were compared on multiple outcome variables: hospital length of stay (LOS), costs, incidence of airway obstruction, unplanned intubations after surgery, tracheotomies, intensive care unit (ICU) admissions, hoarseness, dyspnea, respiratory failure, dysphasia and dysphagia, readmissions, and need for percutaneous endoscopic gastrostomy (PEG) tubes. All outcome variables that were binary in nature were analyzed using linear logistic regression analyses predicting use of BMP. Deaths up to 90 days post surgery were analyzed with a Cox proportional hazards model. Variables significantly related to BMP use were used as covariates in the above analyses.

Results.—Patients that underwent cervical procedures with BMP were noted to have significantly longer hospital stays (7.2 ± 11.1 days vs. 4.3 ± 5.2 days, $p < 0.001$), and greater costs ($129,483 versus $74,974, $p < 0.001$) than the control group (Table 1). Tracheotomies (Odds Ratio = 3.79, p-value = 0.021), unplanned intubations after surgery (2.81, 0.008), dysphagia (8.94, 0.001), dyspnea (2.43, 0.001), and respiratory failure (3.35, 0.001) were all significantly associated with the BMP group (Table 2 & Figure 1). In addition, hospital readmissions (1.96, 0.040), ICU admissions (3.05, 0.001), and 90 day mortality rates (Hazard Ratio = 2.44, p = 0.047) were significantly worse for the BMP group.

Conclusions.—Acute airway obstruction in the postoperative period following cervical spine fusion using BMP is a complication of its use. Due to the degree of obstruction and difficulty with intubation postoperatively, a clinical awareness is necessary to effectively manage these patients. Collaborative efforts between the spine surgeon, anesthesia and the otolaryngologist are required for management of the complications that occur after surgery.

▶ This article reviews the serious and often fatal complications associated with the off-label or physician-directed use of Infuse (recombinant bone morphogenetic protein 2) with anterior cervical spine fusion. Spine surgeons may consider the on-label use of bone morphogenetic protein 2 (BMP-2) to facilitate the fusion or arthrodesis of the lumbar spine. The product has shown to be helpful in the lumbar spine also for the treatment of pseudoarthrosis or in lieu of autologous bone graft when the use of a separate incision is not desirable or possible.[1] Clinically, BMP-2 produces a strong inflammatory response that can lead to radiculitis, wound drainage, and bone formation in the spinal canal. Clinicians have adapted its use to the cervical spine with the reported results of airway management difficulties, dysphagia, dyspnea, and respiratory failure. The authors have described a large cohort study of patients treated with BMP-2 to facilitate cervical fusion that would support restricting the use of BMP-2 in the anterior cervical spine.

P. M. Huddleston III, MD

Reference

1. Wong DA, Kumar A, Jatana S, Ghiselli G, Wong K. Neurologic impairment from ectopic bone in the lumbar canal: a potential complication of off-label PLIF/TLIF use of bone morphogenetic protein-2 (BMP-2). *Spine J.* 2008;8:1011-1018.

Lumbar Interspinous Spacers: A Systematic Review of Clinical and Biomechanical Evidence
Kabir SMR, Gupta SR, Casey ATH (Natl Hosp for Neurology and Neurosurgery, London, UK)
Spine 35:E1499-E1506, 2010

Study Design.—Systematic review.

Objective.—To evaluate the current biomechanical and clinical evidence available on the use and effectiveness of lumbar interspinous devices and to recommend indications for their use.

Summary of Background Data.—Lumbar interspinous spacers (ISPs) have recently become popular as an alternative treatment for lumbar degenerative disease. Several spacers are currently available in the market and there have been various proposed indications. The relevant biomechanical and clinical papers are analyzed.

Methods.—A systematic review of clinical and biomechanical studies was done using the following key words: interspinous implants, interspinous devices, interspinous spacers, dynamic stabilization, X-STOP, Coflex, Wallis, DIAM. The database inclusions were MEDLINE, CINAHL (Cumulative Index to Nursing and Allied Health Literature), and PubMed. The main outcome measure was clinical outcome assessment based on validated patient-related questionnaires. Biomechanical studies were analyzed to evaluate the effects of ISPs on the kinematics of the spine. The methodology of the clinical studies was also analyzed.

Results.—Largest number of studies has been with the X-STOP device. The biomechanical studies with all the devices showed that ISPs have a beneficial effect on the kinematics of the degenerative spine. Apart from 2 randomized controlled trials, the other studies with the X-STOP device were not of high methodologic quality. Nevertheless, analysis of these studies showed that X-STOP may improve outcome when compared to nonoperative treatment in select group of patients aged 50 or over, with radiologically confirmed lumbar canal stenosis and neurogenic claudication, who have improvement of their symptoms in flexion. Studies on the other devices show satisfactory outcome to varying degrees. However, due to small number and poor design of the studies, it is difficult to clearly define indications for their use in lumbar degenerative disease.

Conclusion.—Lumbar ISPs may have a potential beneficial effect in select group of patients with degenerative disease of the lumbar spine. However, further good quality trials are needed to clearly outline the indications for their use.

▶ This comprehensive review by researchers from London, United Kingdom, is a very balanced report of the state of interspinous spacers and their clinical and biomechanical evidence for treatment of lumbar spinal stenosis. The premise for the interspinous device is simple; the extension block of the spacer provides a low morbidity, minimally invasive treatment for patients who might otherwise not be candidates for a more stressful standard spine operation. This editor would ask, "less stressful to whom?" Certainly, most surgeons would not volitionally choose to operate on their patients in the awake state and lateral position. If the most dreaded complication of placing the interspinous spacer occurs, that is, fracture of the spinous process, there is no salvage without aborting the case to reposition, prepare, and drape for a prone general anesthesia. Additionally, it's not clear to me that there is an accepted standard for who is too sick for a standard spine surgery. Aged, obese, and immunocompromised patients routinely undergo complex surgical interventions without pause, so I would suggest that the most important single point going forward to justify these devices' use would be answering the question, "who is truly too sick for general anesthesia?" A second concern would be the cost of the device. I seriously doubt that the current technology will pass the more rigid outcomes standards of showing societal benefit in quality-adjusted life years. Lastly, I have not seen a solution presented that addressed the most common mechanism I see for chronic failure of these devices: subsidence into the osteoporotic adjacent bone.

P. M. Huddleston III, MD

Clinical Accuracy of Computer-Assisted Two-Dimensional Fluoroscopy for the Percutaneous Placement of Lumbosacral Pedicle Screws

Ravi B, Zahrai A, Rampersaud R (Univ of Toronto, Ontario, Canada)
Spine 36:84-91, 2011

Study Design.—Clinical case series.

Objective.—The primary objective of this study was to evaluate the clinical accuracy of computer-assisted two-dimensional fluoroscopy (2D-CAS) for the percutaneous placement of lumbosacral pedicle screws.

Summary of Background Data.—Loss of visual anatomic landmarks and reduced tactile feedback increases the risk of pedicle screw misplacement when using minimally invasive (MIS) percutaneous techniques. However, objective data on screw misplacement in this scenario is lacking.

Methods.—A MIS-2D-CAS technique (FluoroNav) was used for the placement of pedicle screws in 41 consecutive patients undergoing MIS—interbody instrumented fusion. Postoperative computerized tomography (CT) was obtained in all patients at 6 months after surgery and was evaluated by 3 observers. The relative position of the screw to the pedicle was graded regarding pedicle breach (I, no breach; II, <2 mm; III, 2−4 mm; IV, >4 mm), breach direction, vertebral body perforation and screw trajectory. Interobserver reliability of CT grading was assessed with kappa statistics.

Results.—A total of 161 screws were placed. No neurologic, vascular, or visceral injuries occurred. About 37 (23%) screws breached the pedicle. The majority (83.8%, 31/37) of breaches were graded II. There were 5 Grade III and 1 Grade IV breaches. Medial *versus* lateral breaches occurred in 30% (11/37) and 60% (22/37), respectively; 10% (4/37) of the breaches were superior. Overall, 8 (5%) vertebral body breaches occurred.

Of the pedicle screws, 19 (12%) had trajectories that deviated from acceptable, with the majority being medial (16/19, 84%). Fluoroscopy time for screw placement was typically less than 20 seconds total per case. There was 1 clinically significant breach at L5 (III, medial) which resulted in a L5 radiculopathy. Kappa statistics showed excellent overall agreement between reviewers (k = 0.73−0.92; 90%−96% agreement).

Conclusion.—The two-dimensional (2D) virtual fluoroscopy is a clinically acceptable option for percutaneous placement of pedicle screws. However, this technique requires cautious application and is particularly vulnerable to axial trajectory errors.

▶ A continuing commentary on the rapid growth of minimally invasive surgery will always be incomplete without the mention of improved imaging. The authors from the Department of Orthopaedics in Toronto, Ontario, Canada, have confirmed what practitioners in the trade know well: minimally invasive techniques compromise classical visualization of the spinal anatomy and increase the use of fluoroscopy time during a spine instrumentation without guaranteeing a safe placement of all implants. In this particular study, the implants in the series, when misplaced, tended to be so in the axial plane.

Medial breaches of the pedicle were common, and many screw trajectories were deemed unacceptable. While there will be a learning curve for any surgeon on using new techniques, in this instance, I believe that either techniques that use no radiation, such as the electrophysiologic stimulation of the spinal implants in vivo, or newer imaging techniques that specifically address the axial imaging question, such as the O-arm, will prove superior. I personally still verify the safety of screw placement with electrical stimulation postplacement on all cases to identify implants adjacent to all neural elements and minimize radiation exposure to the patient and myself.

P. M. Huddleston III, MD

Appropriateness Criteria for Surgery Improve Clinical Outcomes in Patients With Low Back Pain and/or Sciatica
Danon-Hersch N, Samartzis D, Wietlisbach V, et al (Univ of Lausanne, Switzerland; Univ of Hong Kong, Hong Kong SAR, China; Schulthess-Clinic, Zürich, Switzerland)
Spine 35:672-683, 2010

Study Design.—Prospective, controlled, observational outcome study using clinical, radiographic, and patient/physician-based questionnaire data, with patient outcomes at 12 months follow-up.

Objective.—To validate appropriateness criteria for low back surgery.

Summary of Background Data.—Most surgical treatment failures are attributed to poor patient selection, but no widely accepted consensus exists on detailed indications for appropriate surgery.

Methods.—Appropriateness criteria for low back surgery have been developed by a multispecialty panel using the RAND appropriateness method. Based on panel criteria, a prospective study compared outcomes of patients appropriately and inappropriately treated at a single institution with 12 months follow-up assessment. Included were patients with low back pain and/or sciatica referred to the neurosurgical department. Information about symptoms, neurologic signs, the health-related quality of life (SF-36), disability status (Roland-Morris), and pain intensity (VAS) was assessed at baseline, at 6 months, and at 12 months follow-up. The appropriateness criteria were administered prospectively to each clinical situation and outside of the clinical setting, with the surgeon and patients blinded to the results of the panel decision. The patients were further stratified into 2 groups: appropriate treatment group (ATG) and inappropriate treatment group (ITG).

Results.—Overall, 398 patients completed all forms at 12 months. Treatment was considered appropriate for 365 participants and inappropriate for 33 participants. The mean improvement in the SF-36 physical component score at 12 months was significantly higher in the ATG (mean: 12.3 points) than in the ITG (mean: 6.8 points) $(P = 0.01)$, as well as the mean improvement in the SF-36 mental component score (ATG mean: 5.0 points; ITG mean: -0.5 points) $(P = 0.02)$. Improvement was also significantly higher in the ATG for the mean VAS back pain (ATG mean: 2.3 points; ITG mean: 0.8 points; $P = 0.02$) and Roland-Morris disability score (ATG mean: 7.7 points; ITG mean: 4.2 points; $P = 0.004$). The ATG also had a higher improvement in mean VAS for sciatica (4.0 points) than the ITG (2.8 points), but the difference was not significant ($P = 0.08$). The SF-36 General Health score declined in both groups after 12 months, however, the decline was worse in the ITG (mean decline: 8.2 points) than in the ATG (mean decline: 1.2 points) ($P = 0.04$). Overall, in comparison to ITG patients, ATG patients had significantly higher improvement at 12 months, both statistically and clinically.

Conclusion.—In comparison to previously reported literature, our study is the first to assess the utility of appropriateness criteria for low back surgery at 1-year follow-up with multiple outcome dimensions. Our results confirm the hypothesis that application of appropriateness criteria can significantly improve patient outcomes.

▶ Although appropriateness criteria have been present in many disciplines such as cardiology and spine surgery for more than a decade, they still have not been widely adopted. As patient selection for any procedure of therapeutic benefit is probably the strongest predictor of ultimate outcome, it is complicated, of course, to explain why a tool with such promise to improve patient care has not been adopted widely, but the simplest explanation may be that the current system has not been incentivized to facilitate this result. In this editor's geographic area, state, region, and organization, mandates supporting greater transparency, both in the selection of patients for surgery and their treatment outcomes, are being developed and implemented as funded and unguided mandates. Although I believe that the efforts will be marred by challenges in their formation, execution, and implementation, I believe they will evolve into useful tools to educate the public and hopefully improve decision making for patients, physicians and surgeons.

This prospective observational study performed in Lausanne, Switzerland, documented improved outcomes in patients whose treatment was consistent with a multidisciplinary guideline of appropriateness criteria for surgery. While I believe that there may be some very real differences in style, preference, and philosophy between the standard orthopedic private or group practice in the United States and government-run institutions in Europe, I believe this appropriateness tool can be a powerful way for physicians to build consensus in their groups or clinics, and the evidence would suggest to also improve their patients' outcomes. The next logical step for the Swiss authors would be to prospectively implement their appropriateness tool as a real-time clinical tool and report its effects and their patients' outcomes.

P. M. Huddleston III, MD

Efficacy of Prophylactic Placement of Inferior Vena Cava Filter in Patients Undergoing Spinal Surgery
Ozturk C, Ganiyusufoglu K, Alanay A, et al (Florence Nightingale Hosp, Istanbul, Turkey)
Spine 35:1893-1896, 2010

Study Design.—Retrospective case series.

Objective.—To evaluate the safety and efficacy of prophylactic inferior *vena cava* filter (IVCF) to prevent pulmonary embolism (PE) in high risk patients undergoing major complex spinal surgery.

Summary of Background Data.—PE has been reported to be the major cause of death after spinal reconstructive surgery. Mechanical prophylaxis alone is often not sufficient whereas anticoagulation therapy carries a significant risk of bleeding complications. Prophylactic IVCF placement is advocated in high-risk patients.

Methods.—A total of 129 high-risk patients undergoing complex spine surgery, having prophylactic IVCF were compared to a matched cohort of age, diagnosis, and risk factors of 193 patients for whom only mechanical prophylaxis was used. Patients were observed for potential complications related to the IVCF and also for clinical signs and symptoms of PE.

Results.—Eight cases (4.2%) of symptomatic PE were detected in the matched cohort control group (5 cases having combined anterior + posterior surgery and 3 patients having only posterior surgery). One of them died due to massive PE (0.5%). Symptomatic PE was detected in only 2 patients (1.5%), having combined anterior + posterior surgery due to lumbar spinal stenosis in IVCF group who responded well to medical treatment $(P < 0.05)$. No complications were associated with filter insertion.

Conclusion.—Prophylactic IVCF is effective and safe in prevention of pulmonary embolism in patients with risk factors for PE.

▶ Besides the horrific complications of perioperative blindness or paralysis, death from pulmonary embolism (PE) may be one of the most dramatic complications that can occur following spine surgery. This case-control series reported from Florence Nightingale Hospital, Istanbul, Turkey, describes the outcomes of 129 patients who received a preoperative inferior vena cava filter (IVCF) in an attempt to prevent sudden death from PE. There were 5 symptomatic PEs with 1 death in the historical control group treated by the mechanical prophylaxis of thromboembolic disease (TED) stockings and sequential compression devices. This contrasted to the 2 symptomatic PEs in the IVCF group who suffered no deaths and were reported to do well. Notwithstanding the obvious lack of a more detailed assessment of thromboembolic incidence, such as an ultrasound or venogram, this limited report supports the use of prophylactic IVCF use in high-risk patients. This intervention would be a highly desirable alternative to more intensive medical interventions such as anticoagulation. Warfarin or low—molecular weight heparin can be very effective in prophylaxing TED, but they have the potential risk for catastrophic neurovascular complications secondary to hemorrhage and hematoma. While the removal of the IVCF is not without incident, it may allow the surgeon to mitigate PE risks in oncologic, sedentary, or other high-risk patients undergoing spinal surgery and extended hospitalization. Why, even as early as 1859, the hospitals' namesake stated, "It may seem a strange principle to enunciate as the very first requirement in a Hospital that it should do the sick no harm" (Florence Nightingale).

P. M. Huddleston III, MD

Clinical Examination Is Insufficient to Rule Out Thoracolumbar Spine Injuries

Inaba K, DuBose JJ, Barmparas G, et al (Los Angeles County Med Ctr–Univ of Southern California, CA; Wilford Hall Med Ctr, Lackland AFB, TX)
J Trauma 70:174-179, 2011

Purpose.—The role of clinical examination in the diagnosis of thoracolumbar (TL) spine injuries is highly controversial. The aim of this study was to assess the sensitivity and specificity of a standardized clinical examination for diagnosing TL spine injuries after blunt trauma.

Methods.—This was a prospective observational study conducted at a level I trauma center from March 2008 to September 2008. After Institutional Review Board approval, all evaluable blunt trauma patients older than 15 years were evaluated by a senior resident or attending surgeon for TL spine deformity, tenderness to palpation, and neurologic deficits. Patients were followed through their hospital course to capture all TL spine injury diagnoses, all imaging performed, and any immobilization or stabilization procedures.

Results.—Of the 884 patients enrolled, 81 (9%) had a TL spine injury. More than half (55.6%) had two or more fractures with 30.9% having three or more. Isolated L-spine fractures occurred in 56.8%, T-spine fractures occurred in 34.6% only, and combination injuries sustained in 8.6%. The most commonly identified fractures were of the transverse process (67.9%) followed by the verterbral body (30.9%) and spinous process (12.3%). Among the 666 patients who were evaluable, 56 (8%) had a TL spine fracture. Of these, 29 (52%) had a negative clinical examination, of which 2 (7%) had clinically significant compression fractures. For evaluable patients who had localized pain or tenderness elicited on examination, although the finding triggered imaging appropriately, the site of pain correlated to the site of actual injury in only 61.5% of cases. The sensitivity and specificity of clinical examination for TL spine fractures were 48.2% and 84.9%, respectively, for all fractures and 78.6% and 83.4% for those that were clinically significant.

Conclusion.—Clinical examination as a stand-alone screening tool for evaluation of the TL spine is inadequate. In this series, all the clinically significant missed fractures were diagnosed on computed tomography (CT) obtained for evaluation of the visceral torso. A combination of both clinical examination and CT screening based on mechanism will likely be required to ensure adequate sensitivity with an acceptable specificity for the diagnosis of clinically significant injuries of the TL spine. Further research is warranted, targeting the at-risk patient with a negative clinical examination, to determine what injury mechanisms warrant evaluation with a screening CT.

▶ This is a well-done prospective study of patient screening for thoracolumbar (TL) spine fractures at Los Angeles County and University of Southern California Medical Center, a large level I trauma center. The study was selected because it is a meaningful contribution to the literature in the area of imaging for spinal fractures, specifically thoracic and lumbar. Although evidence exists for the trauma screening of the cervical spine,[1,2] there is not consensus for TL fractures. Although the easiest way to screen for TL injuries may be CT, some have expressed concerns over cost and unnecessary radiation exposure and stressed the importance of clinical examination. This study places grave doubts in my mind about the ability to diagnose TL fractures by examination alone. The authors have generated data supporting the use of injury mechanism as a cue to obtaining spinal imaging and using the scans generated from screening the chest, abdomen, and pelvis to screen the spine. Interestingly, this suggested that even when an injury was suspected, the imaging localized the injury to a different, not necessarily adjacent, level of the spine 38.5% of the time.

P. M. Huddleston III, MD

References

1. Hoffman JR, Mower WR, Wolfson AB, Todd KH, Zucker MI. Validity of a set of clinical criteria to rule out injury to the cervical spine in patients with blunt trauma. National Emergency X-Radiography Utilization Study Group. *N Engl J Med.* 2000;343:94-99.
2. Canadian CT Head and C-Spine (CCC) Study Group. Canadian C-Spine Rule study for alert and stable trauma patients: II. Study objectives and methodology. *CJEM.* 2002;4:185-193.

Measuring spine fracture outcomes: Common scales and checklists
Schoenfeld AJ, Bono CM (Texas Tech Univ Health Sciences Ctr; Harvard Med School, Boston, MA)
Injury 42:265-270, 2011

Introduction.—Although outcome instruments have been used extensively in spine surgical research, few studies at present specifically address their use in investigations regarding spine trauma. In this review we provide a summary of the outcome instruments used most frequently in spine trauma research, identify the unique challenges of studying outcomes of spine trauma patients, and propose an integrated approach that may be beneficial for future studies.

Methods.—We reviewed the use of outcome instruments applicable to spine trauma research, including generic health measures, inventories of back-specific function, pain scales, health related quality of life (HRQOL) instruments, and radiographic determinants of outcome.

Results.—Several inventories have been utilised to measure clinical outcomes following spinal trauma. Excluding measures of neurological function (e.g. ASIA motor score), none have been specifically validated for use with spine fractures. The SF-36, RMDQ, and ODI are amongst the most commonly used instruments. Importantly, the use of validated functional outcome measures in spine trauma research is hampered by the fact that the pre-morbid state of patients who sustain spine trauma may not be accurately represented by normative values established for the general population. The VAS is used most frequently to assess degree of neck and back pain. Most studies have relied on non-validated measures to determine radiographic results of treatment, although more elegant radiographic metrics exist.

Conclusions.—Functional outcome measurement of traumatically injured spine patients is challenging because available generic and spine-specific instruments were not designed for or validated in this population. Furthermore, no single inventory is capable of capturing global data necessary to evaluate results following these injuries. Investigations seeking to quantify outcomes following spine trauma should consider the use of a combination of existing surveys in a complementary fashion that should include a generic health survey, a measure of back-specific function, and determinants of bodily pain and work-related disability (Table 1).

▶ This review from authors at William Beaumont Army Medical Center and Harvard Medical School is a very helpful review of commonly used spine patient outcomes instruments and their relevance to spine trauma patients. The article makes several good points supporting the use of a physician-directed and

TABLE 1.—Descriptions of Outcome Instruments Commonly Used in Assessing Results Following Spinal Trauma

Spine Related Outcome Instrument	Dimensions Considered
RMDQ	Back function, physical ability, mobility, pain
ODI	Back function, physical ability, mobility, pain, sexual function
SF-36/SF-12	Overall quality of health: physical and mental
VAS pain scale	Pain intensity
SF-36 pain scale	Pain intensity, limitations due to pain
McGill pain questionnaire	Sensory, affective, and intensity features of pain
Low back outcome score	Back function, physical ability, mobility, pain, sexual function
EQ-5D	Overall quality of health
QUALEFFO	Overall quality of life including pain, physical, social and mental function
EVOS	Health impact, back pain and functional capacity of vertebral compression fractures
AAOS/NASS questionnaire	Pain/disability, physical health, co-morbidities, neurogenic symptoms, treatment expectations, satisfaction

institutionally relevant combination of existing spine surveys. Practically, the execution of this could be problematic. I remember hearing stories from the corresponding author about the difficulty of trying to obtain follow-up in the classic spine trauma article by Wood et al.[1] Obtaining these measures in a preinjury state is not often possible unless the patient has been seen for another spine problem in the recent past. Patients tend to be younger, more resistant to regular follow-up, and often noncompliant. The challenge of reliably obtaining postinjury or surgical measurements requires a significant system process that may not be available for the solo or small-group practitioner. It may be that a custom spine trauma outcomes measure is indicated to achieve a compromise between increasing payer demand for patient-reported outcomes measures and the practical need to minimize reporting burden on the patient to increase outcome measure yield. I agree with the authors that using some type of hybrid between an existing set of validated and commonly used tools (Table 1) is probably ideal.

P. M. Huddleston III, MD

Reference

1. Wood K, Buttermann G, Mehbod A, et al. Operative compared with nonoperative treatment of a thoracolumbar burst fracture without neurological deficit. A prospective, randomized study. *J Bone Joint Surg Am.* 2003;85-A:773-781.

Maggot Debridement Therapy for Postsurgical Wound Infection in Scoliosis: A Case Series in Five Patients
Hwang J-H, Modi HN, Suh S-W, et al (Korea Univ Guro Hosp, Seoul, South Korea; et al)
Spine 36:313-319, 2011

Study Design.—Case series of 5 patients who developed resistant wound infection after scoliosis surgery.

Objective.—To present maggot debridement therapy (MDT) as an effective alternative to the conventional treatment in postsurgical infection in scoliosis.

Summary of Background Data.—Numerous clinical reports have been published that describe outstanding effects of MDT, most notable on debridement, cleansing, disinfection, and healing of indolent wounds, many of which have previously failed to respond to conventional treatment. However, till date no reports have been found in the literature describing its use for the treatment of wound infection after scoliosis surgery, which has relatively longer and deeper wound.

Methods.—A total of 5 patients (2 females and 3 males) who developed wound infection after scoliosis correction surgery were included in this study. All were operated for neuromuscular scoliosis using posterior approach with pedicle screw fixation. All developed deep wound infection within 2 to 6 weeks of surgery, which was resistant to all kinds of conventional therapy. MDT applied in all using prepared commercially available maggot bags, and dressing was changed twice a week till wound shows signs of healing. After confirming negative culture, MDT was stopped and routine dressings or secondary closure was done. During the treatment, wound appearance, size, and development of healing were observed. *Results.*—There were 1 patient with paralytic scoliosis and 4 with cerebral palsy. All wound healed completely within 5.2 ± 1.8 weeks of MDT or 8.8 ± 3.8 cycles of MDT. There was no recurrence on final follow-up of 21.6 ± 5.9 months. Wound size was also decreased from 24.2 ± 3.3 cm of pre-MDT to 11.8 ± 4.5 cm post-MDT showing 51.2% reduction in wound size. There was partial implant removal in 2 cases before MDT; however, no further implant extraction was needed in any case after MDT. Treatment was tolerated well by all patients without any obvious complications due to MDT.

Conclusion.—We would propose to use MDT for the treatment of wound infection after scoliosis surgery as an effective alternative to conventional treatment. In this way, implant extraction could be avoided without losing any correction.

▶ The authors from South Korea actually performed this study, although the title may not seem so dramatic with a reading of the patient characteristics and indications. This article is included in the reviews as a sobering reminder to ourselves that the continuing rise of multidrug-resistant infections will continue as long as there continues to be a widespread indiscriminate use of antibiotics. Does the idea of using medicinal maggots sound repulsive and extreme? Possibly, but what would you do for your patient who is a compromised host after multiple surgical debridements that had failed over 8 months of antibiotic treatment, including prolonged wound vacuum treatment and soft tissue management? While I believe that the authors have showed us a radical solution to the problem of resistant implant-associated spinal infection, I think removing the foreign body (implants) would be a wise move prior to such heroic interventions as the use of disinfected larvae of *Phaenicia* (*Lucilia*) *sericata.*

P. M. Huddleston III, MD

C-Reactive Protein, Erythrocyte Sedimentation Rate and Orthopedic Implant Infection
Piper KE, Fernandez-Sampedro M, Steckelberg KE, et al (Mayo Clinic College of Medicine, Rochester, MN)
PLoS One 5:e9358, 2010

Background.—C-reactive protein (CRP) and erythrocyte sedimentation rate (ESR) have been shown to be useful for diagnosis of prosthetic hip and knee infection. Little information is available on CRP and ESR in patients undergoing revision or resection of shoulder arthroplasties or spine implants.

Methods/Results.—We analyzed preoperative CRP and ESR in 636 subjects who underwent knee (n = 297), hip (n = 221) or shoulder (n = 64) arthroplasty, or spine implant (n = 54) removal. A standardized definition of orthopedic implant-associated infection was applied. Receiver operating curve analysis was used to determine ideal cutoff values for differentiating infected from non-infected cases. ESR was significantly different in subjects with aseptic failure infection of knee (median 11 and 53.5 mm/h, respectively, p = <0.0001) and hip (median 11 and 30 mm/h, respectively, p = <0.0001) arthroplasties and spine implants (median 10 and 48.5 mm/h, respectively, p = 0.0033), but not shoulder arthroplasties (median 10 and 9 mm/h, respectively, p = 0.9883). Optimized ESR cutoffs for knee, hip and shoulder arthroplasties and spine implants were 19, 13, 26, and 45 mm/h, respectively. Using these cutoffs, sensitivity and specificity to detect infection were 89 and 74% for knee, 82 and 60% for hip, and 32 and 93% for shoulder arthroplasties, and 57 and 90% for spine implants. CRP was significantly different in subjects with aseptic failure and infection of knee (median 4 and 51 mg/l, respectively, p<0.0001), hip (median 3 and 18 mg/l, respectively, p<0.0001), and shoulder (median 3 and 10 mg/l, respectively, p = 0.01) arthroplasties, and spine implants (median 3 and 20 mg/l, respectively, p = 0.0011). Optimized CRP cutoffs for knee, hip, and shoulder arthroplasties, and spine implants were 14.5, 10.3, 7, and 4.6 mg/l, respectively. Using these cutoffs, sensitivity and specificity to detect infection were 79 and 88% for knee, 74 and 79% for hip, and 63 and 73% for shoulder arthroplasties, and 79 and 68% for spine implants.

Conclusion.—CRP and ESR have poor sensitivity for the diagnosis of shoulder implant infection. A CRP of 4.6 mg/l had a sensitivity of 79 and a specificity of 68% to detect infection of spine implants (Table 3).

▶ The article by Sampedro et al[1] details the increased sensitivity and specificity of accurate diagnosis of spine implant-associated infection by culture of surgically explanted peri-implant tissue followed by culture and subsequent polymerase chain reaction of the ultrasonicate of the implants. But this article provides the clinician with information confirming infection after the act of revision surgery has taken place. But what of aiding the decision-making process before surgery? This article by Piper et al provides valuable information of 3 relatively standard tests: a complete blood count with differential, a sedimentation rate, and a C-reactive protein. This study, as does the article by Sampedro et al, serves as an intellectual bridge between the knowledge gained by infectious disease research and orthopedic appendicular surgery to the axial skeleton. It is interesting to note the differences in sensitivity and specificity in patients between different anatomic areas. The authors show statistically significant differences between spine and knee surgeries and hip and shoulder implant infections. Weaknesses of the study include the lack of a gold standard for definition of implant-associated infection and variations in the timing of preoperative serology testing screening for infection. In my practice, all patients will receive testing with infection labs prior to surgical intervention. The results

TABLE 3.—Sensitivity and Specificity of CRP (>10 mg/l) and/or ESR (>30 mm/h) for the Detection of Infected Knee, Hip and Shoulder Arthroplasty and Spinal Instrumentation

	Sensitivity	Specificity	PPV	NPV	Area Under the ROC Curve	p-Value from Logistic Regression
Knee ESR >30 mm/h	71 (58/82)	89 (191/215)	71 (58/82)	89 (191/215)	0.80	<0.0001
Knee CRP >10 mg/d	83 (68/82)	79 (170/215)	60 (68/113)	92 (170/184)	0.81	<0.0001
Knee ESR >30 mm/h or CRP >10 mg/l	87 (71/82)	75 (161/215)	57 (71/125)	94 (161/172)	0.81	<0.0001
Hip ESR >30 mm/h	47 (16/34)	84 (158/187)	36 (16/45)	90 (158/176)	0.66	<0.0001
Hip CRP >10 mg/l	74 (25/34)	78 (146/187)	38 (25/66)	94 (146/155)	0.76	<0.0001
Hip ESR >30 mm/h or CRP >10 mg/l	76 (26/34)	71 (132/187)	32 (26/81)	94 (132/140)	0.74	<0.0001
Shoulder ESR >30 mm/h	16 (3/19)	98 (44/45)	75 (3/4)	73 (44/60)	0.57	0.0764
Shoulder CRP >10 mg/l	42 (8/19)	84 (38/45)	53 (8/15)	78 (38/49)	0.63	0.0269
Shoulder ESR >30 mm/h or CRP >10 mg/l	42 (8/19)	82 (37/45)	50 (8/16)	77 (37/48)	0.62	0.0455
Spine ESR >30 mm/h	64 (9/14)	83 (33/40)	56 (9/16)	87 (33/38)	0.73	0.0021
Spine CRP >10 mg/l	57 (8/14)	85 (34/40)	57 (8/14)	85 (34/40)	0.71	0.0038
Spine ESR >30 mm/h or CRP >10 mg/l	79 (11/14)	75 (30/40)	52 (11/21)	91 (30/33)	0.77	0.0013

allow for optimizing the preoperative counseling for the patient and preparing the operative team. In the possible event that perioperative tissue cultures are not helpful in making the postoperative diagnosis, the results of the preoperative testing may be one of the only bits of evidence supporting the diagnosis of spine implant-associated infection and justifying a prolonged antimicrobial treatment.

P. M. Huddleston III, MD

Reference

1. Sampedro MF, Huddleston PM, Piper KE, et al. A biofilm approach to detect bacteria on removed spinal implants. *Spine (Phila Pa 1976)*. 2010;35:1218-1224.

A Biofilm Approach to Detect Bacteria on Removed Spinal Implants

Sampedro MF, Huddleston PM, Piper KE, et al (Mayo Clinic College of Medicine, Rochester, MN; et al)
Spine 35:1218-1224, 2010

Study Design.—This is a prospective study comparing the diagnosis of spinal implant infection by conventional peri-implant tissue culture with a technique which uses a combination of vortexing and bath sonication to dislodge bacteria growing as a biofilm on the surface of retrieved spinal implants.

Objective.—We hypothesized that the biofilm-sampling technique would be more sensitive than peri-implant tissue culture.

Summary of Background Data.—Culture of peri-implant tissue is inaccurate for the diagnosis of orthopedic device-related infection; cultures taken from the implant may be more sensitive. We have developed a technique which uses vortexing-bath sonication to sample bacterial biofilms on the surface of retrieved hip and knee implants, and shown that it is more sensitive than periprosthetic tissue culture for the microbiologic diagnosis of prosthetic knee, hip, and shoulder infection.

Methods.—We compared peri-implant tissue culture to the vortexing-bath sonication technique which samples bacterial biofilm on the surface of retrieved spinal implants, for the diagnosis of spinal implant infection. In addition, we compared detection of *Staphylococcus* and *Propionibacterium acnes* by rapid cycle real-time polymerase chain reaction with culture of sonicate fluid.

Results.—A total of 112 subjects were studied; 22 had spinal implant infection. The sensitivities of peri-implant tissue and sonicate fluid culture were 73% and 91% ($P = 0.046$), and the specificities were 93% and 97%, respectively. *P. acnes* and coagulase-negative staphylococci were the most frequent microorganisms detected among subjects with spinal implant infection, with *P. acnes* detected in 56 and 45%, and coagulase-negative staphylococci detected in 31 and 40% of peri-implant tissue and sonicate fluid cultures, respectively. Compared with the culture of sonicate fluid, polymerase chain reaction was 100 and 67% sensitive for the detection of culture-positive *Staphylococcus* and *P. acnes* spinal implant infection, respectively.

Conclusion.—Implant sonication followed by culture is more sensitive than peri-implant tissue culture for the microbiologic diagnosis of spinal implant infection (Fig 1).

▶ The work of Sampedro and colleagues from the Infectious Diseases Laboratory at the Mayo Clinic continues to define the standard for identification of organisms in implant-associated spine infection. All too often, I have seen my patients and others suffering from chronic pain and discomfort without an obvious etiology. A patient with a computed tomography demonstrating a solid arthrodesis with trabecular bone in the interbody space, normal infection laboratory test results (complete blood cell count with differential, sedimentation rate, and C-reactive protein level), and continued pain presents a diagnostic dilemma. Carefully documenting any wound issues immediately postoperatively may hint at a latent indolent implant-associated infection. Previous work in the hip and knee literature has definitively demonstrated the role of organisms such as *Staphylococcus epidermidis* and *Propionibacterium* sp to cause symptomatic infected arthroplasties. The mechanism involves colonization of the foreign body surface with bacteria protected within a defensive biofilm. In the spine, implants may be contaminated at the time of surgery or postoperatively from a seemingly insignificant local infection. These organisms may contribute to otherwise unattributable symptoms of pseudoarthrosis, implant loosening, and chronic unexplained pain. The results of this study adapt the techniques learned from successful treatments of other areas of implant infection: define the organism, remove the foreign body, and threaten the host with effective antimicrobials.

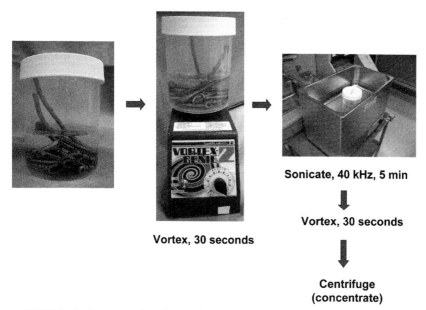

Sonicate, 40 kHz, 5 min

⬇

Vortex, 30 seconds

Vortex, 30 seconds

⬇

Centrifuge
(concentrate)

FIGURE 1.—Sonication procedure. The container was vortexed for 30 seconds (Vortex Genie, Scientific Industries Inc., Bohemia, NY), and then subjected to sonication in an Aquasonic Model 750T ultrasound bath (VWR Scientific, Weschester, PA) for 5 minutes, followed by additional vortexing for 30 seconds. For the first 40 subjects studied (January 2005–December 2005), 0.5 mL of sonicate fluid was plated onto aerobic and anaerobic sheep blood agar plates which were incubated at 35°C in 5% CO_2 aerobically and anaerobically for 5 and 7 days, respectively. For the last 72 subjects studied (January 2006–April 2007), a concentration step was added. Fifty milliliters of sonicate fluid was placed into each of 8 conical 50 mL tubes; tubes were centrifuged at 3150g for 5 minutes. The supernatant was aspirated leaving 0.5 mL remaining in each tube (100-fold concentration). A 0.1-mL aliquot of the sediment was plated onto aerobic and anaerobic sheep blood agar plates which were incubated at 35°C in 5% CO_2 aerobically and anaerobically for 2 and 14 days, respectively. Microorganisms were enumerated and identified using routine techniques. (Reprinted from Sampedro MF, Huddleston PM, Piper KE, et al. A biofilm approach to detect bacteria on removed spinal implants. *Spine.* 2010;35:1218-1224, with permission from Lippincott Williams & Wilkins.)

While few would argue that routine cultures should be performed in the face of an obvious infection, the infrastructure to perform more than 3 tissue cultures, to culture the ultrasonicate removed from the extracted implants, and to perform polymerase chain reaction assays to further define the presence of bacteria may not be present in most facilities (Fig 1). Nevertheless, Sampedro et al have demonstrated an increased diagnostic benefit with each additional step of their method. The physician should have an awareness of the significance of the study and acknowledge that in a postoperative patient with no other obvious etiology of pain, the final answer may not be apparent until all metals have been removed and implant-associated infection has been ruled out or treated.

P. M. Huddleston III, MD

Article Index

Chapter 1: General Orthopedics

Meta-Analysis Comparing Arthroplasty with Internal Fixation for Displaced Femoral Neck Fracture in the Elderly   1

Cost-effectiveness analyses of elective orthopaedic surgical procedures in patients with inflammatory arthropathies   2

Do "Premium" Joint Implants Add Value?: Analysis of High Cost Joint Implants in a Community Registry   3

IOC consensus paper on the use of platelet-rich plasma in sports medicine   4

Improving Injection Accuracy of the Elbow, Knee, and Shoulder: Does Injection Site and Imaging Make a Difference? A Systematic Review   6

A Proximal Strengthening Program Improves Pain, Function, and Biomechanics in Women With Patellofemoral Pain Syndrome   7

Co-existent medial collateral ligament injury seen following transient patellar dislocation: observations at magnetic resonance imaging   8

A clinical prediction rule for identifying patients with patellofemoral pain who are likely to benefit from foot orthoses: a preliminary determination   9

Anatomy of Lateral Patellar Instability: Trochlear Dysplasia and Tibial Tubercle–Trochlear Groove Distance Is More Pronounced in Women Who Dislocate the Patella   10

A Prospective Study of 80,000 Total Joint and 5000 Anterior Cruciate Ligament Reconstruction Procedures in a Community-Based Registry in the United States   11

Is Physical Activity a Risk Factor for Primary Knee or Hip Replacement Due to Osteoarthritis? A Prospective Cohort Study   13

Arthroscopic femoral osteochondroplasty for cam lesions with isolated acetabular chondral damage   15

Open Surgical Dislocation Versus Arthroscopy for Femoroacetabular Impingement: A Comparison of Clinical Outcomes   17

Comparative Systematic Review of the Open Dislocation, Mini-Open, and Arthroscopic Surgeries for Femoroacetabular Impingement   19

Assessment of peritrochanteric high T2 signal depending on the age and gender of the patients   20

Analysis of the microbial load in instruments used in orthopedic surgeries   22

A Prospective, Randomized Clinical Trial Comparing an Antibiotic-Impregnated Bioabsorbable Bone Substitute With Standard Antibiotic-Impregnated Cement Beads in the Treatment of Chronic Osteomyelitis and Infected Nonunion   23

Increased cancer risks among arthroplasty patients: 30 year follow-up of the Swedish Knee Arthroplasty Register   24

Are Dropped Osteoarticular Bone Fragments Safely Reimplantable in Vivo?   27

Chapter 2: Basic Science

Perivascular Lymphocytic Infiltration Is Not Limited to Metal-on-Metal Bearings 29

Lymphocyte Proliferation Responses in Patients with Pseudotumors following
Metal-on-Metal Hip Resurfacing Arthroplasty 30

Mechanical Loading Increased BMP-2 Expression which Promoted Osteogenic
Differentiation of Tendon-Derived Stem Cells 32

Novel Nanostructured Scaffolds as Therapeutic Replacement Options for Rotator
Cuff Disease 33

Ibuprofen Upregulates Expressions of Matrix Metalloproteinase-1, -8, -9, and -13
without Affecting Expressions of Types I and III Collagen in Tendon Cells 35

Autologous Chondrocyte Implantation Using the Original Periosteum-Cover
Technique Versus Matrix-Associated Autologous Chondrocyte Implantation:
A Randomized Clinical Trial 36

Development of simulated arthroscopic skills: A randomized trial of virtual-reality
training of 21 orthopedic surgeons 37

Experimental Knee Pain Reduces Muscle Strength 38

Influence of icing on muscle regeneration after crush injury to skeletal muscles in
rats 40

Chapter 3: Trauma and Amputation

Atypical Fractures as a Potential Complication of Long-term Bisphosphonate
Therapy 41

Bisphosphonates and Fractures of the Subtrochanteric or Diaphyseal Femur 42

East Practice Management Guidelines Work Group: Update to Practice
Management Guidelines for Prophylactic Antibiotic Use in Open Fractures 48

The Relationship Between Time to Surgical Débridement and Incidence of
Infection After Open High-Energy Lower Extremity Trauma 48

Osteoporosis as a Risk Factor for Distal Radial Fractures: A Case-Control Study 50

Ultrasound-guided reduction of distal radius fractures 52

Traumatic and Trauma-Related Amputations: Part I: General Principles and
Lower-Extremity Amputations 55

Is Surgery Necessary for Femoral Insufficiency Fractures after Long-term
Bisphosphonate Therapy? 57

Femoral Insufficiency Fractures Associated with Prolonged Bisphosphonate
Therapy 59

Cumulative Alendronate Dose and the Long-Term Absolute Risk of
Subtrochanteric and Diaphyseal Femur Fractures: A Register-Based National
Cohort Analysis 61

Immediate Spica Casting of Pediatric Femoral Fractures in the Operating Room
Versus the Emergency Department: Comparison of Reduction, Complications, and
Hospital Charges 64

Femoral Fractures in Adolescents: A Comparison of Four Methods of Fixation 66

Analysis of Postoperative Knee Sepsis After Retrograde Nail Insertion of Open Femoral Shaft Fractures — 69

Comparison of RIA and conventional reamed nailing for treatment of femur shaft fractures — 70

Femoral Malrotation After Unreamed Intramedullary Nailing: An Evaluation of Influencing Operative Factors — 73

Functional Outcome After Antegrade Femoral Nailing: A Comparison of Trochanteric Fossa Versus Tip of Greater Trochanter Entry Point — 75

Risk Factors for Femoral Nonunion After Femoral Shaft Fracture — 78

Outcomes of acetabular fracture fixation with ten years' follow-up — 78

Outcomes of Posterior Wall Fractures of the Acetabulum Treated Nonoperatively After Diagnostic Screening with Dynamic Stress Examination Under Anesthesia — 80

External Fixation for Stable and Unstable Intertrochanteric Fractures in Patients Older Than 75 Years of Age: A Prospective Comparative Study — 81

The Value of an Organized Fracture Program for the Elderly: Early Results — 82

Iron Supplementation for Anemia After Hip Fracture Surgery: A Randomized Trial of 300 Patients — 85

Intramedullary nailing appears to be superior in pertrochanteric hip fractures with a detached greater trochanter: 311 consecutive patients followed for 1 year — 86

Long-term outcome after 1822 operatively treated ankle fractures: A systematic review of the literature — 88

Outcomes of Ankle Fractures in Patients with Uncomplicated Versus Complicated Diabetes — 89

Shock Wave Therapy Compared with Intramedullary Screw Fixation for Nonunion of Proximal Fifth Metatarsal Metaphyseal-Diaphyseal Fractures — 91

Outcomes of Suture Button Repair of the Distal Tibiofibular Syndesmosis — 92

A Systematic Review on the Treatment of Acute Ankle Sprain: Brace versus Other Functional Treatment Types — 93

Timing of Definitive Fixation of Severe Tibial Plateau Fractures With Compartment Syndrome Does Not Have an Effect on the Rate of Infection — 96

Effect of Calcium Phosphate Bone Cement Augmentation on Volar Plate Fixation of Unstable Distal Radial Fractures in the Elderly — 97

Medial and Lateral Pin Versus Lateral-Entry Pin Fixation for Type 3 Supracondylar Fractures in Children: A Prospective, Surgeon-Randomized Study — 98

A Prospective Study on the Effectiveness of Cotton Versus Waterproof Cast Padding in Maintaining the Reduction of Pediatric Distal Forearm Fractures — 101

The Effects of Surgical Delay on the Outcome of Pediatric Supracondylar Humeral Fractures — 102

The effect of haematoma aspiration on intra-articular pressure and pain relief following Mason I radial head fractures — 104

Comminuted fractures of the radial head and neck: is fixation to the shaft necessary? — 106

Comparison of Plates versus Intramedullary Nails for Fixation of Displaced
Midshaft Clavicular Fractures   107

Elastic stable intramedullary nailing is best for mid-shaft clavicular fractures
without comminution: Results in 60 patients   109

Functional bracing of humeral shaft fractures. A review of clinical studies   111

Locking Intramedullary Nails and Locking Plates in the Treatment of Two-Part
Proximal Humeral Surgical Neck Fractures: A Prospective Randomized Trial with
a Minimum of Three Years of Follow-up   114

Wrist function recovers more rapidly after volar locked plating than after external
fixation but the outcomes are similar after 1 year: A randomized study of 63 patients
with a dorsally displaced fracture of the distal radius   116

Should unstable extra-articular distal radial fractures be treated with fixed-angle
volar-locked plates or percutaneous Kirschner wires? A prospective randomised
controlled trial   118

Long-Term Outcomes of Fractures of Both Bones of the Forearm   119

Complications of K-Wire Fixation in Procedures Involving the Hand and Wrist   121

Successful Reconstruction for Complex Malunions and Nonunions of the Tibia
and Femur   122

Optimized Perioperative Analgesia Reduces Chronic Phantom Limb Pain Intensity,
Prevalence, and Frequency: A Prospective, Randomized, Clinical Trial   123

Outcomes Associated with the Internal Fixation of Long-Bone Fractures Proximal
to Traumatic Amputations   124

Chapter 4: Total Hip Arthroplasty

A Population-Based Study of Trends in the Use of Total Hip and Total Knee
Arthroplasty, 1969-2008   127

Choice of Hospital for Revision Total Hip Replacement   129

Hospital Economics of Primary THA Decreasing Reimbursement and Increasing
Cost, 1990 to 2008   130

Adverse reaction to metal debris following hip resurfacing: The influence of
component type, orientation and volumetric wear   131

Acetabular UHMWPE Survival and Wear Changes With Different Manufacturing
Techniques   132

Aseptic Lymphocyte-Dominated Vasculitis-Associated Lesion: A Clinicopathologic
Review of an Underrecognized Cause of Prosthetic Failure   134

Catastrophic failure due to aggressive metallosis 4 years after hip resurfacing in
a woman in her forties — a case report   135

Arthroprosthetic Cobaltism: Neurological and Cardiac Manifestations in Two
Patients with Metal-on-Metal Arthroplasty: A Case Report   138

Do Ion Levels In Hip Resurfacing Differ From Metal-on-metal THA at Midterm?   140

A Prospective Randomized Trial of Mini-Incision Posterior and Two-Incision Total
Hip Arthroplasty   141

A comparison of hemiarthroplasty with total hip replacement for displaced intracapsular fracture of the femoral neck: A randomised controlled multicentre trial in patients aged 70 years and over   142

Comparison of Bipolar Hemiarthroplasty with Total Hip Arthroplasty for Displaced Femoral Neck Fractures: A Concise Four-Year Follow-up of a Randomized Trial   143

Cemented Versus Cementless Total Hip Replacements in Patients Fifty-five Years of Age or Older with Rheumatoid Arthritis   145

Hip Dislocation: Are Hip Precautions Necessary in Anterior Approaches?   146

A Monoblock Porous Tantalum Acetabular Cup Has No Osteolysis on CT at 10 Years   147

Cementless Femoral Fixation in Total Hip Arthroplasty   148

Association of Osteonecrosis and Failure of Hip Resurfacing Arthroplasty   149

Does morbid obesity affect the outcome of total hip replacement?: An analysis of 3290 THRS   150

Cementless revision for infected total hip replacements   151

Acetabular Reconstruction with Impaction Bone-Grafting and a Cemented Cup in Patients Younger than Fifty Years Old: A Concise Follow-up, at Twenty to Twenty-Eight Years, of a Previous Report   152

Chapter 5: Total Knee Arthroplasty

Hospital Economics of Primary Total Knee Arthroplasty at a Teaching Hospital   155

Preoperative Predictors of Returning to Work Following Primary Total Knee Arthroplasty   156

Do Residents Perform TKAs Using Computer Navigation as Accurately as Consultants?   157

What is the Evidence for Total Knee Arthroplasty in Young Patients?: A Systematic Review of the Literature   158

A Prospective Randomized Study of Minimally Invasive Total Knee Arthroplasty Compared with Conventional Surgery   160

Changes in hip fracture rate before and after total knee replacement due to osteoarthritis: a population-based cohort study   161

Fast-track surgery for bilateral total knee replacement   162

Comparison Between Standard and High-Flexion Posterior-Stabilized Rotating-Platform Mobile-Bearing Total Knee Arthroplasties: A Randomized Controlled Study   163

A Second Decade Lifetable Survival Analysis of the Oxford Unicompartmental Knee Arthroplasty   165

Wear Damage in Mobile-bearing TKA is as Severe as That in Fixed-bearing TKA   166

The John Insall Award: Control-matched Evaluation of Painful Patellar Crepitus After Total Knee Arthroplasty   167

Management of Intraoperative Medial Collateral Ligament Injury During TKA   168

Deep Vein Thrombosis After Total Knee Arthroplasty in Asian Patients Without
Prophylactic Anticoagulation — 169

The Mark Coventry Award: Diagnosis of Early Postoperative TKA Infection Using
Synovial Fluid Analysis — 170

Chapter 6: Shoulder

Measuring shoulder injury function: Common scales and checklists — 173

Frozen shoulder: the effectiveness of conservative and surgical interventions—
systematic review — 175

Cigarette Smoking Increases the Risk for Rotator Cuff Tears — 176

Platelet-Rich Plasma Augmentation for Arthroscopic Rotator Cuff Repair:
A Randomized Controlled Trial — 176

The Arthroscopic Management of Partial-Thickness Rotator Cuff Tears:
A Systematic Review of the Literature — 178

Pathomechanisms and Complications Related to Patient Positioning and
Anesthesia During Shoulder Arthroscopy — 180

Position and Duration of Immobilization After Primary Anterior Shoulder
Dislocation: A Systematic Review and Meta-Analysis of the Literature — 181

Pain Relief for Reduction of Acute Anterior Shoulder Dislocations: A Prospective
Randomized Study Comparing Intravenous Sedation With Intra-articular Lidocaine — 183

Arthroscopic Capsulolabral Revision Repair for Recurrent Anterior Shoulder
Instability — 184

Contact Pressure and Glenohumeral Translation Following Subacromial
Decompression: How Much Is Enough? — 185

Chapter 7: Elbow

Revision Arthroscopic Contracture Release in the Elbow Resulting in an Ulnar
Nerve Transection: Surgical Technique — 187

Combination of Arthrolysis by Lateral and Medial Approaches and Hinged
External Fixation in the Treatment of Stiff Elbow — 190

Arthroscopic Restoration of Terminal Elbow Extension in High-Level Athletes — 191

Clinical Assessment of the Ulnar Nerve at the Elbow: Reliability of Instability
Testing and the Association of Hypermobility with Clinical Symptoms — 192

The effect of haematoma aspiration on intra-articular pressure and pain relief
following Mason I radial head fractures — 193

Chapter 8: Sports Medicine

Orthopaedic In-Training Examination: An Analysis of the Sports Medicine Section — 197

Osteochondral Lesions of the Knee: A New One-Step Repair Technique with Bone-
Marrow-Derived Cells — 198

6-year follow-up of 84 patients with cartilage defects in the knee: Knee scores
improved but recovery was incomplete — 202

Cartilage from the edge of a debrided articular defect is inferior to that from a standard donor site when used for autologous chondrocyte cultivation   203

Outcome of Ulnar Collateral Ligament Reconstruction of the Elbow in 1281 Athletes: Results in 743 Athletes With Minimum 2-Year Follow-Up   203

A Systematic Review on the Treatment of Acute Ankle Sprain: Brace versus Other Functional Treatment Types   204

Accuracy of the Anterior Apprehension Test as a Predictor of Risk for Redislocation After a First Traumatic Shoulder Dislocation   206

Does Arthroscopic Partial Meniscectomy Result in Knee Osteoarthritis? A Systematic Review With a Minimum of 8 Years' Follow-up   207

Meniscal Repair for Radial Tears of the Midbody of the Lateral Meniscus   208

Can the Reparability of Meniscal Tears Be Predicted With Magnetic Resonance Imaging?   209

Biological Knee Reconstruction: A Systematic Review of Combined Meniscal Allograft Transplantation and Cartilage Repair or Restoration   210

Anatomic Reconstruction of the Posterolateral Corner of the Knee: A Case Series With Isolated Reconstructions in 27 Patients   212

Posterolateral corner injuries of the knee: A serious injury commonly missed   214

A Comparison of the Effect of Central Anatomical Single-Bundle Anterior Cruciate Ligament Reconstruction and Double-Bundle Anterior Cruciate Ligament Reconstruction on Pivot-Shift Kinematics   215

A Long-Term, Prospective, Randomized Study Comparing Biodegradable and Metal Interference Screws in Anterior Cruciate Ligament Reconstruction Surgery: Radiographic Results and Clinical Outcome   216

Allograft Anterior Cruciate Ligament Reconstruction in the Young, Active Patient: Tegner Activity Level and Failure Rate   217

Factors Explaining Chronic Knee Extensor Strength Deficits after ACL Reconstruction   218

Prompt Operative Intervention Reduces Long-Term Osteoarthritis After Knee Anterior Cruciate Ligament Tear   219

Anterior Cruciate Ligament Reconstruction Improves Activity-Induced Pain in Comparison With Pain at Rest in Middle-Aged Patients With Significant Cartilage Degeneration   221

Cost-Effectiveness of Anterior Cruciate Ligament Reconstruction: A Preliminary Comparison of Single-Bundle and Double-Bundle Techniques   222

Adductor Tenotomy in the Management of Groin Pain in Athletes   223

Chapter 9: Foot and Ankle

Are the feet of obese children fat or flat? Revisiting the debate   225

Autologous Platelets Have No Effect on the Healing of Human Achilles Tendon Ruptures: A Randomized Single-Blind Study   226

The Majority of Patients With Achilles Tendinopathy Recover Fully When Treated With Exercise Alone: A 5-Year Follow-Up   227

Operative versus Nonoperative Treatment of Acute Achilles Tendon Ruptures: A Multicenter Randomized Trial Using Accelerated Functional Rehabilitation   228

Peroneal tendon subluxation: the other lateral ankle injury   230

Tibiotalocalcaneal Arthrodesis With a Curved, Interlocking, Intramedullary Nail   232

Limb Salvage In Severe Diabetic Foot Infection   233

Long-Term Results After Modified Brostrom Procedure Without Calcaneofibular Ligament Reconstruction   234

Total Ankle Replacement Outcome in Low Volume Centers: Short-Term Followup   235

High Rate of Osteolytic Lesions in Medium-Term Followup After the AES Total Ankle Replacement   236

Reconstruction of the Symptomatic Idiopathic Flatfoot in Adolescents and Young Adults   237

Chapter 10: Forearm, Wrist, and Hand

Accuracy of In-Office Nerve Conduction Studies for Median Neuropathy: A Meta-Analysis   241

Comparison of CT and MRI for Diagnosis of Suspected Scaphoid Fractures   242

Osteoporosis as a Risk Factor for Distal Radial Fractures: A Case-Control Study   244

The Distal Radius, the Most Frequent Fracture Localization in Humans: A Histomorphometric Analysis of the Microarchitecture of 60 Human Distal Radii and Its Changes in Aging   245

Ulnomeniscal Homologue of the Wrist: Correlation of Anatomic and MR Imaging Findings   246

Wrist function recovers more rapidly after volar locked plating than after external fixation but the outcomes are similar after 1 year: A randomized study of 63 patients with a dorsally displaced fracture of the distal radius   249

Comparison of united and nonunited fractures of the ulnar styloid following volar-plate fixation of distal radius fractures   250

Volar Locking Plate Implant Prominence and Flexor Tendon Rupture   251

Joint Leveling for Advanced Kienbĭck's Disease   253

Three-point index in predicting redisplacement of extra-articular distal radial fractures in adults   254

The Unstable Nonunited Scaphoid Waist Fracture: Results of Treatment by Open Reduction, Anterior Wedge Grafting, and Internal Fixation by Volar Buttress Plate   256

Color-Aided Visualization of Dorsal Wrist Ganglion Stalks Aids in Complete Arthroscopic Excision   257

The International Registry on Hand and Composite Tissue Transplantation   258

Chemical Denervation with Botulinum Neurotoxin A Improves the Surgical Manipulation of the Muscle–Tendon Unit: An Experimental Study in an Animal Model   259

Injectable Collagenase Clostridium Histolyticum: A New Nonsurgical Treatment for Dupuytren's Disease   260

A Prospective Trial on the Use of Antibiotics in Hand Surgery   262

Avoiding Flexor Tendon Repair Rupture with Intraoperative Total Active Movement Examination   263

Composite Grafting for Traumatic Fingertip Amputation in Adults: Technique Reinforcement and Experience in 31 Digits   264

Arthrodesis as a Salvage for Failed Proximal Interphalangeal Joint Arthroplasty   265

Scope-Assisted Release of the Cubital Tunnel   266

Very Distal Sensory Nerve Transfers in High Median Nerve Lesions   267

Clinical Outcomes Following Median to Radial Nerve Transfers   268

Chapter 11: Orthopedic Oncology

A Comparison of Fine-needle Aspiration, Core Biopsy, and Surgical Biopsy in the Diagnosis of Extremity Soft Tissue Masses   271

Analysis of Nondiagnostic Results after Image-guided Needle Biopsies of Musculoskeletal Lesions   272

Elderly patients with painful bone metastases should be offered palliative radiotherapy   274

Comparative study of whole-body MRI and bone scintigraphy for the detection of bone metastases   275

Joint Space Widening in Synovial Chondromatosis of the Hip   276

Endoprosthetic reconstruction of the distal tibia and ankle joint after resection of primary bone tumours   277

Custom-made endoprostheses for the femoral amputation stump: An alternative to hip disarticulation in tumour surgery   278

Intercalary Allograft Reconstructions Using a Compressible Intramedullary Nail: A Preliminary Report   278

Computer-assisted Navigation in Bone Tumor Surgery: Seamless Workflow Model and Evolution of Technique   279

How Long Do Endoprosthetic Reconstructions for Proximal Femoral Tumors Last?   280

Cemented Endoprosthetic Reconstruction of the Proximal Tibia: How Long Do They Last?   282

Local Recurrence, Survival and Function After Total Femur Resection and Megaprosthetic Reconstruction for Bone Sarcomas   283

A Comparative Study of F-18 FDG PET and ^{201}Tl Scintigraphy for Detection of Primary Malignant Bone and Soft-Tissue Tumors   284

Local Recurrence After Initial Multidisciplinary Management of Soft Tissue Sarcoma: Is there a Way Out?   285

Clinicopathologic Prognostic Factors of Pure Myxoid Liposarcoma of the Extremities and Trunk Wall   286

Extracorporeally Irradiated Autograft-prosthetic Composite Arthroplasty With Vascular Reconstruction for Primary Bone Tumor of the Proximal Tibia   288

Evolution of Surgical Treatment for Sarcomas of Proximal Humerus in Children: Retrospective Review at a Single Institute Over 30 Years   290

Is Humeral Segmental Defect Replacement Device A Stronger Construct than Locked IM Nailing?   291

Femoral diaphyseal endoprosthetic reconstruction after segmental resection of primary bone tumours   292

Joint-sparing or Physeal-sparing Diaphyseal Resections: The Challenge of Holding Small Fragments   293

Late Complications and Survival of Endoprosthetic Reconstruction after Resection of Bone Tumors   294

Extraarticular Knee Resection for Sarcomas with Preservation of the Extensor Mechanism: Surgical Technique and Review of Cases   295

Disparity in limb-salvage surgery among sarcoma patients   296

Factors Predicting Local Recurrence, Metastasis, and Survival in Pediatric Soft Tissue Sarcoma in Extremities   297

Clinical and Treatment Outcomes of Planned and Unplanned Excisions of Soft Tissue Sarcomas   298

Double Ray Amputation for Tumors of the Hand   299

Chondrosarcoma of Bone: Lessons From 46 Operated Cases in a Single Institution   300

Cemented Distal Femoral Endoprostheses for Musculoskeletal Tumor: Improved Survival of Modular versus Custom Implants   301

MFH of Bone and Osteosarcoma Show Similar Survival and Chemosensitivity   302

Does Increased Rate of Limb-sparing Surgery Affect Survival in Osteosarcoma?   303

Curettage and Graft Alleviates Athletic-Limiting Pain in Benign Lytic Bone Lesions   304

Endoscopic Surgery for Young Athletes With Symptomatic Unicameral Bone Cyst of the Calcaneus   305

Curettage and Cryosurgery for Low-grade Cartilage Tumors Is Associated with Low Recurrence and High Function   307

Is Sclerotherapy Better than Intralesional Excision for Treating Aneurysmal Bone Cysts?   309

Giant Cell Tumor of Bone: Risk Factors for Recurrence   310

Chapter 12: Spine

The Economics of Minimally Invasive Spine Surgery: The Value Perspective   314

Trends in the Use of Bone Morphogenetic Protein as a Substitute to Autologous Iliac Crest Bone Grafting for Spinal Fusion Procedures in the United States   315

Quantifying the variability of financial disclosure information reported by authors presenting at annual spine conferences   316

Who's in the Driver's Seat? The Influence of Patient and Physician Enthusiasm on Regional Variation in Degenerative Lumbar Spinal Surgery: A Population-Based Study   319

Surgical Outcomes of Decompression, Decompression with Limited Fusion, and Decompression With Full Curve Fusion for Degenerative Scoliosis With Radiculopathy   320

The Current State of Minimally Invasive Spine Surgery   322

Lumbar Decompression Using a Traditional Midline Approach *Versus* a Tubular Retractor System: Comparison of Patient-Based Clinical Outcomes   323

Minimally Invasive Surgery: Lateral Approach Interbody Fusion: Results and Review   324

Percutaneous Vertebroplasty for Pain Management in Malignant Fractures of the Spine with Epidural Involvement   326

Minimal Access *Versus* Open Transforaminal Lumbar Interbody Fusion: Meta-Analysis of Fusion Rates   327

Adjacent Segment Disease After Interbody Fusion and Pedicle Screw Fixations for Isolated L4–L5 Spondylolisthesis: A Minimum Five-Year Follow-up   329

The Effect of Sacral Decortication on Lumbosacral Fixation in a Calf Spine Model   330

Acute airway obstruction associated with the use of bone-morphogenetic protein in cervical spinal fusion   332

Lumbar Interspinous Spacers: A Systematic Review of Clinical and Biomechanical Evidence   333

Clinical Accuracy of Computer-Assisted Two-Dimensional Fluoroscopy for the Percutaneous Placement of Lumbosacral Pedicle Screws   335

Appropriateness Criteria for Surgery Improve Clinical Outcomes in Patients With Low Back Pain and/or Sciatica   336

Efficacy of Prophylactic Placement of Inferior *Vena Cava* Filter in Patients Undergoing Spinal Surgery   338

Clinical Examination Is Insufficient to Rule Out Thoracolumbar Spine Injuries   339

Measuring spine fracture outcomes: Common scales and checklists   340

Maggot Debridement Therapy for Postsurgical Wound Infection in Scoliosis: A Case Series in Five Patients   342

C-Reactive Protein, Erythrocyte Sedimentation Rate and Orthopedic Implant Infection   343

A Biofilm Approach to Detect Bacteria on Removed Spinal Implants   345

Author Index

A

Aaboe J, 38
Abatzoglou S, 285
Abbaszadegan H, 116, 249
Abrahamsen B, 61
Ackerman DB, 265
Adolphson PY, 116, 249
Adoubali A, 285
Agarwal M, 293
Agel J, 78
Ahlmann ER, 271
Ahmad TS, 183
Ahuja N, 296
Alanay A, 338
Alemdaroğlu KB, 254
Allen RT, 314
Allison DC, 271
Al-Omari AA, 92
Alsousou J, 4
Altchek DW, 187
Amendola A, 228
Ammon J, 10
Andersen C, 37
Anderson DG, 322, 323
Andrews JR, 203
Aponte-Tinao L, 303
Appleyard D, 27
Arai E, 298
Arakawa T, 40
Aretha D, 123
Arthurs SC, 19
Aston W, 278
Aston WJS, 292
Atanásio MJ, 300
Athanasian EA, 299
Attal RE, 109
Aydın N, 262
Aydoğan NH, 254
Ayerza MA, 303
Ayre CA, 214

B

Backx F, 93, 204
Baek MK, 233
Bahney TJ, 185
Bajaj S, 6
Balcarek P, 10
Bales JG, 102
Balliu E, 275
Baptista AM, 300
Barlič A, 203
Barmparas G, 339
Barrett GR, 217

Barsoum WK, 156
Bartl C, 184
Barvencik F, 245
Baumgarten KM, 176
Baur LA, 225
Beck M, 106
Bedair H, 170
Bederman SS, 319
Bedi A, 197, 215
Beil FT, 245
Bell M, 263
Berend KR, 29
Bernthal NM, 209, 280
Bertelli JA, 267
Bishop G, 251
Bisson LJ, 6
Black DM, 42
Blonna D, 191
Boada M, 275
Boakye M, 315
Bollen SR, 214
Bonadies JA, 48
Bono CM, 340
Bosco G, 283
Bot AGJ, 119
Botser IB, 17
Bove J, 266
Briffa N, 78
Brophy R, 210
Brophy RH, 222
Brorsson A, 227
Brothers J, 146
Bruce B, 27
Brudvik C, 50, 244
Bryant D, 228
Buck FM, 246
Buda R, 199
Budnar VM, 232
Buijze GA, 122
Burger B, 235
Burhanoğlu ADY, 262
Busch VJJF, 152

C

Cachecho R, 48
Cain EL Jr, 203
Calfee RP, 192, 253
Callahan MF, 259
Campos S, 274
Cannada LK, 69
Cardona DM, 134
Carlisle JC, 19
Casey ATH, 333
Castricini R, 176

Cates TB, 98
Cavallo M, 198
Cavo M, 210
Chang C-H, 107
Chang H-N, 35
Charron KD, 150
Chen C-F, 169
Chen S-Y, 264
Chen W-M, 169
Cheok CY, 183
Chia W-T, 107
Chinnock B, 52
Chiu R, 307
Cho M-R, 57
Choi N-H, 208
Choi WC, 163
Choi WJ, 233
Christiansen SE, 212
Christodoulou AG, 104, 193
Chung L-H, 169
Citak M, 73
Cleland J, 9
Coleman S, 260
Collins N, 9
Coyte PC, 319
Crawford EA, 304
Cross MB, 197
Curran C, 223

D

Dai Z, 1
Daley EL, 6
Danon-Hersch N, 336
da Silva CB, 22
Davis KE, 132
Dayerizadeh N, 235
De Benedetto M, 176
de Camargo OP, 300
DeGroot H, 92
Della Valle CJ, 141
Denard PJ, 185
Dennis DA, 167
Desai P, 70
de Souza RQ, 22
Devito D, 98
Ditsios KT, 104, 193
Dittle E, 141
Doornberg JN, 119, 242
Downing S, 296
Drosos GI, 111
DuBose JJ, 339
Dubernard J-M, 258
Dugas JR, 203

E

Earl JE, 7
Earp BE, 251
Eastell R, 61
Eiken P, 61
Eilber FC, 282, 301
Ejerhed L, 216
El Ghazaly SA, 92
Ellis SJ, 237
Emori M, 288
Engebretsen L, 4
Enocson A, 143
Eskelinen A, 145
Eunice S, 158
Eysel P, 157

F

Fan C-Y, 190
Farfalli GL, 303
Farrelly C, 8
Favejee MM, 175
Fayad L, 272
Fernandez-Sampedro M, 343
Field J, 118
Fraser JF, 327
Frassica FJ, 272
Friedman SM, 82
Fu J-P, 264
Fu RH, 166
Fuchs B, 295
Fujita N, 40
Furia JP, 91

G

Galatz LM, 176
Ganiyusufoglu K, 338
Gardeniers JWM, 152
Garfin SR, 314
Gaston RG, 98
Gebauer M, 245
Gelberman RH, 192
Gerlach D, 176
Ghate R, 147
Gheno R, 246
Ghizoni MF, 267
Ghoneim A, 256
Gikas PD, 278
Gilpin D, 260
Gioe TJ, 3
Gjesdal CG, 50, 244

Goddard MS, 148
Gordon WT, 124
Gozani SN, 241
Grimshaw CS, 80
Gulia A, 293
Gupta SR, 333
Gyuricza C, 253

H

Ha Y-C, 57
Haliloglu N, 20
Hall S, 260
Ham J, 290
Hamada K-I, 288
Hanna SA, 277, 292
Harmsen WS, 127
Harries WG, 232
Harris IA, 59
Harris JD, 210
Härtl R, 327
Hashimoto N, 288
Haviv B, 15
Healy WL, 130, 155
Heck R, 291
Hedbeck CJ, 143
Heir S, 202
Henriksen M, 38
Hepple S, 232
Higgins A, 263
Hill AM, 78
Hilverdink EF, 142
Hoch AZ, 7
Hoff WS, 48
Holme I, 202
Hoque M, 140
Hsu C-C, 35
Hsu LP, 121
Huddleston PM, 345
Hüfner T, 73
Huisstede BMA, 175
Husted H, 162
Hwang J-H, 342

I

Ikävalko M, 236
İltar S, 254
Inaba K, 339
Inceoglu D, 20
Innami K, 305
Inwards CY, 310
Iorio R, 130, 155
Irenberger A, 109
Isaacs JD, 59

J

Jacovides C, 170
Jakobsen BW, 212
Jameson SS, 131
Janda H, 291
Janicki JA, 66
Javaid MK, 161
Jeon D-G, 302
Jiang D, 1
Jiang JJ, 101
Johnson DR, 167
Jones DB Jr, 265
Joseph A, 89
Joyce TJ, 131
Ju BL, 316
Juliano PJ, 91
Jung K, 10
Jupiter JB, 122

K

Kabir SMR, 333
Kabo JM, 282, 301
Kalainov DM, 121
Kalson NS, 278
Karanikolas M, 123
Karikis J, 81
Kasraeian S, 271
Kates SL, 82
Katz JN, 129
Kawaguchi Y, 284
Kawase Y, 284
Keating EM, 132
Keeling JJ, 55
Keeney JA, 158
Kelly G, 8
Kelly NH, 166
Kemler E, 93, 204
Kepler CK, 330
Kercher J, 178
Kerkhoffs GMMJ, 88
Khaletskiy A, 52
Khan SA, 309
Khanuja HS, 148
Khoury JG, 101
Kim BS, 233
Kim CW, 322
Kim DJ, 250
Kim J-S, 151
Kim JK, 97, 250
Kim JS, 234
Kim KH, 329
Kim RH, 167
Kim S-H, 221

Kim S-J, 221
Kim T-H, 208
Kim Y-H, 151
Kirby SB, 185
Klenke FM, 310
Kocheida EM, 326
Koes BW, 175
Koester M, 181
Koh YD, 97
Kokkonen A, 236
Kong C-B, 302
König DP, 157
Koo K-H, 276
Kook SH, 97
Krasheninnikoff M, 86
Kreder HJ, 319
Kregar-Velikonja N, 203
Krishnan C, 218
Kristiansen IS, 2
Kühnel SP, 295
Kuo K, 52
Kvamme MK, 2
Kvist J, 226
Kwon Y-M, 30
Kymes SM, 222

L

Lad SP, 315
Lalonde DH, 263
Lam Y-L, 279
Lambermont JP, 160
Langton DJ, 131
Lanzetta M, 258
Lapidus G, 143
Lee G-C, 168, 191
Lee KT, 234
Lee S, 163
Lee S-H, 329
Lehmann P, 326
Li Y, 1
Li-Bland EA, 23
Lidgren L, 24
Lindenhovius ALC, 119
Liu H-H, 107
Liu S, 190
Løken S, 202
Lombardi AV Jr, 29
Longo UG, 176
Lotke PA, 168
Lu Y, 114
Luber K, 217
Lubowitz JH, 207, 219
Lui PPY, 32
Lund B, 212

Lundberg M, 227
Lynch JR, 78
Lysén C, 86

M

MacDonald SJ, 150
Mackinnon SE, 268
Mak K-L, 279
Mäkelä KT, 145
Malawer M, 294
Maletis GB, 11
Maličev E, 203
Maliogas G, 81
Mallee W, 242
Maltenfort M, 323
Manfrini M, 290
Mannava S, 259
Manske PR, 192
Mansour AA III, 64
Mansour AS, 64
Marcus KJ, 297
Marinescu R, 291
Maskell J, 161
Matsuda DK, 19
McAfee PC, 324
McCaffrey N, 223
McCalden RW, 150
McCall DA, 307
McCann P, 118
McFadyen I, 118
McKee MD, 23
Meding JB, 132
Mehbod AA, 320
Mendelson DA, 82
Menon KS, 134
Meyers K, 330
Milgrom C, 206
Miller BJ, 278
Miller CP, 316
Mirza A, 266
Miyamoto W, 305
Modi HN, 342
Moed BR, 80
Moein CA, 75
Moen TC, 147
Mohamad JA, 183
Mohler DG, 307
Moretti VM, 304
Moric M, 141
Morlock MM, 149
Moroni A, 140
Mortazavi SMJ, 146
Motamedi K, 209
Musahl V, 215

N

Nair LS, 33
Nakashima H, 286
Namba RS, 11
Nasser R, 17
Nathan JK, 315
Neumann M, 106
Ng VY, 29
Ni M, 32
Nico MAC, 246
Nierhoff C, 36
Nishida Y, 286, 298
Norrman H, 226
Noveau J, 294
Nukavarapu SP, 33
Nyffeler R, 106

O

Oakes DA, 280
Oberle D, 36
O'Brien FP, 124
O'Driscoll SW, 191
Oey L, 75
Oh I, 237
O'Loughlin P, 215
Olsson H, 24
Osbahr DC, 197
Osnes-Ringen H, 2
O'Toole RV, 69
Otte KS, 162
Øyen J, 50, 244
Oyetunji TA, 296
Ozturk C, 338

P

Pacheco RJ, 214
Pala E, 283
Palm H, 86
Papasoulis E, 111
Park J-W, 151
Park K-H, 221
Park KH, 57
Park YU, 234
Parker MJ, 85
Pashos G, 158
Patel A, 323
Paterson WH, 181
Patty CA, 324
Paul J, 184
Paxton ES, 222
Paxton EW, 11

Pearce R, 78
Peláez I, 275
Petruzzo P, 258
Petsatodis G, 81
Petty CA, 207
Pinto FMG, 22
Piper KE, 343, 345
Poehling GG, 219
Pollak AN, 48
Presutti R, 274
Price AJ, 165
Prieto-Alhambra D, 161
Puhaindran ME, 299
Pulkkinen P, 145
Puri A, 293

Q

Quinlan JF, 8

R

Radeva-Petrova DR, 206
Rains DD, 180
Rampersaud R, 335
Ramseier LE, 66
Rana AJ, 130, 155
Raphael BS, 187
Rastogi S, 309
Ravi B, 335
Ray WZ, 268
Reinhart MK, 266
Replogle WH, 217
Restrepo C, 146
Reuver JM, 235
Richardson S, 122
Riche K, 69
Richmond JC, 219
Riddiford-Harland DL, 225
Ring D, 242
Robert CE, 101
Robertson IJ, 223
Rooke GA, 180
Rosager S, 38
Roth JA, 230
Ruan H-J, 190
Ruggieri P, 283
Rui YF, 32
Ryan M, 89

S

Sacchetti L, 160
Safran O, 206
Sahin G, 20
Salata MJ, 178
Salaz N, 147
Saliou G, 326
Samartzis D, 336
Sammer DM, 265
Sampedro MF, 345
Sanzén L, 135
Sauter G, 149
Savarino L, 140
Sawamura C, 297
Schepull T, 226
Schnurr C, 157
Schoenfeld AJ, 340
Schumann K, 184
Schwartz AJ, 280, 282, 301
Schwartz EG, 121
Seeger LL, 209
Sellmeyer DE, 41
Seong SC, 163
Sernert N, 216
Sewell MD, 277, 292
Sharma A, 3
Shawen SB, 55
Shehadeh A, 294
Sheibani-Rad S, 27
Shekkeris AS, 277
Shen J, 114
Shidiak L, 59
Shim CS, 329
Siemionow K, 322
Sierevelt IN, 142
Silbernagel KG, 227
Simpson JA, 13
Singh JA, 127
Singh PJ, 15
Slobogean BL, 173
Slobogean GP, 173
Slotcavage RL, 304
Smekal V, 109
Smith TW Jr, 17
Smyth KA, 156
So TYC, 279
Somers M, 332
Son K-M, 208
Song WS, 302
Soong M, 251
Spencer HT, 102

Springfield DS, 297
Stavridis SI, 104, 193
Steckelberg KE, 343
Steele JR, 225
Steffen K, 4
Stener S, 216
Strauss EJ, 178
Strauss JE, 124
Streubel PN, 70
Strickland JW, 241
Stufkens SAS, 88
Styron JF, 156
Suero EM, 73
Suh S-W, 342
Suk M, 70
Summer B, 30
Svard U, 165

T

Taitsman LA, 78
Takagi R, 40
Takao M, 305
Takla A, 15
Tatman P, 3
Taylor ED, 33
Taylor WC, 230
ten Duis H-J, 75
Thomas A, 330
Thomas P, 30
Throckmorton TW, 181
Tiihonen R, 236
Ting N, 170
Tintle SM, 55
Tiwari A, 290
Toma M, 332
Topp R, 320
Tower SS, 138
Trach SM, 259
Transfeldt EE, 320
Trindade MCD, 257
Troelsen A, 162
Tsai W-C, 35
Tsolakis I, 123
Tsukushi S, 286, 298
Turcotte RE, 285

U

Uraloğlu M, 262

V

Vakil JJ, 148
van den Bekerom MPJ, 88, 142
van de Port I, 93, 204
Vannini F, 198
Van Steyn MO, 253
Varshney MK, 309
Verdonschot N, 152
Ververidis AN, 111
Vessely MB, 127
Vesterby MS, 37
Vicenzino B, 9
Virkus WW, 278
von Schewelov T, 135

W

Wade AM, 91
Wagner P, 24
Wahl CJ, 180

Wang C-H, 264
Wang Y, 13
Watters TS, 134
Weiland AJ, 187
Weir S, 66
Wenger DE, 310
Whalen J, 230
Whang PG, 316
Wietlisbach V, 336
Wilcke MKT, 116, 249
Wild LM, 23
Williams BR, 237
Williams GN, 218
Willits K, 228
Wilmoth JC, 64
Winding TN, 37
Wluka AE, 13
Wong MA, 102
Wright EA, 129
Wright J, 129
Wright TM, 166
Wu RH, 327
Wukich DK, 89
Wülker N, 160

Y

Yamamoto Y, 284
Yang J, 272
Yao J, 257
Yaremchuk K, 332
Yoo JJ, 276
Yoon PW, 276
Youssef JA, 324
Yun Y-H, 250

Z

Zahrai A, 335
Zeifang F, 36
Zhang L, 274
Zhu Y, 114
Zura RD, 96
Zustin J, 149
Zwolak P, 295

Printed and bound by CPI Group (UK) Ltd, Croydon, CR0 4YY

08/05/2025

01864677-0014